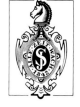

G. Dallenbach-Hellweg

Histopathology of the Endometrium

Translation by F.D. Dallenbach

Fourth, Revised and Enlarged Edition

With 176 Figures and 2 Color Plates

Springer-Verlag
Berlin Heidelberg New York
London Paris Tokyo

Dr. med. GISELA DALLENBACH-HELLWEG, FIAC
form. Professor for General Pathology and
Pathological Anatomy at the University Hospital for Women of Mannheim
University of Heidelberg
Head of the Division of Gynecological Pathology
Institute of Pathology, A2, 2, D-6800 Mannheim

Translated from the German Edition by:
Dr. med. FREDERICK D. DALLENBACH, MD
Professor for General Pathology and Pathological Anatomy
Head of the Institute of Pathology, A2, 2, D-6800 Mannheim

German
1st edition 1969
2nd edition 1981

English
1st edition 1971
2nd edition 1975
3rd edition 1981
4th edition 1987

Spanish edition published by
   Salvat Editores, Barcelona 1985
Italian edition published by
   Piccin Editore S.A.S., Padova 1986

ISBN 3-540-18156-3 4th edn. Springer-Verlag Berlin Heidelberg New York Tokyo
ISBN 0-387-18156-3 4th edn. Springer-Verlag New York Berlin Heidelberg Tokyo
ISBN 4-431-18156-3 4th edn. Springer-Verlag Tokyo Berlin Heidelberg New York

ISBN 3-540-10658-8   3rd edn. Springer-Verlag Berlin Heidelberg New York
ISBN 0-387-10658-8   3rd edn. Springer-Verlag New York Heidelberg Berlin

Library of Congress Cataloging-in-Publication Data. Dallenbach-Hellweg, G. (Gisela) Histopathology of the endometrium. Translation of: Endometrium. Bibliography: p. . Includes index. 1. Endometrium – Diseases – Diagnosis. 2. Endometrium – Histopathology. I. Title. [DNLM: 1. Cytodiagnosis. 2. Endometrium – pathology. 3. Genital Diseases, Female – diagnosis.
WP 141 D146e] RG316.D3413 1987   618.1'4   87-23412
ISBN 0-387-18156-3 (U.S.)

This work is subject to copyright. All rights are reserved, whether the whole or part of the material is concerned, specifically the rights of translation, reprinting, reuse of illustrations, recitation, broadcasting, reproduction on microfilms or in other ways, and storage in data banks. Duplication of this publication or parts thereof is only permitted under the provisions of the German Copyright Law of September 9, 1965, in its version of June 24, 1985, and a copyright fee must always be paid. Violations fall under the prosecution act of the German Copyright Law.

© Springer-Verlag Berlin Heidelberg 1971, 1975, 1981, and 1987
Printed in Germany

The use of registered names, trademarks, etc. in this publication does not imply, even in the absence of a specific statement, that such names are exempt from the relevant protective laws and regulations and therefore free for general use.

Product liability: The publisher can give no guarantee for information about drug dosage and application thereof contained in this book. In every individual case the respective user must check its accuracy by consulting other pharmaceutical literature.

Reproduction of the figures: Gustav Dreher GmbH, D-7000 Stuttgart
Typesetting, printing, and bookbinding: Universitätsdruckerei H. Stürtz AG, D-8700 Würzburg
2123/3130-543210

Preface to the Fourth Edition

Since the last edition of this monograph the use of new techniques and the increased exchange of interdisciplinary and international information have greatly advanced our understanding of endometrial histopathology.

Immunocytochemistry has helped to clarify specific aspects of the molecular biology of cells and of complex interrelationships between cellular form and function. The intracellular localization of intermediate filaments, of steroid hormone receptor-associated proteins, and of tumor-associated antigens has proved increasingly important for the histogenetic recognition and subclassification of tumors and the monitoring of their therapy. As a result of the enhanced interdisciplinary and international cooperation, the classification of endometrial tumors has had to be revised. Increased longevity, modern ways of living, new life-styles, and the latest methods of treatment have modified, increased, or changed many of the clinical and diagnostic problems confronting us.

Accordingly, therapy with hormones and intrauterine contraception receive special attention in this monograph, commensurate with the importance afforded them today. Under the precept *nil nocere,* the almost unlimited uses for these agents warrant that their effects be carefully monitored by precise morphological studies, a prerequistite that succeeds only when clinician and pathologist work together.

The sections on the preparation of endometrial specimens, on steroid receptors, on functional disturbances, on intrauterine pregnancy have been changed and brought up-to-date to incorporate the results of recent investigations that appear significant. Only time, however, will prove their true value. Much of historical interest in the text has been left intact, for "who wants to read into the future, must consult the past" (André Malraux).

To the correspondents and consultants who have contributed valuable observations and suggestions and brought to my attention errors or omissions in the last edition, I gladly acknowledge my cordial thanks. Again, the staff of Springer-Verlag has earned my gratitude for their patience, generosity, and skill in preparing this new edition.

Mannheim/Heidelberg, September 1987   GISELA DALLENBACH-HELLWEG

Foreword to the First German Edition

During life form changes. From the form seen we can often interpret function. From such correlation *functional morphology* has developed. When applied to the endometrium it means we use histological features existing at the time of biopsy to diagnose functional changes. What we try to detect are the local reactions induced by hormones under control of higher centers. Correlation of form with function succeeds only when the clinician and morphologist work together. Of the many factors that are important, the time of biopsy is decisive, since the target tissues need time before they can react and change in response to the hormonal stimulus. In our interpretations we must always take such reaction-times into account. By using functional morphology as a method of study, we can determine what type of hormonal dysfunction exists, how intense it is, and how it changes with time. More important, we are able to evaluate the biological effects of the hormonal stimuli on the peripheral target tissues with greater accuracy than if we were to measure the hormones biochemically. Although the advantage may shift in favor of biochemical analyses, as our knowledge progresses in the practice of medicine today the morphological change in the target organ remains the basis by which we recognize disease processes and decide how to treat them.

Besides the changes of functional morphology, we must also evaluate other local changes we find in the histological sections, which, from present-day knowledge, may or may not be induced by hormonal stimuli. Whether certain morphological changes in target organs, particularly the precancerous or carcinomatous transformations, may be brought about be excessive hormonal stimulation or may become refractory to such influences, are questions of extreme importance in learning about the biology of these changes.

In gynecology every morphology must be functional morphology, a principle that particularly applies to the interpretation of the endometrium. My associate, Dr. DALLENBACH-HELLWEG, is an authority on the diagnosis of endometrial changes. Brought up in the HAMPERL school where she became familiar with both general and gynecological pathology, she finished her training under A.T. HERTIG in Boston. By coming to a women's hospital she finally found her way to applied gynecological pathology. Consequently, she is in the position to represent the interests of the clinician as well as those of the morphologist. In this monograph she has recorded her vast experience and thorough knowledge of both disciplines. Her book serves as a bridge between clinician and pathologist, its purpose – to facilitate an exchange of information and ideas in both directions. May the conditions prevail to encourage such trade, hopefully leading to collaboration and teamwork between these specialists.

Mannheim, November 1969   PETER STOLL

Preface to the First German Edition

The endometrium differs from all other tissues of the body in that it rhythmically changes its structure and function. For many years the meaning of these changes remained puzzling and obscure. At about the turn of the century some investigators held the physiological fluctuations of the menstrual cycle to be inflammatory changes. Later, when stricter criteria for the pathology of the endometrium were applied, morphologists misinterpreted pathological fluctuations in the cycle either as physiological variations, or they overlooked them entirely. Today as previously the pathologist is often confronted with the dilemma that he is unable to adequately diagnose the endometrium merely from the structural changes. Accordingly, the gynecologist finds the pathological report of little value. In like manner, if the clinical information given the pathologist is incomplete, then he cannot form a clear notion of the clinical problem.

Although the detection of focal lesions of the endometrium is important, of much greater consequence is the recognition of functional (hormonally controlled) variations and their cyclic course, for it is from these that the clinician is guided in deciding what therapy he should use. The ability to detect such functional changes requires not only that the morphologist possess a thorough knowledge of the physiological and pathological anatomy of the endometrium but also that he receive exact information about the patient's menstrual history and have insight into clinical problems. Prerequisites of that kind make it possible to relate morphology with function, a synthesis essential for the optimal diagnosis of the endometrium. Such a correlation is the purpose of this monograph. It attempts to bridge the gap between pathologist and clinician; it is designed for both. Should these pages stimulate the pathologist's interest for clinical problems or aid the clinician in understanding why the pathologist needs clinical information, thus fostering close cooperation between the two, then the book has achieved its purpose.

The numerous photographs depict most of the endometrial variations that one might encounter. I thank the publishers for accepting so many illustrations and particularly for reproducing halftones of such high quality. Although addressed primarily to the practicing pathologist, this book is intended as well for the gynecologist or research pathologist who, it is hoped, will find among its pages stimulating suggestions and information. May the numerous references cited facilitate further study of special problems. The bibliography, albeit comprehensive, is hardly complete. Every effort was made, however, to cull from the boundless wealth of literature precisely those works that have contributed significantly in their time to the solution of a specific problem.

My special thanks go to Professor Dr. med. PETER STOLL for his critical review of my manuscript, for his invaluable suggestions and advice, as well as for his helpful and understanding support. I am most indebted to Mrs.

G. SANKOVIC for her untiring and dedicated devotion in typing the manuscript and in preparing the bibliography. To Miss B. MERKEL I gladly acknowledge my gratitude for reading the manuscript and for her valued support in overcoming technical problems. Again, I express my sincere thanks to the publishers for their care and efficiency in preparing the text and illustrations, and their willingness to fulfill my many requests.

Mannheim/Heidelberg, November 1969　　　　　GISELA DALLENBACH-HELLWEG

Contents

A. Methods of Obtaining, Preparing, and Interpreting the Endometrium . . 1

   1. Indications for Curettage 1
   2. Selection of the Proper Time for Curettage 2
   3. Procedures for Obtaining Endometrial Tissue 4
   4. Preparation of the Endometrial Specimen 7
      a) Fixation 7
      b) Embedding 10
      c) Orientation 10
      d) Staining 11
      e) Immunocytochemistry with Monoclonal Antibodies 15
      f) Quantitative and Experimental Methods 16
   5. Components of Curettings and Their Diagnostic Value 17
   6. Statistical Analysis of the Histological Results 23

B. The Normal Histology of the Endometrium 25

   1. The Individual Structures 25
      a) The Glandular Epithelium 25
      b) The Superficial Epithelium 29
      c) The Stromal Cells 29
      d) The Reticulum Fibers 36
      e) The Ground Substance 36
      f) The Vessels 39
      g) The Nerves 41
   2. Histochemical Localization of Enzymes; the Reciprocal Action Between Enzymes and Hormones 42
   3. Structural Changes Induced in the Endometrium by the Physiological Action of the Ovarian Hormones 45
      a) Molecular Biology of Steroid Hormones 45
      b) Endometrial Steroid Receptors 48
      c) Estrogen 50
      d) Progesterone 51
      e) Relaxin 51
   4. Changes in Structures in the Endometrium During Nidation . . . 53
   5. The Endometrium Before Puberty 54
   6. The Normal Menstrual Cycle and Its Possible Variations 55
      a) The Normal Proliferative Phase 57
      b) The Normal Secretory Phase 64
      c) Menstruation 77
      d) Regeneration 84

e) Possible Variations in the Endometrium During the Normal
   Cycle 84
7. The Endometrium in the Climacterium and After the Menopause 86

C. The Histopathology of the Endometrium 93

1. Morphological Effects of Circulatory and Coagulation Disturbances 94
   a) Edema 94
   b) Chronic Passive Hyperemia; Hemorrhage Caused by
      Extragenital Diseases 96
2. Functional Endogenous (Hormonal) Disturbances 99
   a) Atrophic Endometrium from Non-Functioning Ovaries 99
   b) Resting Endometrium Resulting from Inadequate Ovarian
      Function (Ovarian Insufficiency, Hypofolliculinism) 101
   c) The Endometrium Associated with a Persistent Follicle 102
      α) The Anovulatory Cycle 103
      β) Glandular-Cystic Hyperplasia 108
      γ) Adenomatous Hyperplasia 120
      δ) Special Forms of Hyperplasia (Focal Hyperplasia, Polyps,
         Glandular, and Stromal Hyperplasias) 129
   d) The Deficient Secretory Phase Associated with Deficiency or
      Premature Regression of the Corpus Luteum 136
   e) The Endometrium Associated with a Persistent Corpus Luteum 143
      α) Irregular Shedding 143
      β) Dysmenorrhea Membranacea 148
      γ) Secretory Hypertrophy 149
   f) The Endometrium Associated with Infertility 149
   g) Functional Disturbances During the Climacteric 156
   h) The Effect of Hormone-Producing Ovarian Tumors on the
      Endometrium 157
   i) The Functional Disturbances of the Endocervical Mucosa . . . 158
3. Exogenous (Iatrogenic) Changes of the Endometrium 158
   a) After Hormonal Therapy 158
      α) Estrogens 159
      β) Gestagens 161
      γ) Both Hormones 165
      δ) Oral Contraceptive Agents 166
      ε) Gonadotropins 186
      ζ) Clomiphene 186
   b) After Intrauterine Contraceptive Device 190
   c) After Intrauterine Instillation 197
   d) Regeneration after Curettage 198
   e) With In Vitro Fertilization 200
4. Endometritis 200
   a) Acute Endometritis 201
   b) Chronic Non-Specific Endometritis 203
   c) Tuberculous Endometritis 205

    d) Specific Endometritis Caused by Rare Microorganisms 208
    e) The Foreign Body Granuloma 212
    f) Endocervicitis 213
 5. Metaplasias and Related Changes 214
    a) Epithelial Metaplasia 214
       α) Squamous Metaplasia, Morules, and Ichthyosis 215
       β) Mucinous (Endocervical) Metaplasia 216
       γ) Serous Papillary Metaplasia 219
       δ) Ciliated Cell Change 220
       ε) Clear Cell Change 222
    b) Stromal Metaplasia 222
 6. Neoplasms 223
    a) Benign Tumors 223
    b) Carcinoma of the Endometrium 226
       α) Carcinomas with Endometrial Differentiation 232
       β) Carcinomas Which Originate from Pluripotent Müllerian
           Epithelium 238
       γ) Histochemical Results 245
       δ) Precursors of Endometrial Carcinoma 254
       ε) Etiological Concepts 259
       ζ) Progesterone Treatment of Endometrial Carcinoma 272
    c) Sarcoma of the Endometrium 275
    d) Malignant Mixed Mesodermal Tumors 283
    e) Metastatic Tumors 291
    f) Primary Carcinomas of the Ecto- and Endocervix
       as Components of Curettings 294

D. The Diagnosis of Normal and Pathologic Pregnancy from Curettings 298

 1. The Early Intrauterine Pregnancy and Its Disturbances 298
    a) Therapeutic Abortion (Induced Abortion) 298
    b) Spontaneous Abortion 300
       α) Causes 300
       β) Microscopic Changes 304
    c) Partial Hydatidiform Mole 315
    d) Complete Hydatidiform Mole, Invasive Mole, and
       Choriocarcinoma 317
    e) Placental Site Trophoblastic Tumor 323
    f) Late Endometrial Changes Following Intrauterine Abortion . . 324
 2. The Endometrium Associated with Extrauterine Pregnancy 328
 3. The Postpartum Endometrium 331

References 337

Subject Index 403

A. Methods of Obtaining, Preparing, and Interpreting the Endometrium

The diagnosis of changes in endometrium obtained by curettage depends not only on a thorough microscopic examination of the histological preparations; the diagnosis actually starts in the clinic. The close interplay between structure and function that is so apparent in the human endometrium requires we ask about or determine what the patient's hormonal state is. We need to know about her menstrual history, previous pregnancies, basal temperature, and any hormones she may have received. What we learn will help us in evaluating the microscopic sections and in detecting abnormal changes.

1. Indications for Curettage

A curettage may be indicated for diagnostic or therapeutic reasons. Before a diagnostic curettage is performed, two questions should be answered: will the curettage contribute to the diagnosis, what dangers are there in the procedure? Although large statistics indicate the mortality rate for the operation is 0%, in rare instances the uterus may be perforated. On the other hand, with well-founded indications a curettage is especially recommended after the menopause since it often leads to discovery of a carcinoma; or it may also be used to exclude the presence of such a tumor, thereby sparing the patient a more extensive operation (DAICHMAN and MACKLES 1966).

Complete curettage of the endometrium for histological study is indicated:

a) Only rarely, in conjunction with other methods of study (clinical history, measurement of basal temperature, cytological examination, determinations of hormones), *for diagnosing the functional state when the menstrual cycles are regular,* as for example, in infertility or in monitoring hormone therapy. Instead, a simple ("stingle stroke" or "strip") endometrial biopsy suffices here and may be carried out in the outpatient clinic or office without dilatation of the cervix.

b) Most often *for the diagnosis and treatment of all types of abnormal bleeding,* where the functional (hormonal) or morphological cause needs to be clarified. Here, a complete curettage including the tubal recesses is desirable. To perform it the cervix must be dilated under anesthesia.

c) *When a carcinoma is suspected with or without bleeding;* a complete curettage should be made including the tubal recesses. To insure a thorough and accurate examination the endocervical canal should be curetted separately from the endometrial cavity, and the fragments from each region collected separately. Only enough tissue should be scraped away as is needed for diagnosis if a possibility exists of perforating the uterine wall.

d) In an *abortion* with bleeding and a patent endocervical canal. A complete curettage is indicated here, usually carried out with a large blunt curette. If it can be easily inserted into the endocervical canal, anesthesia is not required.

It becomes apparent that a curettage sometimes serves to supplement or complete a functional diagnosis. At other times, however, curettage becomes necessary as a life-saving procedure. When used for purely diagnostic reasons, then it should be performed at a time optimal for histological study, insuring that the most information will be gained.

2. Selection of the Proper Time for Curettage

The best time depends on the *functional disturbance* presented by the patient and on the diagnosis that the gynecologist anticipates from the histological study. For example, if the clinical signs and symptoms suggest an anovulatory cycle, then a curettage during the proliferative phase would be of little value. A diagnosis of an anovulatory cycle is possible only during the secretory phase, by recognizing that the typical secretory changes have failed to appear in the epithelial cells and stroma. Since the proliferative phase may be prolonged, even normally, and since the first secretion by the glandular cells can be detected with routine stains not before 36–48 h after ovulation, the curettage should be performed shortly before menstruation. It should certainly be done no earlier than 12 days before the last date for onset of menstruation, as calculated from the clinical history. A diagnosis that ovulation took place can readily be made during the last days of the secretory phase or even on the 1st day of menstruation, not, however, directly after ovulation. For most of the functional diagnoses, particularly for evaluating the function of the corpus luteum and for diagnosing sterility, the late secretory phase is the best and occasionally the only time for curettage to insure a useful histological diagnosis. Admittedly, in patients under study for infertility the danger exists that a pregnancy might be interrupted by curettage in the secretory phase (ARRONET et al. 1973). Such a risk, however, may be circumvented by postponing the curettage until the basal temperature falls; that is, from 2 days before to just before menstruation starts, provided the basal temperature has been elevated indicating ovulation had probably occurred. In rare instances an endometrial biopsy taken during the "conception cycle" may not disturb the implanting blastocyst and may in fact promote a better decidual reaction (KAROW et al. 1971; ROSENFELD and GARCIA 1975). Another advantage of curettage in the late secretory phase or just before menstruation, even though the menstrual cycle is irregular, is that the secretory changes should be maximal by then. Thus the degree and extent of luteal differentiation reached can best be evaluated.

Intense hemorrhage but also even *mild atypical bleeding* represent exceptions to the rule of late curettage. Such hemorrhages are an indication for prompt curettage, not only from a clinical standpoint but also from that of the pathologist, since the longer the bleeding continues, the less the amount of tissue to be found in the uterus. Consequently, the changes the histological study will prove worthwhile diminish with the duration of the hemorrhage. Because of the greater danger of cancer after the menopause, if appropriate clinical signs exist, it is highly advisable to perform a curettage promptly. WINTER (1956) was able to make a pathological diagnosis in 74% of his patients when the endometrial curettage was performed during the period of abnormal bleeding. When he performed the curettage after the bleeding had ceased, he was able to make a diagnosis in only 34%.

Waiting until bleeding has stopped is justifiable in only a few instances: 1. When irregular shedding is suspected – the histological changes typical of that condition are difficult to recognize in curettings obtained on the 1st day of menstruation. Rather, the histological diagnosis here depends on finding fragments of involuted, though well-preserved endometrium several days after bleeding starts. 2. For diagnosing a hypomenorrhea, the curettage is best performed shortly before or 3–5 days after the onset of menstrual bleeding. If the endometrium is still highly secretory before the bleeding begins, or if only superficial fragments of endometrium are discharged after bleeding has commenced and these reveal involution, then there is no ovarian insufficiency. The changes described more likely represent scanty menstrual shedding with intense shrinkage within normal limits (HINZ 1953). In rare instances menstrual bleeding fails to occur although ovarian function apparently is normal (PHILIPPE et al. 1966). Since amenorrhea may have various causes, if the endometrium discloses no characteristic changes it is advisable to repeat the curettage; a single strip biopsy suffices.

In summary, the guidelines in Table 1 are valid.

Table 1. Guidelines for the best time for curettage. (Based on HINZ 1953)

Clinical diagnosis	Best time for curettage
Infertility with suspicion of a corpus luteum insufficiency or an anovulatory cycle	Shortly before or at the onset of menstruation; 26th–28th day of a regular cycle
Hypomenorrhea	Shortly before or 3–5 days after onset of menstruation
Oligomenorrhea	On the 1st day of menstrual bleeding
Menorrhagia with suspicion of irregular shedding	According to clinical history of bleeding, from 5–10 days after onset of menstruation
Amenorrhea (pregnancy must be excluded)	Endometrial biopsy repeated at short intervals
Metrorrhagia	Best done without delay

Equally as important as selecting the most favorable time for curettage is the **reporting to the pathologist** about the patient's menstrual history and any hormone therapy she may have received. Besides the patient's name and age, the clinical report sent with the curettings should include: the date of curettage, the date on which the last menstruation started, a schema describing the menstrual cycles, an account of the menstrual flow, details of previous hormonal therapy, a statement about the patient's constitution including any endocrine disturbances, the clinical diagnosis, and questions to be answered (LAU and STOLL 1963). The pathologist can make an accurate functional diagnosis only if he is sent the pertinent clinical information. For example, it is self-evident why an anovulatory cycle or a shortened or prolonged cycle can be diagnosed only when the phase of the patient's cycle is known, or why secretory change of the endometrium can be interpreted as deficient only when the day of the cycle is stated. Lack of information about previous therapy with hormones may lead to false interpretations of histological changes and to false conclusions about the patient's ovarian function. Consequently, a purely morphological description of endometrial structure is worthless without correlation with clinical information. Some clinicians maintain that only they are in a position to interpret the histological diagnoses made by the pathologist. I regard such a viewpoint to be wrong. The close interplay between form and function becomes apparent only during the study of a histological preparation, not a posteriori from a histological report. Clinicians and pathologists should endeavor to work together (LETTERER and MASSHOFF 1941; STOLL 1949; HINZ 1953; LAU and STOLL 1963).

3. Procedures for Obtaining Endometrial Tissue

From the pathologist's standpoint it would be ideal to have a *complete curettage* performed lege artis in every patient, since an examination of only all endometrial tissue will insure that no important changes are overlooked. If the slightest suspicion of carcinoma exists, then the entire endometrial cavity should be curetted. In doing so, it is often advisable to collect the tissue from the corpus separately from that of the endocervical canal, making it possible to localize the tumor. On the other hand, if the purpose of the curettage is to determine the changes brought about by hormonal therapy, that is, to make a functional diagnosis, then duplicate curettages should be employed. Such a study involves repeating an *endometrial biopsy* (strip or single stroke) during a menstrual cycle; it provides more information than a single, complete curettage. In addition, a simple biopsy is usually enough if only a functional diagnosis of the mucosa is sought, for example, in the diagnosis of infertility (SILLO-SEIDL 1967). Although the amount of tissue obtained with a strip biopsy is relatively scanty, that does not compromise the accuracy of the diagnosis made from it, since the endometrium of the uterine cavity usually develops homogeneously. NOYES (1956) was able to prove that fact by comparing biopsies of the right and left anterior and posterior walls. The decision of what type of procedure to use as well as when to perform the operation will depend upon the patient and the problems involved. If the curettage is indicated for therapeutic reasons, then only a complete curettage will suffice.

Whether a complete curettage is decided upon, or only a biopsy, what is important is that tissue be removed from the endometrial cavity, since all the normal and pathological changes in question take place in the endometrial cavity, not however (or only very slightly) in the isthmic portion (of the lower uterine segment). A careful curettage of the tubal recesses (cornua) is important, since these are sites of predilection for carcinoma and benign polyps, and they often shelter the last remnants of placental tissue. When the mucosa of the cornua is normal it is particularly high and well developed, superbly suited for diagnosing functional changes.

In the last few years the histological study of endocervical curettings has become more important for two reasons: 1. Gynecologists have learned the value of collecting endocervical curettings separately from endometrial curettings, and are practicing the procedure with increasing frequency, especially for the exact localization and extension of a malignancy. 2. Therapy with progestational agents, especially certain potent oral contraceptives, induces changes in the endocervix that are characteristic and should be recognized as such.

The Technique of Endometrial Biopsy
The procedure may be carried out in the doctor's office without anesthesia. Preparation: the patient's temperature, leukocyte count and sedimentation rate should be normal. Those with localized or systemic illnesses must be excluded as well as those with a pregnancy as strongly suggested by careful questioning and serological tests. The patient should empty her urinary bladder. After the speculum is inserted and the portio inspected, colposcopy may be done and cytological smears prepared, including wet-mount preparations for phase-contrast microscopy (STOLL 1970). The uterus is palpated to determine its position and size, attention being paid to adjacent structures.

The portio vaginalis (ectocervix) is cleansed with disinfectants. Under direct inspection and without the need of a tenaculum to stabilize the cervix, the biopsy curette is inserted into the endocervical canal and up into the fundus. The biopsy of the endometrium is made with a single stroke, usually along the anterior wall, and the curette is withdrawn.

The Technique of Complete Curettage
The procedure is best performed under a brief inhalation or intravenous anesthesia. Preparation of the patient is the same as for the endometrial biopsy (see above). After the pubic hair is trimmed away with scissors, the vulva is cleansed with disinfectants. The portio vaginalis is grasped with a tenaculum and pulled lightly to stretch the uterus. A probe is inserted and the endometrial cavity carefully explored and evaluated. The endocervical canal is then enlarged with Hegar dilators up to size No. 10. A sharp curette is inserted into the endometrial cavity and strips of endometrium gently scraped from the anterior, posterior, right and left uterine walls. The strips of tissue are collected on a linen cloth on the instrument table, examined, and promptly placed in an appropriate fixative. A more thorough curettage may be made by ensuring the strokes of the curette parallel one another and reach the tubal recesses.

When a carcinoma is suspected the endocervix should be scraped first before the curette is inserted into the endometrial cavity: the fragments of endocervical mucosa should be collected separately and fixed. If friable, soft, gray-white tissue is removed from the corpus, highly suggestive of a carcinoma, then the curettage should be discontinued to insure the uterus is not inadvertently perforated by additional scraping.

Emptying the endometrial cavity in imminent or incipient abortion. If the products of conception have not been discharged and ultrasonic studies indicate the amnion is empty, curettage is performed after prostaglandin priming has dilated the endocervical canal. If in *incomplete abortion* the cervical os is found dilated a finger's breadth, permitting insertion of a curette, then no anesthesia is required unless to spare the patient possible psychic trauma. The vulva is cleansed with disinfectants. The position, size and consistency of the uterus and neighboring structures are determined by careful palpation. A speculum is inserted and the portio carefully inspected, paying special attention to evidence of disease. The cervix is seized and held fast with a tenaculum and the endometrial cavity explored with the largest blunt curette possible. To stimulate uterine contraction 3 IU of oxytocin are injected i.v. before the curettage is begun. The curettage is performed gently to make sure the soft trophoblastic tissue is removed but not the underlying basal layer of the endometrium or the myometrium. Curettage is completed when the uterus contracts well.

Procedure with a hydatidiform mole – occasionally with a hydatidiform mole two curettages become necessary, the first being limited to partial removal of the mole to allow the uterus to contract. Later, a second and complete curettage is performed. The procedure used depends on the severity of bleeding. It is advisable to inject oxytocin during the curettage.

Besides biopsing the endometrium with a curette, *biopsy by suction* (vacuum aspiration) has been introduced mainly for office practice because it does not require anesthesia or endocervical dilatation.

For such a suction biopsy NOVAK (1935, 1937) and RANDALL (1935) employed a thin, hollow probe with a saw-toothed rim. It has subsequently been modified in various ways by numerous other investigators. NUGENT (1963) compiled the results of several series of studies made with the suction biopsy and calculated that among 1434 biopsies cancer was overlooked in 7.9%. With the probe designed for suction biopsy by FREI-SCHÜTZ and JOPP (1964), however, the use of vacuum suction and sharp excision with a retractable ring-knife within the hollow probe make it possible to remove larger pieces of endometrium. The jet-washer introduced by GRAVLEE in 1969 combines suction with a system for flushing the uterine cavity with physiological saline. The method has proved fairly popular. Since then, further technical improvements have been described and introduced for collecting endometrial tissue suitable for diagnosis (HALE et al. 1976; INGLIS and WEIR 1976; FERENCZY et al. 1979). Numerous investigators have tested the reliability of many of these methods, especially those used for detecting carcinoma, by comparing the histological diagnoses of them with those made of an ensuing complete curettage or a hysterectomy specimen. The diagnoses agreed in a little over 80% of the patients (KAHLER et al. 1969; DENIS et al. 1973; COHEN et al. 1974; HATHCOCK et al. 1974; MUENZER et al. 1974; LIU et al. 1975; WALTERS et al. 1975; WEBB and GAFFEY 1976; GREENWOOD and WRIGHT 1979). With the jet-wash method HENDERSON et al. (1975) were able to collect enough tissue for diagnosis in only 58% of their studies but increased the diagnostic accuracy to 92% when they performed simultaneous cytological studies of the perfusion fluid. LUKEMAN (1974) found that agreement in diagnoses for his patients was 89.8%. According to many authors, the diagnostic reliability of the suction and jet-wash methods is equally good (DOWLING et al. 1969; SO-BOSITA et al. 1970; HIBBARD and SCHWINN 1971; KANBOUR et al. 1974; RODRIGUEZ et al. 1974; BIBBO et al. 1982). Generally the suction biopsy is recommended for screening asymptomatic women at risk for carcinoma, for patients who are in poor general health or are anesthetic risks (HALLER et al. 1973), and for functional diagnoses in young women (ENGELER et al. 1972; MATHEWS et al. 1973).

From our experience the diagnostic value of the tissue obtained either by suction or by jet-washing depends primarily on the amount of intact tissue that can be collected. Because the interrelationships between gland and stroma are so important in evaluating the quality of neoplastic and preneoplastic hyperplasias, without these interrelationships important distinctions cannot be made. Consequently, we prefer the suction method to the pure washing methods (see also VASSILAKOS et al. 1975). For diagnosing endometrial *function,* the strip or suction biopsy is adequate in most instances and well recommended as a method that saves time and expense (see also ANSARI and COWDREY 1974). Although a complete curettage performed afterwards may at times contain polyps which escaped the suction biopsy, these contribute no important information needed for the functional diagnosis.

Despite all the encouraging reports about the diagnostic reliability of detecting asymptomatic endometrial cancer by suction biopsy, a warning should be issued against placing too much reliance on that method which has the same limitations as does endometrial strip biopsy with the curette. Under optimal conditions a carcinoma may be diagnosed with both methods. Failure to find carcinoma in the tissue removed with these two methods, however, does not prove that there is no carcinoma in other parts of the endometrium. That holds true especially for the early stages, since endometrial carcinoma generally develops in the basalis or in tubal recesses which are difficult to reach by suction.

For purposes of thoroughness we should mention the use of *whole uteri* in the study and diagnosis of the endometrium. For the pathologist, whole uteri represent ideal specimens for study. When properly examined, they present no problems in diagnosis, nor do they require such detailed diagnoses as do curettings, except when a carcinoma is present.

Besides providing tissue for histological studies, freshly extirpated uteri are a source of material for *cytological smears* and tissue culture. Desquamated, viable epithelial and stromal cells may be examined in wet-mount preparations under the phase-contrast microscope, or in fixed smears stained after the Papanicolaou method or other techniques (SCHÜLLER 1961; DALLENBACH-HELLWEG and JÄGER 1969). In some respects the study of living cells with phase-contrast yields information that histological sections cannot provide; for example, knowledge about ciliary motion of the columnar epithelium, or about motility of bacteria or protozoa.

Cytological studies alone are unsuitable for evaluating endometrial function or for diagnosing carcinomas (LÜDINGHAUSEN and ANASTASIADIS 1984; SCHNEIDER 1985). They fail to provide the cellular interrelationships of the tissue so important for making a definitive diagnosis. Since the study of material obtained by sponge and brush techniques is based on cytologic criteria, these techniques have proved unsatisfactory. The strip or suction biopsy are preferred, particularly because they are easiest for patient and physician. If, however, cytologically scored atypias of endometrial cells are found in smears of postmenopausal women, they should serve as a guideline for further investigation (ZUCKER et al. 1985; SKAARLAND 1986).

4. Preparation of the Endometrial Specimen

a) Fixation

Since the endometrium is exceedingly soft and undergoes rapid autolysis, it should be carefully handled and promptly fixed. Before fixation, however, it is best to remove clots of blood and mucus. These may be separated either by rinsing the fragments of tissue gently in physiological saline or by spreading them on a fine-meshed sieve or fabric, from which they may be transferred into the fixing solution with one arm of a blunt forceps, exercising care to avoid squeezing or pinching them. If the curettings are left in the gauze or tampon for delivery to the pathologist, then subsequent drying and squeezing will make it difficult for the pathologist to remove the now sticky fragments from the meshes of the gauze. Consequently, we recommend that endometrial curettings never be wrapped in fabric.

In selecting a fixative one should be guided by the principle of trying to preserve intravital structures as completely as possible. To obtain the finest preservation, however, it would be best to forgo a fixative entirely, and instead prepare *sections of unfixed, rapidly frozen tissues* with the *cryostat*. Such sections preserve most structural details, are free from artefacts owing to shrinkage, and provide a fair facsimile of the living state (KERN-BONTKE and WÄCHTER 1962). Since, however, knowledge in histopathology has been acquired through the use of fixatives and embedding techniques, and since the diagnoses we make depend in part on the artefacts produced in the tissues during its processing, frozen sections free of such artefacts are usually more difficult to interpret. An example of the difficulty one might encounter is the absence in frozen sections of basal vacuoles in the glandular epithelium during the early secretory phase. In preparing paraffin sections the accumulations of glycogen in these cells dissolve away, leaving instead diagnostically important vacuoles behind. In frozen sections, however, the glycogen remains and no prominent vacuoles form. Further, only a few dyes stain frozen tissue at all well; the structures of the tissue usually display much less contrast of color (eosinophilia, basophilia) than they do in fixed tissues. The greatest disadvantage of frozen sections is that to prepare them one needs special equipment not always found in a routine histological laboratory. The tissues must be rapidly frozen in liquid nitrogen or on dry ice to prevent large ice crystals from forming. If not sectioned directly, they must be stored at low temperatures until later. Submitting tissue by mail for study virtually precludes frozen sections, which are best used for emergency or rapid diagnoses and for investigative studies, especially for enzyme histochemistry and immunocytochemistry (see p. 15). Frozen sections are essential for detecting specific cellular proteins with monoclonal antibodies, such as hormone receptors.

Fixatives may be classified into coagulants, which denature the proteins of tissue, and non-coagulants, which stabilize the proteins by chemical bonding (BAKER 1963). The best known coagulant fixative is *ethyl alcohol*. By extracting water, it induces substantial shrinkage of tissues and cells. It coagulates nuclei and cytoplasm, destroys mitochondria and chromosomes, dissolves lipids or causes them to diffuse. In brief, with alcohol fixation much of the fine structure of the cell is lost.

The most commonly employed non-coagulant is the aqueous solution of formaldehyde (H_2CO), *formalin*. It preserves the hydrophilic groups of proteins, and probably links chains of proteins together by reacting with the $-NH_2$ of the side groups of certain amino acids (BAKER 1963). The majority of the formaldehyde-protein linkages are reversible by washing the fixed tissue in water. Consequently, proteins are not denaturated, and any shrinkage of tissue that develops is followed by expansion. DNA, mitochondria and the fine structures of cells remain well preserved. In general, formalin does not dissolve lipids. Although it does not fix soluble carbohydrates, it does impede the solution of glycogen from tissues by fixing the proteins. The ideal concentration for almost all staining methods used in the diagnosis of the endometrium is a 4% neutral solution of formaldehyde (that is, a 10% solution of the strong commercial 40% formalin). For routine use in the clinic and in office practice formalin has the advantage of being inexpensive, easy to handle, and fairly stable, especially when buffered at pH 7.0. We use a buffered solution since the best linkage of formaldehyde to the tissue proteins takes place around pH 7.0–8.0. As the pH of the formalin rises to pH 10 or more the number of protein-formaldehyde linkages falls. Tissue may be left in the fixative for weeks without harm; thus, it is ideal for fixing specimens to be mailed, or suited for storage of excess tissue for long periods if such becomes necessary. Fixation with formalin enables the pathologist to use almost all important stains that he might need for differentiating tissues, cells and cellular structures. Most cytoplasmic constituents remain well preserved, except for some enzymes and a small amount of glycogen. Lipids (particularly neutral fats) and some glycogen may be dissolved from the tissue during its dehydration for paraffin embedding. To expedite the fixation and reporting of fresh gynecological tissues sent to our laboratory, we promptly examine and describe the specimens on receipt, select representative portions for study, trim these to no thicker than 3 mm, and fix them in buffered 4% formalin at 70° C for 90 min. To prevent formalin precipitates from forming, we wash the tissue samples (now in capsules) in running cold tap water for at least 10 min.

Mixtures of fixatives, made by combining two or more primary fixatives, have advantages derived from the good properties of each component as well as from the favorable and unfavorable reactions of the additives with one another. One usually selects a compound fixative for a special purpose; for example, for preserving chromosomes or specific cytoplasmic inclusions. For such purposes the compound fixatives are generally superior to the primary fixatives.

If, in addition to fixation for routine diagnostic work, one wishes to carry out enzyme studies, for example, of acid phosphatase, he may add *calcium chloride* to the formaldehyde solution without fear its fixative properties will be impaired. The formula for such a fixative, as given by BAKER (1946), is: 10 ml 10% formalin, 10 ml 10% aqueous solution of $CaCl_2$, 80 ml distilled water. Fixation is carried out at 4° C, and to preserve enzyme activity fixation should not be prolonged more than 12–18 h.

Many other solutions or mixtures, named after the men who invented them (STIEVE, BOUIN, ZENKER, SAN FELICE, CARNOY) fix tissues particularly well, rendering excellent preservation of histological structures and superb retention of nuclear details. These fixatives, however, are more difficult to prepare and they limit the number of staining methods that may be used. Therefore, these mixtures are generally reserved for research studies. All other types of fixatives should be employed only in emergencies when nothing else is available. Thus, as mentioned above, alcohol is unsuitable as a fixative in any concentration since it causes the loose and fluid-rich endometrium to shrink, badly distorting most of its structures.

b) Embedding

Although *paraffin* may not be the best *embedding* medium, it is at least good, easy to use, and inexpensive. An alternative medium would be the polyester waxes, which are convenient but more expensive. If the techniques of dehydration and embedding are carried out properly, by insuring that the various solutions are frequently replenished and that dehydration is not unduly prolonged, shrinkage of the tissue may be minimized.

To facilitate processing of the specimens we receive each day, we use a computerized tissue processor that automatically carries the tissue specimens through the following solutions during the night:

80% ethyl alcohol – No. 1 for 30 min.
80% ethyl alcohol – No. 2 for 1 h.
96% ethyl alcohol – No. 1 for 1 h.
96% ethyl alcohol – No. 2 for 1 h.
100% isopropyl alcohol – No. 1 for 2 h.
100% isopropyl alcohol – No. 2 for 2 h.
100% isopropyl alcohol – No. 3 for 2 h.
Xylol-isopropyl alcohol 1:1 for 1 h.
Xylol – No. 1 for 30 min.
Xylol – No. 2 for 30 min.
Paraplast at 60° C – No. 1 for 2 h.
Paraplast at 60° C – No. 2 for 2 h.

In the morning the tissues are ready for embedding in Paraplast.

Frozen sections of endometrium are no more difficult to make than those of other fragmented soft tissues. Fresh unfixed endometrial curettings should be used, since material fixed in formalin is less easy to handle and is unsuitable for immunohistological studies, such as the demonstration of hormone receptors. The remaining fragments should be fixed, embedded, and sectioned as usual, since the study of all tissue is important if one wants to avoid overlooking an early carcinoma or small remnants of decidua.

c) Orientation

When possible, the fragments of endometrium should be placed in the paraffin so the mucosal surface is perpendicular to the plane at which the block will be sectioned. If the entire uterus is available then there will be no difficulty in properly orienting the tissue or in selecting specimens from specific regions of the endometrial cavity and numbering them accordingly. Since we generally receive endometrial curettings in small fragments, it is virtually impossible to orient their mucosal surfaces properly. What we must do then is to place as many fragments on the bottom of the paraffin well as is feasible to insure all are sectioned. Only when curettings are extraordinarily plentiful is it safe to embed only part of them. Abundant curettings usually come from advanced pathological conditions that are easy to diagnose, as for example, a large endometrial carcinoma, extensive glandular-cystic hyperplasia, or an abortion. Carcinomatous tissue, characteristically yellow-white, firm but crumbly and granular, can usually be grossly recognized by these features. In contrast, fragments of a glandular-cystic hyperplasia are softer, smoother, edematous and consequently translucent. Remnants of a placenta can be distinguished by their sponginess. Inspite of careful blocking and sectioning of the curettings, if a satisfactory diagnosis of them cannot be made, then it is advisable to re-embed the fragments by turning them 90°. The practice of preparing step-sections of curettings, as routinely followed at some institutes, insures a more thorough study of the tissue and affords a better chance for detecting small, localized lesions. The disadvantage of step-sections is that the tissue cut away between them is lost forever. Therefore, we find it advisable to section first at only one level. Then, depending on the case and how unclear or complicated the tissue changes are, we decide whether to re-embed the curettings or to section the block at deeper levels.

d) Staining

For the experienced pathologist the standard *hematoxylin-eosin stain* is adequate for diagnosing all important pathological changes of the endometrium. Since one should endeavor, however, to gain as much information from the occasionally scanty curettings as possible by making not only a pathological diagnosis but a functional diagnosis as well, we find it worthwhile to employ two additional stains routinely. These are the periodic acid-Schiff (PAS) reaction and the van Gieson stain.

The *PAS reaction* (method: ROMEIS 1968, §§ 1120–1122) is particularly helpful in making functional diagnoses by staining smallest amounts of glycogen or mucus that normally are inapparent with other stains (AUGUSTIN 1952); with the reaction, finely dispersed droplets of glycogen can be detected in the glandular epithelium as early as the second half of the proliferative phase. Glycogen persisting in the glandular epithelium long after a pregnancy and invisible with hematoxylin-eosin stains may be colored with the PAS reaction, enabling one to diagnose that there had been a pregnancy, although it may have gone clinically unrecognized (CRAMER 1957). Hyalinized remnants of decidua retained post partum or post abortum give a positive PAS reaction and therefore can be readily distinguished from the surrounding unstained structures. In contrast, with hematoxylin-eosin the decidual remnants stain like all other parts, making their recognition difficult (ELSTER and SPANKNEBEL 1959). During the secretory phase if glycogen is found in only some of the glands, that disparity in distribution indicates ovarian function is abnormal. The PAS reaction may also aid one in recognizing and classifying mucoepidermoid carcinomas or mucus-secreting adenocarcinomas, since these tumors at times produce scanty amounts of mucus inconspicuous in sections stained with hematoxylin-eosin.

The *van Gieson stain* (method: ROMEIS 1968, § 708) is useful for detecting polyps, for it colors their stroma of delicate collagenous fibers red, making the polyps stand out from the unstained normal endometrial stroma. The van Gieson stain proves particularly helpful in distinguishing polyps when their glands resemble those of the remaining endometrium. Another advantage of the van Gieson stain is its distinctive staining of old placental villi embedded in fibrin. The villi stain bright red, the sheaths of fibrin yellow. In contrast, with the hematoxylin-eosin stain both stain pink, as do other necrotic remnants of tissue, making recognition of the villi difficult.

Because of these advantages we routinely employ the PAS reaction and the van Gieson stain, in addition to the hematoxylin-eosin stain. All are easy to perform on large numbers of sections.

Several other special stains and histochemical reactions have proved worthwhile for clarifying particular defects of the endometrium and for diagnosing functional bleeding and infertility of endometrial origin. These methods should be employed whenever problems in diagnosis arise (STOLL et al. 1954). A few examples of these special stains will be considered here under the discussion of techniques; the reader will find a more detailed account of the uses and advantages of these methods under the discussion of the appropriate pathological conditions.

Special Methods for Demonstrating the Fibers of Connective Tissues
The *Masson-trichome stain* (method: ROMEIS 1968, § 1538) is useful for demonstrating in degenerating decidual cells the collagen inclusions, which may indicate that a pregnancy had occurred some time before (DALLENBACH-HELLWEG 1961). With careful study these inclusions may be recognized even in the van Gieson stain. In sections stained with hematoxylin-eosin they are invisible. – The *demonstration of reticulum fibers* (with, for example, the method of GOMORI: ROMEIS 1968, §§ 1573–1575) may be of diagnostic value in irregular shedding of the endometrium, since in that condition the reticulum fibers fail to undergo normal dissolution in those regions where menstrual shedding is retarded. Occasionally, it is important to demonstrate reticulum fibers when one wishes to differentiate polyps or endometrial tissue from the isthmic region, which are rich in stromal fibers, from the corpus endometrium, which is poor in fibers. Further, it is often possible with the reticulum stain to detect that the patient used oral contraceptive agents since the endometrium under that therapy forms almost no fibers (WAIDL et al. 1968). – As ELSTER and SPANKNEBEL (1959) have shown, the *Goldner* stain may be used to differentiate the connective tissue fibers (they stain green) from other structures of the stroma (nerve fibers, vessels) that stain pink. With the Goldner stain the stroma of polyps stains bright green, distinguishing them from the gray-green of an atrophic endometrium or from the yellow-brown of the myometrium. Moreover, the Goldner stain is useful in detecting regions that have undergone a hyaline change: the amorphous parts of an incompletely desquamated endometrium stain pale green; the thickened hyalinized walls of capillaries found after an abortion are colored bright green; the hyaline thrombi in a glandular-cystic hyperplasia appear gray-brown; the edematous stroma stains from yellow to red.

Histochemical Reactions for Demonstrating Nucleic Acids
In establishing a functional diagnosis it may be important to determine the content of desoxyribonucleic acid (DNA) of the endometrial cells. DNA is stained easily and well with the *Feulgen reaction* (method: ROMEIS 1968, § 1192ff.). Since the content of ribonucleic acid (RNA) in glandular and stromal cells serves as a measure or criterion of the effect of estrogen, it is often worthwhile to stain for RNA. For that we may use either the *methyl green-pyronin* stain (after PAPPENHEIM-UNNA, ROMEIS 1968, §§ 1199–1200) or the *gallocyanin-chromalum* method (after EINARSON, ROMEIS § 1203). With the latter, however, both RNA and DNA are stained, requiring that the DNA be removed by digestion with desoxyribonuclease before we apply the method. Because plasma cells contain abundant RNA and are an important sign of chronic inflammation, both the methyl green-pyronin stain and the gallocyanin-chromalum method may be used to good advantage in detecting them.

Special Staining Reactions Based on Proteinaceous Components of Cells
We can demonstrate proteins of cells with the *tetrazonium reaction*. If we benzoylate the sections first before the reaction, then we can reveal histidine, or if we first treat the sections with "H Acid" (Hoechst, FRG) then we can restrict our staining to tryptophan and arginine (method: PEARSE 1968, p. 612). Certain amino acids may be visualized by coupling them to diazo dyes or to similar reagents. For example, the *Millon reaction* has proved of value in detecting tyrosine (PEARSE 1968, p. 606); tryptophan can be demonstrated with the DMAB-nitrite method of ADAMS (PEARSE 1968, p. 615 or ARNOLD 1968, p. 127); arginine is readily stained with the *Sakaguchi reaction* (PEARSE 1968, p. 617). The reaction of BARRNETT and SELIGMAN (ARNOLD 1968, p. 128) is particularly useful for revealing SH groups. For staining the basic SH groups we use the *aldehyde-fuchsin reaction* (method after CAMERON and STEELE: HUMASON 1962, p. 168). Since the reaction also detects SO_3 groups of acid mucopolysaccharides as well as the aldehyde groups of lipids, we must differentiate our results as outlined in Table 2:

Table 2. Histochemical differentiation of the chemical groups revealed with the aldehyde-fuchsin reaction

	Aldehyde-fuchsin positive		
	SO_3 groups in acid mucopolysaccharides	SH groups in basic proteins	Aldehyde groups in lipids
Aldehyde-fuchsin without oxidation	+	+	−
Metachromasia	+	−	−

Often the occurrence of countless endometrial granulocytes (differentiated stromal cells) in the second half of the secretory phase gives rise to the erroneous diagnosis of endometritis. In questionable cases the HELLWEG (1954) modification of the *phloxine-tartrazine stain* of LENDRUM (1947), an uncomplicated method for demonstrating protein, may be helpful in proving that the cells present are endometrial granulocytes:

Paraffin sections of formalin-fixed tissue are first stained with hematein or iron-hematoxylin (as nuclear stains). Sections are then washed in tap water until blue, and stained for 30 min in the following solution: phloxine (C.I. 45410) 0.5 g, calcium chloride 0.5 g, distilled water 100 ml. Sections are washed in tap water. To differentiate and counterstain, a saturated solution of tartrazine (C.I. 19140) in ethylene glycol (Cellosolve) is dropped onto the sections individually until, as checked under the microscope, all phloxine is washed free from the tissue except from the cytoplasmic granules of the endometrial granulocytes. The differentiation usually takes only 1 min. The sections are then washed in 60% ethyl alcohol and run up through a series of alcohols of increasing strength to xylene. Sections are mounted with Canada balsam.

In sections stained with hematoxylin-eosin the protein-rich cytoplasmic granules of these modified stromal cells are uncolored and inconspicuous. With the phloxine stain, however, the granules turn bright red and contrast sharply from their surrounding yellow cytoplasm. Since granulocytic leukocytes and lymphocytes possess no such granules, it is easy to distinguish the endometrial granulocytes from them. The phloxine-tartrazine stain is also valuable for revealing hornified epithelial squames from a previous pregnancy or keratinized pearl formations of a carcinoma, as well as for differentiating between muscle fibers (red) and connective tissue (yellow).

Special Methods for Demonstrating Polysaccharides
Both the *PAS reaction* (see above) and the *aldehyde-fuchsin reaction* (see above) are suitable for making more precise evaluations of ovarian function (STRAUSS 1963). By means of the distinct, colorful, and contrast-rich staining of the acid mucopolysaccharides we may detect the onset of mucus secretion of the glandular epithelium almost 1 week before glycogen can be demonstrated. If we use the aldehyde-fuchsin stain at that time we notice the apical margin of the epithelial cells is red-violet. Daily fluctuations in the quantity and quality of the secretion as well as in the ratio between mucus and glycogen may point to abnormal ovarian function. The aldehyde-fuchsin reaction is easy to perform and suitable for routine studies. Another stain recommended for demonstrating acid mucopolysaccharides and equally as easy to perform is the *alcian blue stain* (method: ROMEIS 1968, § 2077). When combined with the PAS reaction, the double-staining enables the acid mucopolysaccharides to be distinguished from the neutral mucopolysaccharides and from glycogen (RUNGE et al. 1956).

The Demonstration of Lipids
In paraffin sections of endometrium the total lipids are best stained with *Sudan black B* (method after LISON: ROMEIS 1968, § 1055). The other Sudan stains that require frozen sections are more difficult to perform for routine diagnostic studies, because the soft, endometrial tissue usually comes as many small fragments. Sudan black B is especially useful for staining foam cells in the endometrial stroma; these are a sign of hyperestrogenism. Phosphatides are well demonstrated with BAKER's *acid hematein test* (PEARSE 1968, p. 689) or with the *Luxol-fast blue stain*. Cholesterol and its esters may be detected with SCHULZ's *method* (PEARSE 1968, p. 702) or with polarized light since crystals of cholesterol are doubly refractive.

Many additional histochemical and particularly enzyme-histochemical techniques may be employed that may help to detect or clarify subtle variations in the physiological and pathological behavior of glands and stroma. Before we resort to these intricate methods, however, we should ask pertinent questions or have specific research purposes in mind, since the techniques are all too complicated, expensive and time-consuming to be employed as routine methods for daily diagnostic studies. SCHMIDT-MATTHIESEN (1963) applied these special methods to the normal endometrium and compiled his results for ready reference. Later, when we discuss functional disturbances of the endometrium we shall examine in detail the uses and value of these various techniques for the histological diagnosis of pathological states. In performing the methods we have followed PEARSE's recommendations.

The technique of *fluorochromation with acridine-orange* (SCHÜMMELFEDER 1950; SCHÜMMELFEDER et al. 1957) is too important to go unmentioned. With this technique we can not only follow the daily changes in the menstrual cycle, as with sections stained with hematoxylin-eosin, but we can also detect the first signs of hormonal action: by demonstrating RNA in the nuclei and cytoplasm of endometrial cells we are able to evaluate the effect of estrogen; by demonstrating the first droplets of glycogen in the glandular epithelium we can measure the effect of progesterone (DALLENBACH and DALLENBACH-HELLWEG 1968). The technique, too difficult for routine studies, has value in research work for revealing subtle changes not evident with other methods. If compared with sections stained with hematoxylin-eosin, it induces us to look for equivalent changes in these.

e) Immunocytochemistry with Monoclonal Antibodies

During the past few years, detailed studies of the molecular biology of cells have resulted in the development of monoclonal antibodies against specific proteins of the cytoskeleton. With these antibodies it has become possible to study by immunohistochemical techniques specific cellular functions and to follow cellular differentiation. The following are the most important marker proteins for the histopathology of the endometrium:

Proliferation Markers. The most reliable monoclonal antibody which recognizes all active stages of the cell cycle (G_1, S, G_2 phases and mitoses, but not G_0 phases) is KI-67 which has been detected and developed by GERDES et al. (1983). The antibody can be made visible and evaluated with the immunoperoxidase reaction. The results of these evaluations are much more precise than previous data gained by mitotic counts, DNA measurements, etc. The proliferating activity detected with KI-67 gives important additional information for evaluating the proliferative activity of endometrial tumors, for judging their prognosis and for selecting the best therapy.

Markers for Intermediate Filaments. The intermediate filaments constitute an important part of the cytoskeleton of epithelial and mesenchymal cells since they characterize the nature and histogenesis of each cell type: epithelial cells contain cytokeratin filaments, which can be subdivided into at least 19 different polypeptides, mesenchymal cells vimentin filaments, myogenic cells desmin filaments, neuronal cells neurofilaments and astrocytes glial filaments. Because of the complexity of the various epithelial and stromal (mesenchymal) cells of the normal and neoplastic endometrium, a study of these filaments, especially in poorly differentiated tumors, is of particular interest. Such studies can be performed with indirect immunofluorescence microscopy using monoclonal antibodies directed against the individual filaments according to the techniques described by MOLL et al. (1983) and CZERNOBILSKY et al. (1984).

The Detection of Specific Receptor Sites for Estrogen and Progesterone in the Nuclei of the Target Cells. For this purpose an estrogen receptor immunocytochemical assay (ER-ICA) has been developed using monoclonal antibodies against receptor-associated proteins (GREENE et al. 1980, 1984; KING et al. 1985); (cf. p. 48f.). This assay method is more accurate than the biochemical (RIA) assay in which the cytosol fraction of a mixture of various disrupted cells is measured for receptor content (BAULIEU 1979; JENSEN 1979). With the ER-ICA assay, the precise localization, number, and concentration of occupied and unoccupied receptor sites can be visualized and determined histologically. The results gained are particularly important for the diagnosis of changes in the endometrium in infertility and for the evaluation of the hormonal responsiveness of endometrial tumors. Very recently, a progesterone receptor immunocytochemical assay (PR-ICA) has been developed which can now be used in parallel with the ER-ICA assay.

Monoclonal Antibodies Against Epithelial Surface Antigens. This technique may also become more important in the future. At present various methods using these antibodies are still in the developmental stage.

f) Quantitative and Experimental Methods

Besides the histochemical methods, quantitative techniques such as *morphometry* (BISWAS and FINBOW 1975; BAAK and DIEGENBACH 1977), *karyometry* (WITT 1963) or *cytometry* (KAISERLING 1950; STÄHLER 1950) may be of diagnostic value. Inspite of recent optimistic reports (BAAK 1984; Ausems et al. 1985; SKAARLAND 1985), the measurements obtained with these methods must be carefully and critically evaluated since various endometria often shrink differently although embedded under like conditions. Furthermore, there are individual variations in the tumor-host interaction that may not influence nuclear size or shape, but will interact to define the outcome. In addition, the lack of aneuploidy is not a decisive criterion against malignancy, since up to 30% of carcinomas have hypodiploid or peridiploid nuclear values (NORRIS 1985). In general, with practice in studying cellular details one can do without these measurements in routine diagnostic studies.

The *culture of endometrium in vitro* is mainly of scientific interest (for review of literature see HELLWEG and SHAKA 1959). Nonetheless, by adding hormones in various concentrations and combinations to cultures and comparing these with untreated controls it is possible to gain valuable information about the sensitivity of endometrial tissue as it grows isolated from ovarian influences. When combined with other research methods, endometrial organ culture in particular can be ideally used to study hormonal binding and mode of action (CSERMELY et al. 1969). After *subcutaneous transplantation* into nude mice, human endometrium reacts in the same way to hormonal stimuli as eutopic human endometrium (BERGQVIST et al. 1985).

Among the many techniques for *chromosome analysis* (HUGHES and CSERMELY 1965; SHERMAN 1969), three were found to be reasonably useful in obtaining cells for karyotyping: (a) the direct squash preparation of endometrium; (b) the tissue culture squash preparation; and (c) the air-dried cell suspension. One must be cautious about making or accepting diagnoses of aneuploidy with these techniques since the cells are badly disrupted during the squashing procedure. Skepticism is also warranted for the modern trend to employ *computer programs* for evaluating single parameters, since such studies tend to place the diagnoses from individual patients in question (BEZEMER et al. 1977).

5. Components of Curettings and Their Diagnostic Value

The histological diagnosis of curettings is much more difficult than that of endometrium intentionally selected from a definite region of a surgically removed uterus. We must not only decide from what parts of the uterine cavity and endometrial layers the haphazardly admixed curettings came, we must also be able to diagnose the stage of endometrial development, for from that we date the endometrium (determine as accurately as possible what day of the menstrual cycle the endometrial changes represent), and make our functional diagnosis accordingly. Such goals presuppose a thorough knowledge of the histology of the normal endometrium and its layers in the fundic, isthmic and cervical regions, as well as a knowledge about how reliable these different regions are for establishing accurate diagnoses. Only endometrium from the fundus is suitable for diagnosis; the whole layer of the *functionalis*, consisting of the superficial compacta and the basal spongiosa, is particularly ideal. In contrast, the *basalis* is generally of little diagnostic value except in two diseases: in carcinoma or its precursors and in irregular shedding of the endometrium. In most endometria the functionalis is distinct and easy to recognize. We should remember, however, that neighboring glands and stroma may vary somewhat in development without these variations implying that ovarian function is abnormal. In addition, the fragments of mucosa are often from different layers or regions of the endometrium (cornual, fundic, isthmic) that normally show variances in their development. Irregular development is best detected in larger fragments of tissue where the structural units retain their relationships.

Endometrium from the *isthmic portion* of the uterus is unsuited for functional diagnosis since its glands fail to undergo changes during the menstrual cycle (DANFORTH and CHAPMAN 1949) or only in exceptional instances (STIEVE 1928; OBER et al. 1958) and then only slightly. The isthmic mucosa may also give the false impression that the endometrium is atrophic or deficient, or only from the basalis. An experienced investigator will easily recognize and know how to evaluate the uniformly low, relatively avascular mucosa of the isthmic region, with its characteristic flattened, slit-like glands and dense fibrous stroma of small cells. Its glands are only occasionally cystic. Their cytoplasm contains no mucous substances, but histochemically shows, compared with the adjacent endocervical and endometrial glands, a surprisingly high enzymatic activity

(PFLEIDERER 1974). In contrast, the glands of the basalis branch more, and the supporting stroma about them is more irregular since the collagenous fibers anchoring the basalis to the myometrium extend in all directions. In addition, the stromal cells of the basalis remain refractory to hormones, whereas the stromal cells of the isthmic mucosa may at times undergo slight cyclic changes like the stromal cells in the functionalis of the corpus endometrium. When studying entire uteri we should remember that during life the mucosa of the uterine isthmus undergoes physiological displacement, moving with the advance (eversion) and retraction (inversion) of the cervical mucosa (OBER et al. 1958). Accordingly, in the reproductive years fragments of isthmic mucosa should be found among curettings from the cervix (since the isthmus has shifted below the internal uterine os). In the postmenopause, however, portions of the isthmic mucosa will be among the endometrial curettings since the isthmus has retracted above the internal os.

Recognition of the *endocervical mucosa* presents no problem because its glands and stroma characteristically differ from those of the endometrium. In contrast to the endometrium, the endocervix is furrowed with glands that branch widely and continuously secrete mucus (LANG and SCHNEIDER 1960). The endocervical mucosa undergoes either no changes during the menstrual cycle (TOPKINS 1949; DUPERROY 1951) or at most only slight changes (WOLLNER 1937; SJÖVALL 1938). These are mainly quantitative differences in the stages of secretion. All stages, however, may be found at any time of the cycle. Usually during the early secretory phase most glands disclose basal vacuolation, whereas in the late secretory phase most are dilated, distended with inspissated mucus. Histochemically, the glandular cytoplasm discloses its greatest enzymatic activity during the 2nd week of the cycle (PFLEIDERER 1974).

Fragments of squamous epithelium from the *portio vaginalis,* often caught up among the curettings, should be carefully inspected and reported in the diagnosis, a principle that well applies to all constituents of the curettings. The height of the squamous epithelium may provide information about the patient's hormonal state or point to a hormonal disturbance, especially when the endometrium is unremarkable, perhaps because its cells are refractory to hormones owing to their inability to make hormonal receptors. In addition, a dysplastic change of the epithelium of the portio may incidentally be discovered in a curetting.

The pathologist should also notify the clinician how much *myometrium* is included with the curettings, for such information helps the gynecologist to draw conclusions about the consistency of the uterine tissues or about his technique of curettage. Further, portions of myometrium may be important in evaluating the extent of a pathological change as, for example, with inflammation of the endometrium or with invasion by trophoblastic cells. At times the myometrial tissue in curettings originates from a *submucosal leiomyoma,* and in some instances the entire tumor, if small, may be included in the curettings (Fig. 1). For deciding whether the muscular tissue is from the myometrium or from a leiomyoma, we apply the same criteria as used with larger pieces of tissue. The muscle fibers of leiomyomata are more compact, arranged in tight, whorled bundles bound by condensed interstitial collagenous tissue. If mucosa still ad-

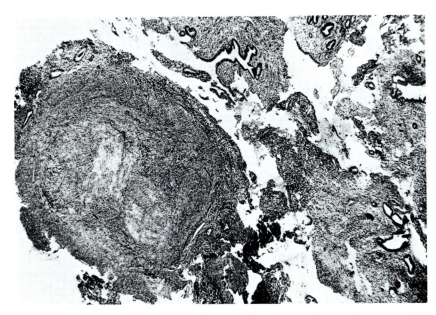

Fig. 1. Submucosal leiomyoma included in curettings, covered in part by a stretched-out and compressed mucosa

heres to the fragment of leiomyoma, then it is usually stretched out and flattened with its glands compressed and narrow, running almost parallel to the surface. In contrast, the mucosa adherent to fragments of myometrium more commonly consists of portions of basalis.

Extensive *regions of necrosis* in curettings may have various causes. Therefore, when endometrial structure in these regions is totally effaced, we are able to reach a diagnosis only if enough preserved endometrial tissue is also present for study. Common examples in which extensive necrosis may be found are: a degenerating carcinoma, an infected (septic) abortion, a degenerated submucosal myoma, and an infarcted polyp. Special stains may occasionally be used in establishing a diagnosis (see above). After a partial abortion the curettings of the retained products of conception may disclose not only variably degenerated or necrotic remnants of *placenta and decidua* but may also reveal several fetal structures at various ages of development or at different stages of maceration. Such fetal parts, surrounded by actively proliferating endometrium, may often be demonstrated weeks or even months after the abortion, serving as proof that an abortion had occurred although it may have been missed clinically. Of all fetal structures the *bony parts* persist the longest and may ultimately induce an endometritis. Such cases, however, are rare. The parts of the products of conception most frequently retained after an abortion are the necrotic or hyaline remnants of decidua. These usually appear as vague, shadowy outlines of the original decidual cells. In the differential diagnosis we must distinguish these remnants from the hyaline thrombi of glandular-cystic hyperplasia that are always devoid of a fibrous network, as a reticulum stain will prove. Moreover, the thrombi stain pale violet with the PAS reaction, whereas the decidual remnants stain bright red (ELSTER and SPANKNEBEL 1959).

Foreign bodies brought into the uterine cavity from the outside belong to the group of rather rare constituents of curettings. The extraneous material may become embedded and "healed into" the endometrium, inducing a foreign-body, granulomatous reaction around it. From the character or age of that reaction we may be able to judge when the foreign material entered the uterus. A foreign-body reaction follows contamination of the uterine cavity with non-soluble particulate matter, for example with talcum crystals. These may be identified under polarized light as the cause of a granulomatous reaction since they are double-refractive. A foreign-body reaction may occasionally develop in the endometrium after intrauterine instillation of a liquid tissue adhesive for sterilization.

We must take care not to misinterpret *artefacts*. Not infrequently artifical changes are produced in the soft endometrial tissue by the squeezing and tearing of curettage and subsequent handling; as a result, the endometrial structures become greatly distorted. Occasionally when glands are squeezed or compressed, their lining epithelium intussuscepts to lie within the lumen. Only an experienced pathologist can distinguish such an artefact from an adenocarcinoma (Fig. 2). Even the stroma may become so altered by compression that it may at first glance suggest a sarcoma. Severe freezing artefacts occur when the endometrial tissue is allowed to freeze slowly, as may happen when the tissue is sent by postal service in the winter (Fig. 3).

Finally, we must consider *what should not be a component of a curetting*. Occasionally when several curettings are prepared for embedding and placed in perforated tissue capsules to facilitate the diffusion of dehydrating fluids, a small fragment of tissue from one capsule may slip through a perforation and be carried into another capsule. We should always think of that possibility. If we find a single tiny fragment of tissue that seems from its composition to be foreign and unrelated to the other fragments in the section, we must interpret that unique fragment with caution. One should not try to diagnose an abortion from a single placental villus in curettings that show no other evidence of a previous pregnancy. A much more serious error would be to diagnose a carcinoma from a small fragment of tissue that as a contaminant has unknowingly been caught up in the endometrial curettings of another patient. In such instances, however, to avoid overlooking a carcinoma it is advisable to section the tissue block at deeper levels so a search can be made for eventual larger fragments of tumor. If the small fragment is found to unite with a larger piece of endometrium, then it matters little how small it is; it is obviously of diagnostic importance. In like manner, if deeper sections prove a single placental villus is attached to a larger fragment of endometrium, the villus on that account may be used to diagnose a previous abortion. Fragments of tissues that do not belong in curettings, for example fat tissue, *indicate* that *contamination* occurred, provided the uterus was not perforated. If the foreign fragments of tissue are large then it is probable they became mixed with the curettings before the tissues were prepared for embedding.

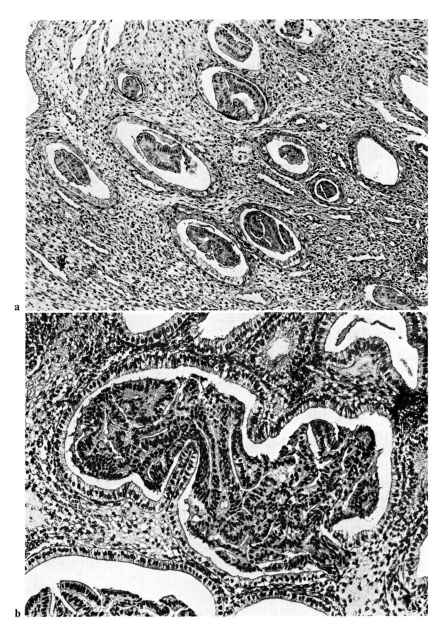

Fig. 2a, b. Artefact: desquamated glandular epithelium has been squeezed into the glandular lumina; **a** low magnification; **b** higher magnification

The **concluding diagnosis** of a histological report of an endometrium should be as comprehensive as possible. That is to say, it should include the pathological diagnosis of the structural changes, and the diagnosis of the corresponding functional state. Provided he has submitted sufficient tissue for study, the gynecologist has a right to expect an explicit pathological report on which he can

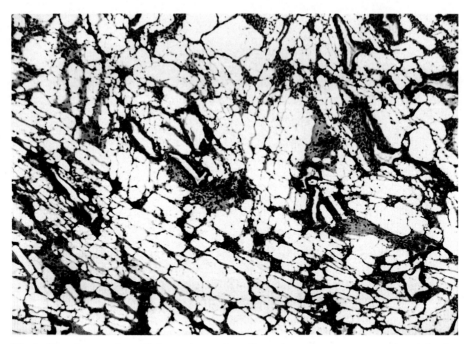

Fig. 3. Freezing artefact of the endometrium. Irregular empty spaces produced by ice crystals separate glands and push stromal cells aside. These spaces have no cellular lining (e.g., endothelial cells)

Table 3. Factors limiting the diagnosis of endometrial curettings

Referring physician	Absent or inaccurate clinical data
	Curettage at the wrong time
	Insufficient curettings
	Incorrect handling or fixation of the material
Pathologist	Inadequate experience
	Incomplete preparation of the material
	Poorly prepared microscopic sections
Endometrial tissue	Changes in morphology lag behind the changes in function (differences in tempo)
	Transition between benign and malignant not clearly detectable (differences in stages)
	Functional changes with no corresponding morphological (histological, histochemical) changes detectable

base his treatment of the patient. The clinician is not benefited by a long account of vague assumptions or a list of the different diagnoses that might be possible. The pathologist should endeavor to reach a precise final diagnosis. With rare exceptions (see Table 3) he will succeed in doing so if he carefully studies the material and uses the appropriate diagnostic aids (special stains and techniques) that are available.

6. Statistical Analysis of the Histological Results

The primary purpose of the histological study of surgically removed tissue is to provide as accurate a diagnosis of the morphological changes present as possible. In addition, however, the study should stimulate scientific interest and encourage questions, and should be employed to investigate these questions. Only with such precepts can a dynamic, intellectually stimulating diagnostic service be guaranteed that will always remain receptive to new scientific information.

With that purpose in mind, our pathology service uses a dual system of cataloguing specimens received for study. The first system consists of an alphabetical registry of the names of all our patients: an index card is used for each patient; it bears the specimen number and code numbers of the final diagnoses of every specimen of tissue received from that patient. The system

Table 4. Statistical analysis of functional changes of the endometrium (altered ovarian function) using the decimal system

	Regeneration	Proliferation	Secretion	Menstrual shedding	No functional changes
Regular cycle	10	20	30	40	50 Resting
Shortened cycle	11	21	31	41	51 Atrophic
Delayed cycle	12	22	32	42	52 Cystic atrophic
Insufficient cycle	13	23	33	43	
Irregular cycle	14	24	34	44	54
Glandular-cystic hyperplasia	15 Adaptation hyperplasia, post partum and post abortum	25 Glandular cystic hyperplasia, resting and active form	35 Hyperplasia with secretory change	45 Remnants of hyperplasia after extensive shedding	55 Regression of hyperplasia
Adenomatous hyperplasia and stromal hyperplasia	16	26	36	46	
Focal hyperplasia and hyperplasia of basalis	17	27	37 Secretory hypertrophy	47	57
Breakthrough bleeding	18	28 Anovulatory cycle	38 (Also ovulatory bleeding)	48 Hormonal withdrawal bleeding	58 Apoplexia uteri

allows a rapid "histological anamnesis" of every patient, for from the record of previous studies one may quickly evaluate the advance or regression of changes, may search for or review possible interrelationships between diseases, or may learn about their final outcome. The second system represents a registry of the diagnoses, using a scheme with decimal numbers that we designed for our clinic. Each diagnosis of normal or functionally disturbed endometrium is given a number of two digits (see Table 4). When contraceptive hormones had been taken by the patient, "ov" is added to the number, when other hormones had been administered, "hz" is added. The diagnoses of organic (primary) diseases of the endometrium, such as endometritis, carcinoma etc., receive numbers of three digits, as do the diagnoses of other gynecological organs (see tables in STOLL and DALLENBACH-HELLWEG 1981; compare with STOLL and RIEHM 1954). As soon as we finish our histological report, we select from our coded list of pathological conditions the appropriate number for the diagnosis. When the secretary writes the report she enters the code number of the patient's card in the alphabetical registry. An alternative is to store these coded data in a computer for instant retrieval. Such a cataloguing system enables us, on the one hand, to collect and utilize the material we have diagnosed for later scientific study. It obviates tedious searching through volumes of bound reports by an assistant or doctoral student who may be working on a research project. On the other hand, it helps in teaching by making it possible for us to plan and prepare demonstrations and clinical-pathological conferences on short notice.

B. The Normal Histology of the Endometrium

1. The Individual Structures

The endometrium of the corpus is composed of two layers: the basalis (the layer from which the endometrium regenerates after menstrual shedding) and the overlying functionalis. In the second half of the menstrual cycle, the functionalis may be differentiated into the superficial compacta and the underlying spongiosa, which extends to the basalis. During the menstrual cycle the endometrium varies from 1 mm (postmenstrual) to about 8 mm at the end of the 3rd week. Every layer consists of two major structures: the epithelial component, either as glands or as superficial epithelium, and the mesenchymal component of stromal cells. Both cellular components are pluripotential and can undergo various metaplastic changes.

As a target organ under the control of the ovarian hormones, the endometrium is rhythmically called upon to rapidly fulfill functional requirements that necessitate frequent remodeling of its structural components, implying rapid and well-adapted changes. To find out how these changes take place and how they are controlled by the ovarian hormones, we shall examine the basic structures of these components involved without, however, going into great detail. For the reader who desires a more thorough discussion of the normal, sexually mature corpus endometrium, I highly recommend SCHMIDT-MATTHIESEN's book (1963). This excellent monograph provides details of normal endometrial histology, karyometry, electronmicroscopy, and histochemistry. Significant new discoveries of recent years are described in the following pages.

a) The Glandular Epithelium

The glandular epithelium is a single layer of columnar epithelial cells. Their height varies, depending on the functional (hormonal) state, from 6 μ postmenstrual to 20 μ at the end of the proliferative phase. The proliferating glandular epithelium remains bipotential as indicated by its immunohistochemical coexpression of vimentin and cytokeratin, whereas the secreting glandular epithelium only expresses cytokeratin (MOLL et al. 1983; DABBS et al. 1986).

During the proliferative phase the *nuclei* of the glandular cells are elongated and have a dense chromatin. Between the 10th and the 16th day of the cycle their DNA content reaches its maximum (VOKAER 1951; HARKIN 1956; MOOKERJEA 1961; FETTIG and OEHLERT 1964; FETTIG 1965; NORDQVIST 1970). During the secretory phase the nuclei become round, vesicular, and gradually lose DNA. The chromosome sets are mostly diploid (79% according to STANLEY 1969), showing a consistant pattern of 46 XX (SHERMAN 1969). Aneuploidy apparently never occurs (WAGNER et al. 1968). Mitoses are most numerous just before ovulation. JOHANNISSON and HAGENFELDT (1971) found an accumulation of nuclei in the S-phase between cycle days 14 and 22 and suggested, therefore, that the synthesis of DNA in the human endometrium was synchronized.

The *nucleoli* contain abundant RNA. In contrast, the RNA of the cytoplasm reaches its greatest concentration after ovulation. The nucleoli of the early proliferative phase are finely granular and compact. They enlarge as mid-cycle is approached and may reach 2.8 µ in diameter (FASSKE et al. 1965). During the 1st week of the secretory phase the nucleoli contain a characteristic tubular or meshwork-like structure, the nucleolar channel system, which is embedded in an electron-dense matrix and contains RNA; some investigators believe it serves the exchange of protein between nucleolus and cytoplasm primarily for enzyme synthesis (DUBRAUSZKY and POHLMANN 1960; CLYMAN 1963; ANCLA and DE BRUX 1965; TERZAKIS 1965; MORE et al. 1974), for example, for the rapid transport of specific, progesterone-induced ribonucleoprotein (ARMSTRONG et al. 1973). The channel system apparently occurs only in human endometrium and seems to depend on adequate levels of progesterone. It may be induced in vitro (KOHORN et al. 1970) or experimentally (NAKAO et al. 1971) when enough gestagen is administered. At the end of the menstrual cycle it is discharged into the cytoplasm and taken up by lysosomes. FELDHAUS et al. (1977) were able to demonstrate the system shortly before ovulation.

During the proliferative phase the *cytoplasm* is unusually rich in RNA, as disclosed by histochemical techniques (WISLOCKI and DEMPSEY 1945; ATKINSON et al. 1949; BREMER et al. 1951; MCKAY et al. 1956; MOOKERJEA 1961; BOUTSELIS et al. 1963; GROSS 1964), by fluorescence microscopy (BONTKE 1960; DALLENBACH and DALLENBACH-HELLWEG 1968) and by autoradiography (FETTIG 1965). Electron-microscopic studies (BORELL et al. 1959; CARTIER and MORICARD 1959; WESSEL 1960; WETZSTEIN and WAGNER 1960; DUBRAUSZKY and POHLMANN 1961; GOMPEL 1962, 1964; THEMANN and SCHÜNKE 1963; MORICARD and MORICARD 1964; MORICARD 1966; WYNN and HARRIS 1967; WYNN and WOOLLEY 1967) indicate the cytoplasm, especially that of the basal parts of the cells, contains abundant ribosomes, some bound to endoplasmic membranes, some free. Bundles of tonofilaments, each about 100 Å in diameter, appear around the 13th day of the menstrual cycle, under the influence of increased estrogen stimulation. Shortly after ovulation, they are redistributed to become incorporated into desmosomal complexes which may be important in stabilizing the rigidity of cells prior to nidation (CLYMAN et al. 1982). Towards the end of the proliferative phase the Golgi complex located above the nucleus becomes visible with secretory granules (probably acid phosphatases; NILSSON 1962). At the base of the cell near the first aggregates of glycogen the mitochondria multiply and enlarge. With the onset of the secretory phase the previously rough endoplasmic reticulum becomes smooth. Abundant basal secretory granules then collect around these smooth endoplasmic membranes, and they in turn gather about the enlarged mitochondria. As glycogen, mucopolysaccharides and proteins accumulate at the lower pole of the nucleus to form cloudy or granular deposits, the large mitochondria nearby swell to giant sizes, and may reach

7 μ in diameter. They have compact cristae and up to eight intramitochondrial filaments of DNA (MERKER et al. 1968; ARMSTRONG et al. 1973). On the 17th day of the menstrual cycle glycogen is found scattered throughout the cytoplasm, and the well-developed Golgi complex with terminal vacuoles is located above the nucleus. With the onset of secretion on the 19th and 20th days the cytoplasm along the luminal surface sends out enlarged microvilli filled with secretory products. Shorty thereafter the apical portion of the cell is discharged into the lumen. Thus, the epithelial cells expel their products by apocrine secretion, thereby becoming smaller. Because minute amounts of glycogen are apparent in the glandular cells with the electron microscope several days before ovulation through to the last week of the cycle (with a distinct maximum between the 16th and 20th days), the glycogen is thought to serve a complex function involving more than pure glandular secretion (SAKUMA 1970; JOHANNISSON and HAGENFELDT 1971). Besides glycogen, the glandular cells also excrete neutral and acid mucopolysaccharides (SALM 1962; STRAUSS 1963) and lipids. Most accumulate at the apical cell border and are either carboxymucins or sulphomucins (SORVARI 1969). Fine droplets of non-double-refractive lipids may be detected during the secretory phase, chiefly in the basal cytoplasm of the glandular epithelium. Since the appearance and quantity of the droplets are influenced by hormones, some investigators believe the lipids indicate increased cellular activity induced by progesterone (ASCHHEIM 1915; BLACK et al. 1941). Other authors (FROBOESE 1924; CRAIG and DANZIGER 1965) regard the lipid droplets as products of degeneration. Their occurrence in the glandular epithelium of the decidua of a young pregnancy, however, favors the first view. By the 22nd day of the cycle only a few secretory granules remain. By the 23rd and 24th days the granular endoplasmic reticulum has involuted.

The apical *surface* of the epithelial cells in the proliferative phase possesses elongated delicate microvilli which contain alkaline phosphatases (BORELL et al. 1959). During the secretory phase, as these microvilli draw back and disappear, the activity of alkaline phosphatase diminishes.

The *substance secreted* by the glandular epithelial cells and found within the glandular lumina is chemically complex, and its composition varies with the phase of the menstrual cycle. During the proliferative phase it consists of a mixture of desquamated superficial glandular cells, RNA, proteins, and acid mucopolysaccharides. During the secretory phase the secretion appears as globules, which contain rounded aggregates of glycogen, acid and neutral mucopolysaccharides, proteins, peptides, neutral lipids, phosphatides and numerous enzymes. During the 4th week of the cycle the globules degenerate; at first they appear amorphous but later they become homogeneous. With that change they take on a β-metachromasia that is resistant to alcohol and ribonuclease. Finally, the glycogen disappears, leaving polysaccharides that are resistant to diastase. The metachromasia thereby increases.

Occasionally it is possible to find a *ciliated cell* among the glandular epithelial cells (MANDL 1911). The ciliated cells initially lie against the basement membrane, and because of their abundant translucent cytoplasm can be readily recognized as "clear cells". Their rounded nucleus is generally located above those of the neighboring epithelial cells (FEYRTER and FROEWIS 1949). In 1950

HAMPERL described a ciliary vesicle in these cells which, he explained, moved upwards through the cell to protrude at the upper surface, releasing its cilium to the outside. Later the ciliary border is shed by apocrine mechanisms. With the electron microscope it is possible to follow the development of the cilia from the basal corpuscles within the cytoplasm. The corpuscles form as the centrioles replicate and migrate to the cell surface where the vesicle develops. Each cell always has just eleven cilia. Their ultrastructure varies more than that of cilia in other organs (HANDO et al. 1968). They can be easily demonstrated with FEYRTER's "thionine-enclosure stain" because their content of mucoprotein makes them appear dark.

The number of ciliated cells fluctuates considerably from patient to patient, probably depending on the functional state of the endometrium (that is, on ovarian function). DAZO et al. (1970) report ciliated cells are more abundant close to the tubal cornua and the endocervical mucosa. "Clear cells" as possible precursor cells are commonest in the proliferative phase and in glandular-cystic hyperplasia. Fully developed ciliated cells are most numerous around mid-cycle and in hyperplastic endometria (MADDI and PAPANICOLAOU 1961; SCHUELLER 1968, 1973). In atrophic endometrium they are virtually non-existent (PAPADIA 1959; FLEMING et al. 1968). From these facts we could assume that estrogen stimulates the cilia to develop (SCHÜLLER 1961, 1968, 1973). No clear concepts exist regarding their function. Some investigators have postulated that the cilia aid in removing the secretions discharged by the neighboring cells. In their electron-microscopic studies of endometrium of the secretory phase, MORE and MASTERSTON (1975) described a transformation of ciliated cells into secretory cells, a change that would explain the apparent decrease in ciliated cells during the second half of the cycle.

In addition to the ciliated clear cells, apparently other *clear cells* become visible in the glandular epithelium. Cells in the early prophase of mitosis (FUCHS 1959) or degenerating cells with karyorrhexis (ROTTER and EIGNER 1949) may also appear as clear cells. Further, lymphocytes and polymorphonuclear leukocytes that migrate through the glandular epithelium may swell up, their cytoplasm becoming conspicuous and clear. FUCHS points out that the nuclear changes found in some of the clear cells, with the disappearance of the nucleoli and the increase in chromatin, are characteristic of the onset of mitosis. The great increase of clear cells in glandular-cystic hyperplasia found by all investigators parallels the rise in mitotic rate of the hyperplastic epithelium. In contrast, SARBACH (1955) believes some of the clear cells represent degenerating forms developing after an unsuccessful mitosis caused by excessive stimulation with estrogen. MÜLLER (1951) and FEYRTER (1952) assumed the clear cells were active as endocrine cells. FEYRTER even included them among the clear cells of the "generalized endocrine organ of epithelia" which he described. Several facts, however, oppose his assumption. The cells contain only meager amounts of RNA, suggesting they are inactive. Their Golgi apparatus is poorly developed (WESSEL 1960) and they possess few enzymes, secretory granules or lipids. They are neither chromaffin, argentaffin, nor argyrophilic.

b) The Superficial Epithelium

During the proliferative phase the superficial epithelium closely resembles the glandular epithelium, although it contains greater numbers of ciliated cells than does the glandular epithelium (FERENCZY et al. 1972). At the onset of the secretory phase, however, it lacks the apical accumulation of acid mucopolysaccharides (LEWIN 1961; SCHMIDT-MATTHIESEN 1963). Neutral mucopolysaccharides are also very sparse. Yet, glycogen appears in the superficial epithelium earlier, in larger amounts, and remains longer than it does in the glandular epithelium. Its acid phosphatase activity is lower then in the glandular epithelium but its phosphatide content is higher (SCHMIDT-MATTHIESEN 1968). Noteworthy is the uniformly high RNA content in its cytoplasm and nucleoli during the whole cycle (BREMER et al. 1951), suggesting that a synthesis of protein persists. Thus, the superficial epithelium also differs from the glandular epithelium functionally. This difference is easy to understand when we consider how important its secretion might be for the adherence and implantation of the blastocyst. As revealed by scanning electron microscopy, the ciliated cells accumulate about the mouths of the glands (HAFEZ et al. 1975). During the secretory phase the cilia degenerate, and as the apical surface of the cell continues to bulge into the uterine cavity, the size and number of its microvilli decrease (JOHANNISSON and NILSSON 1972).

c) The Stromal Cells

The endometrial stroma consists of pluripotential mesenchymal cells, which at the beginning of the menstrual cycle are uniformly spindle shaped, poorly differentiated, and joined to one another by cytoplasmic processes. The cells lie firmly anchored within a delicate network of reticulum fibers. Their elongated nuclei have abundant chromatin and they show in radioautographic studies a well defined synthesis of DNA (FETTIG and OEHLERT 1964), reflecting the DNA-controlled synthesis of RNA (MORE et al. 1974). At the beginning of the menstrual cycle the cytoplasm of the cells forms a narrow rim about the dark nuclei. Near the end of the proliferative phase the nuclear substance becomes less dense, the nucleoli grow larger and more conspicuous, and the nuclear membrane becomes wrinkled. The RNA accumulates in the cytoplasm of the more superficial stromal cells, and their smooth and rough endoplasmic reticulum expand. The Golgi apparatus and mitochondria remain poorly developed. Microfibrils of collagen become apparent, not only within the cells but particularly just outside them (WETZSTEIN and WAGNER 1960; DUBRAUSZKY and POHLMANN 1961; WYNN and WOOLLEY 1967; WIENKE et al. 1968; MORE et al. 1974). During the secretory phase the mitochondria and smooth endoplasmic reticulum increase in number and size, and the Golgi apparatus enlarges, whereas the ribosomes decrease (LIEBIG and STEGNER 1977). Vacuoles and granules begin to appear in the expanding but shortened cytoplasmic microvilli. From the 20th day of the cycle on, glycogen and glycoproteins in diffuse and granular form can be demonstrated in the cytoplasm of the stromal cells with electron-microscopic and histochemical methods (McKAY et al. 1956). Some stromal cells contain lipids as fine droplets (ASCHHEIM 1915; FROBOESE 1924; BLACK et al. 1941; CRAIG and DANZIGER 1965) which, in contrast to the lipids of the glandular epithelium, are double-refractive and appear after stimulation with estrogen. When the lipids accumulate in large amounts the stromal cells may reach the size of decidual cells and acquire a foamy cytoplasm. Consequently, they have been mistaken for macrophages or lipophages. It seems more likely they develop because of an overproduction of estrogen, and the lipids may represent a storage form of that hormone or a metabolite of it (DALLENBACH-HELLWEG 1964). If we consider the experimental studies of FROEWIS and ULM (1957) and GELLER and LOHMEYER (1959) on the endocrine function of the endometrium, it is understandable why they suggested that the stromal cell might be able to produce estrogen. Certainly its fine structure does not exclude such a possibility. Studies by DALLENBACH and RUDOLPH (1974), however, failed to show that endometrial tissues can produce and secrete estrogenic substances (cf. p. 124ff.).

During the second half of the secretory phase the stromal cells of the compacta cease their mitotic activity and differentiate in two directions (Figs. 4 and 5, Color Plate IIb): about one half of the cells enlarge to plump, circular *predecidual cells* with vesicular nuclei and abundant clear cytoplasm. Other cells contract to small rounded *endometrial granulocytes,* which are distinguished by their characteristic and bizarre nuclear shapes and by the phloxinophilic granules in their cytoplasm (HAMPERL 1954; HELLWEG 1954). Their dark, chromatin-rich nuclei apparently account for the rise in stromal DNA at this time (NORDQVIST 1970; see Color Plate IIa). As indicated by histochemical studies (HELLWEG 1956) and ultraviolet microspectrophotometric measurements (HELL-

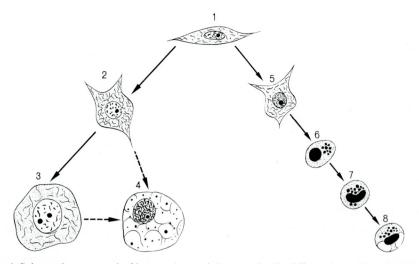

Fig. 4. Schematic portrayal of how endometrial stromal cells differentiate. *1* Poorly differentiated stromal cell, *2* Stromal cell becoming larger and more globular, *3* Decidual cell, *4* Foamy decidual cell ladened with metachromatic granules, *5* Stromal cell becoming smaller and more rounded, *6, 7, 8* Various stages in the development of endometrial granulocytes

WEG and SANDRITTER 1956) these granules contain a large polypeptide molecule rich in tyrosine and tryptophan. The UV absorption curve of the polypeptide molecule is virtually identical with that of relaxin. Immunhistological techniques indicated relaxin was probably present in the granules of endometrial granulocytes (DALLENBACH and DALLENBACH-HELLWEG 1964). Electron-microscopically the cytoplasm of these cells has a well-developed, smooth endoplasmic reticulum. The granules develop within preformed sacculi, which most probably represent dilated cisternae of the endoplasmic reticulum or Golgi complex (CARDELL et al.

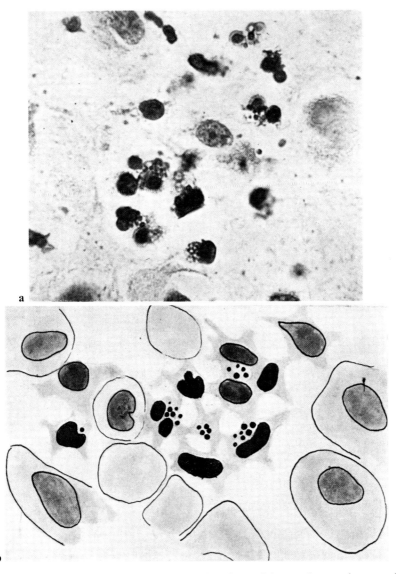

Fig. 5a, b. Decidua, 2nd month. A group of endometrial granulocytes between large decidual cells. **a** Phloxine-tartrazine stain; **b** schematic facsimile

1969; JAEGER and DALLENBACH-HELLWEG 1969; SENGEL and STOEBNER 1972) (Fig. 6). The activity of esterase and acid phosphatase found in human granulocytes (JIRASEK and DYKOVA 1964; personal results) is analogous to the esterase

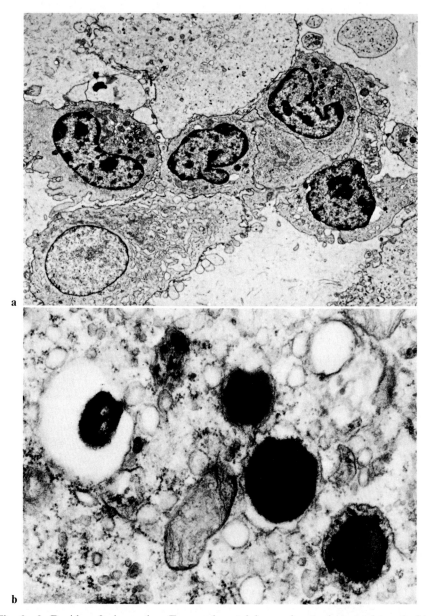

Fig. 6a, b. Decidua, 2nd month. **a** Four endometrial granulocytes between large decidual cells. Lobated nucleus of coarse chromatin network; granules of various sizes in the nuclear recess. **b** Segment of the cytoplasm of a granulocyte with granules of various sizes within cisternae. **a** ×4000; **b** ×46000

activity demonstrated in the granulocytic cells of the myometrial gland of the rat (BULMER 1965), also related to relaxin, and to the activity of acid phosphatase detected in the endometrial granulocytes of the monkey (MANNING et al. 1967). These results suggest the granules containing relaxin are possibly bound to lysosomes. That union would guarantee that relaxin stored in the cells would be released at a definite time. Such is the case. The liberation of relaxin takes place premenstrually and is dependent on the fall of progesterone, for with the decrease in progesterone the lysosomal membranes become permeable (BITENSKI and COHEN 1965) (cf. p. 43). As shown by histochemical and electronmicroscopic studies, the relaxin liberated in the upper layers of the endometrium leads to dissolution of the fibrous network, faciliating thereby the dissociation and disintegration of these parts.

If pregnancy results, then the small, motile granulocytes accumulate in large numbers around the site where the blastocyst begins to embed. As nidation proceeds, proteolytic enzymes become activated (STRAUSS 1964; SCHMIDT-MATTHIESEN 1967). Relaxin is then released locally for a brief period, inducing a local breakdown of the fibrous network, making it easier for the blastocyst to implant. Thus, the endometrium appears to participate actively in the process of implantation, facilitating and setting limits to the invasion by the trophoblasts (DALLENBACH and DALLENBACH-HELLWEG 1964; SCHMIDT-MATTHIESEN 1968). The numerous granulocytes in the remaining stroma, which develops into a decidua, retain their relaxin during the first months of pregnancy (HELLWEG 1957).

Initially, the young decidual cells exhibit no signs of regression as do the predecidual cells, but contain many slender mitochondria and a prominent endoplasmic reticulum (WYNN and WOOLLEY 1967). Histochemically they reveal high activities of enzymes (VACEK 1965); particularly the carbonic anhydrase is incresed. Many decidual cells become binucleated, thereby incresing their nuclear surface and indicating they have become more active.

The endometrial granulocytes, about as numerous premenstrually as the predecidual cells, were originally mistaken for polymorphonuclear leukocytes until studies disclosed their true nature. During the normal menstrual cycle the polymorphonuclear leukocytes infiltrate the dissociated endometrium only after menstruation has set in. No leukocyte infiltration of normal endometrium takes place before menstruation begins.

A special type of predecidual cell that occasionally may be seen is the *metachromatic cell* (ASPLUND and HOLMGREN 1947; McKAY 1950; RUMBOLZ and GREENE 1957; HELLWEG 1959; Fig. 4). It is distinguished by its foamy cytoplasm with loosely scattered metachromatic granules. Its nucleus is denser then that of the decidual cells and is often seen in mitosis. The significance of the metachromatic cell remains unclear. That it occurs rarely and in sparse numbers suggests some decidual cells are particularly capable of adapting to special demands or stimuli. It may merely represent an aberrant differentiation.

In summary, the endometrial stromal cell differentiates into two main forms, the endometrial granulocyte and the predecidual cell. In the secretory phase both dominate the histological picture in about equal numbers. In comparison, all other cells of the stroma under normal conditions are rare. Among them are the poorly differentiated, pluripotential stromal cells that originated from the Müllerian duct or those derived from the primitive mesenchyme (the vascular and perivascular cells, mast cells, cells of perineurium).

Lymphocytes frequently appear in the normal, non-inflamed endometrium. Since they lack the characteristic ploxinophilic granules they may be easily distinguished from the endometrial granulocytes with special stains. FEYRTER (1957) included the lymphocytes among the "resting wander-cells" and named them the "histiogenic lymphocytic round cells". Although they morphologically resemble the lymphocytes in the circulating blood, it seems likely that the majority arise locally from lymphoid tissue in the endometrium. *Lymphoid follicles in the endometrium are not unusual* (MÖNCH 1918; SEITZ 1923; NEUMANN 1930; MASSEL 1947; PAYAN et al. 1964; SEN and FOX 1967). Most probably they merely represent an exaggerated but physiological reaction of a locally well developed lymphatic tissue. RAHN and UEBEL (1965) and RAHN (1968) found lymphoid follicles with germinal centers in 50% of normal endometria from woman in the reproductive years (SEITZ reported in 20%). They regarded the follicles as a mechanism of defense against noxious agents, not only exogenous but endogenous as well. Immunohistological studies with monoclonal antibodies have shown that the occasional intraepithelial and interstitial lymphocytes as well as those in the lymphoid follicles are mainly T lymphocytes, with only very few B lymphocytes intermingled (MORRIS et al. 1985). These findings suggest that the endometrial lymphoid tissue is related to that of the intestine and bronchus. The lymphoid follicles appear in all layers of the endometrium and during every phase of the menstrual cycle (Fig. 7). Prepubertal and postmenopausal endometria, however, lack lymphoid follicles (IRWIN 1956).

The so-called monocytic round cells or *histiocytes* (FEYRTER and KLIMA 1958) perhaps originate from perivascular connective tissues of the endometrium or from wandering monocytes from the blood. They may give rise to various types of phagocytic cells that may occasionally be found in the endometrium, depending on the local requirements or conditions that develop. Thus, we may find lipophages, siderophages, mucophages, cytophages, and others.

Mast cells may also be found in the endometrium. FEYRTER (1957) believed they arose from the stroma. It seems more likely, however, that they infiltrate the endometrium from the circulating blood. Mast cells have been reported by some authors to be more common during the proliferative phase (VON NUMERS 1942; MCKAY 1950; RUNGE et al. 1956); by others, more common in the secretory phase (SYLVEN 1945; RUMBOLZ and GREENE 1957; GUPTA and SCHUELLER 1967). According to VARA (1962) their number runs parallel with the height of the endometrium during the endometrial cycle. Presumably the granules the mast cells form during the secretory phase are discharged just before menstruation. Perhaps the differences of opinion about mast cells have arisen because some authors confuse these cells with the metachromatic predecidual cells. ASPLUND and HOLMGREN pointed to that possibility in 1947 and endeavored to establish criteria for differentiating the two types of cells. Most investigators believe the function of the mast cells in the human endometrium is to release heparin and mucopolysaccharides; precise and definite information about their function is lacking, however.

Plasma cells and eosinophils appear in the normal endometrium only rarely (VON NUMERS 1942; FEYRTER 1957). Increased numbers of these cells, as well

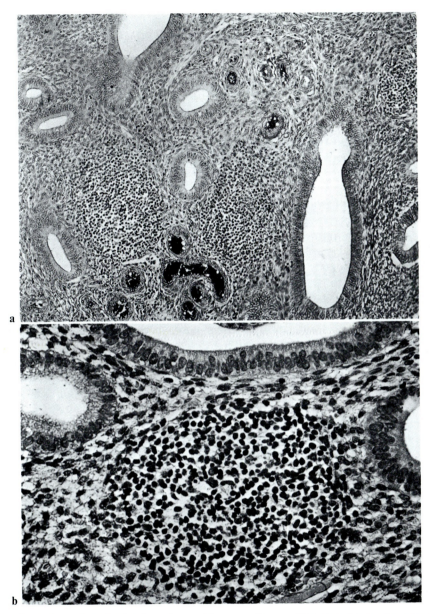

Fig. 7a, b. Lymphoid follicle in endometrial stroma, late proliferative phase. **a** Low magnification; **b** higher magnification

as of polymorphonuclear leukocytes, indicate an inflammatory reaction; all three types infiltrate the endometrium from the blood stream. It is indeed possible, however, that in chronic inflammation lymphocytes locally transform into macrophages or plasma cells, depending upon the kind of inflammatory or antigenic stimulus.

d) The Reticulum Fibers

In contrast to collagen fibers, the reticulum fibers may be reformed within a few days, giving rise again to a dense reticular network. While the stroma of the basalis and the isthmic mucosa remains uniformly dense, the fiber content in the functionalis fluctuates considerably during the menstrual cycle (HÖRMANN 1908; SEKIBA 1924; WERMBTER 1924; CENTARO and SERRA 1949; STAEMMLER 1953; DUBRAUSZKY and SCHMITT 1958; HOFFMEISTER and SCHULZ 1961). HÖRMANN distinguished between elongated cytoplasmic processes of the cell and an extracellular network of fibers in which the stromal cells are suspended. In electronmicroscopic studies HOFFMEISTER and SCHULZ were able to show that the connective tissue fibrils formed within the cells from the 1st to the 4th days of the proliferative phase; thereafter the fibrils matured extracellularly. With the light microscope, however, only occasional delicate reticulum fibers can be made out during the first 8 days of the proliferative phase (Fig. 8a). As ovulation approaches, these fibers become denser and thicker. During the secretory phase they are temporarily pulled apart by the transitory edema that develops. By the 4th week of the cycle, however, they enmesh each predecidual cell and form a dense network about the glands and the spiral arterioles (Fig. 8b). When progesterone decreases and the liberation of relaxin follows, the reticulum fibers disintegrate, at first locally where the granulocytes are located (Fig. 9a), then shortly thereafter throughout the entire compacta. As a result, the glands separate from the stroma and the stromal cells dissociate from one another. As long as the corpus luteum continues to produce progesterone, however, the reticulum fibers remain intact; in young decidua they form a dense fibrous network. The fibers undergo dissolution only about the site of implantation of the blastocyst where granulocytes accumulate. Since the zone containing the great numbers of granulocytes is limited, a relative deficiency of progesterone, which acts as the stimulus for the release of relaxin, must develop locally on the day of implantation. Hence, we see that the structure of the reticulum network is subjected to functional variations just like other components of the endometrium. From the appearance and quality of the reticulum network we are able to evaluate the functional state of the endometrium, and to determine whether a physiological balance in hormones exists or not (see also VACZY and SCIPIADES 1949).

e) The Ground Substance

The ground substance of the endometrial stroma that bathes the cellular and fibrous components generally receives little attention, although it is particularly important in the processes of implantation (SCHMIDT-MATTHIESEN 1962, 1963). During the normal menstrual cycle the ground substance seems to pass through three phases: in the early and midproliferative phase it chiefly contains high-molecular, neutral and acid mucopolysaccharides, which because of their metachromasia may be demonstrated with the alcian blue-PAS reaction (RUNGE et al. 1956). In the late proliferative phase the ground substance begins to resolve

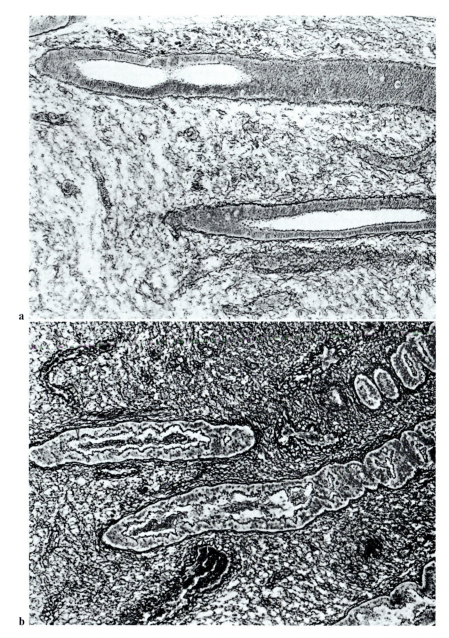

Fig. 8a, b. Reticular fibers of the endometrial stroma. **a** Midproliferative phase; **b** midsecretory phase. Silver impregnation after GOMORI

into subgroups of low molecular size that elude histochemical analysis. During the 1st week of the secretory phase the stroma becomes looser; as the time for implantation approaches in the midsecretory phase it becomes edematous. Directly thereafter, during the 4th week, high-molecular, neutral and acid muco-

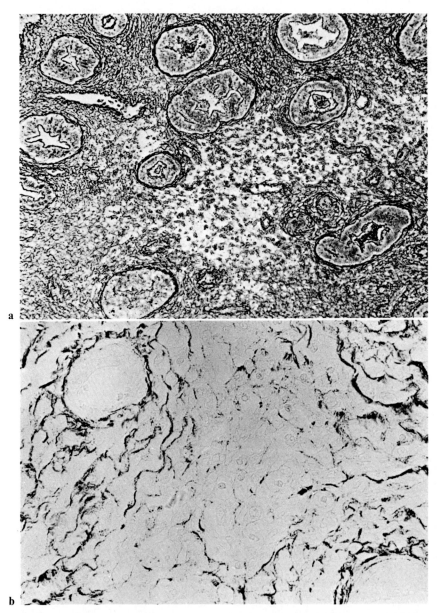

Fig. 9a, b. Predecidual transformation of the endometrium. Focal dissolution of the reticular fibers: **a** in the human endometrium after release of relaxin from the local granulocytes; **b** in the rhesus monkey after injection of relaxin. Silver impregnation after GOMORI

polysaccharides reaccumulate, but only in the compacta and about the spiral arterioles. These changes, it seems, make it easier for the blastocyst to implant and the trophoblast to invade and grow, since the ground substance is at its lowest viscosity and the stromal edema is at its peak. On the other hand, the increase in viscosity that occurs immediately after implantation promotes the adherence of the penetrating blastocyst. Closely integrated with all of these processes are the formation and disintegration of the reticulum fibers, the local release of relaxin, and the activation of fibrinolytic enzymes.

f) The Vessels

The vessels of the functionalis of the endometrium differ from vessels of other organs and tissues by their unique structure, their sensitivity to hormones and their ability to respond quickly to such stimuli (RAMSEY 1955; NIEMINEN 1962). In contrast, the vessels of the basalis are influenced little by hormonal changes of the cycle.

The *spiral arterioles* of the functionalis that branch from the arteries of the basalis finally attain the upper reaches of the endometrium at the end of the proliferative phase. Progesterone stimulates the vessels to grow larger and longer, hence leading to an increase in their tortuosity. Such changes are especially evident during the second half of the secretory phase when the ratio of the height of the endometrium to the length of the spiral arteries is 1:15 (MARKEE 1950). In other words, the arteries undergo intense spiraling because they grow faster than the endometrium. Their walls, thin in the early proliferative phase, grow progressively thicker (WIEGAND 1930; FARRER-BROWN et al. 1970). The lining endothelial cells, originally flat, swell and soon contain large, vesicular nuclei (KELLER 1911). Electron-microscopically they disclose a well-developed Golgi apparatus, abundant ergastroplasm, free ribosomes, mitochondria, and pinocytotic vesicles (ANCLA and DE BRUX 1964). Ultimately the endometrial granulocytes aggregate to form broad mantles about the spiral arterioles. In addition to the changes induced by the humoral stimulation, the spiral arterioles located beneath the implanting blastocyst undergo marked hypertrophy. The endothelial cells of their most superficial and terminal portions (those branches of the precapillary arterioles nearest the trophoblast) proliferate intensely, piling up into several layers (WISLOCKI and STREETER 1938; RAMSEY 1949, 1955). Some investigators have explained these changes by postulating that hormones are acting locally (BORELL et al. 1953). Several studies in animals indicate that the most likely hormones to cause these changes is relaxin, which, owing to the fall in progesterone, is released at this time from the endometrial granulocytes aggregated around the implantation site. By injecting monkeys with estrogen and relaxin, or by giving high doses of relaxin alone (DALLENBACH-HELLWEG et al. 1966) we were able to induce a comparable hypertrophy of the spiral arterioles and intense proliferation of their endothelial cells (Fig. 10). Most probably the reason why the premenstrual release of relaxin fails to induce similar changes in the spiral arterioles is because the estrogen levels fall at that time, or because the amount of relaxin available is much less than that released at the implantation site.

The *capillaries* of the functionalis also respond to cyclic variations of the ovarian hormones. The widely branching, interstitial and periglandular capillaries extend through the compacta to pass just beneath the superficial epithelium.

Their lumina, initially narrow, dilate irregularly during the secretory phase (BOHNEN 1927; WILKIN 1960; FANGER and BARKER 1961), becoming largest in premenstrual endometria and particularly in young decidua of pregnancy. Often lacuna-like sinusoids form (the so-called anastomosing lacunae of SCHMIDT-MATTHIESEN 1962). At the same time their endothelial cells become greatly swollen (KELLER 1911; MAUTHNER 1921; OKKELS 1950).

The *veins* of the functionalis react to the hormonal stimuli of the secretory phase in like manner (KÜSTERMANN 1930; BARTELMEZ 1931; DEBIASI 1962).

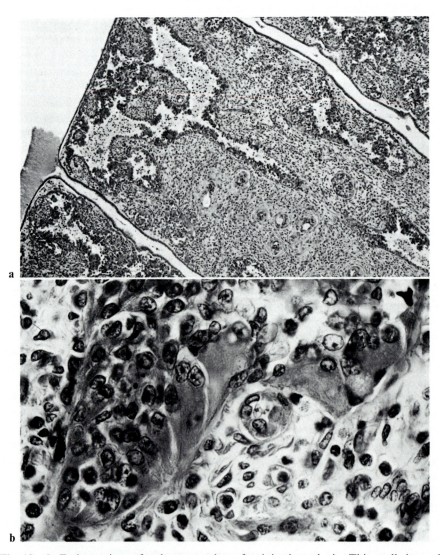

Fig. 10a, b. Endometrium of a rhesus monkey after injecting relaxin. Thin-walled vessels in the compacta are dilated and the endothelial cells strikingly proliferated. **a** Low magnification; **b** higher magnification

The venous network in the endometrium is strikingly dense and in injection studies is much more prominent than the arterial vasculature. The main veins course downwards between the glands to enter the myometrium; they connect with each other, however, by numerous cross-anastomoses (FARRER-BROWN et al. 1970). As OBER (1949) was able to show in serial sections, the thin-walled "lakes" beneath the superficial epithelium are merely localized sinusoidal dilatations of veins otherwise normally distended. Because of their extremely thin walls, these venous dilatations are difficult to dinstinguish from the lacuna-like sinusoids of the capillaries. Such a differentiation, however, would be of theoretical interest only. On the other hand, the equally dilated, thin-walled vessels lined by several layers of proliferated endothelial cells are arterioles, as RAMSEY (1949) was able to prove in serial sections.

After menstruation, if the dilated vessels are not lost by desquamation, they rapidly shrink and revert to their original size.

Lymphatic capillaries end blindly just beneath the surface epithelium and the epithelial cells of glands. Ultrastructurally, they are lined by small, flat endothelial cells and have no basal membrane (BLACKWELL and FRASER 1981). Their number and distribution varies individually from 0-20 per square millimeter. As the lymphatics descend to the basalis they merge to form collecting channels and lacunae, which run either parallel to the myometrium or penetrate it.

g) The Nerves

Despite intensive studies, opinions about the innervation of the endometrium differed greatly until recently. Some investigators reported finding branches of nerves in the basalis accompanying the arteries, and nonmyelinated nerve fibers extending from these branches a short distance into the functionalis where they supposedly terminate about arterioles or glands (STATE and HIRSCH 1941) or end free in the stroma (OKKELS 1950; PRIBOR 1951; KRANTZ 1959). In contrast, KOPPEN (1950) was unable to demonstrate nerve fibers beyond the basalis although he searched for them. Using the osmium-zinc iodide method on the endometrium of the rhesus monkey, LASSMANN (1965) reported seeing nerve fibers that extended to beneath the superficial epithelium where they ended with net-like fibrils. The fibers in his illustrations, however, appear more like those of the reticulum. Since the reticulum network of the endometrium is usually impregnated by all the techniques employed for demonstrating nerves, the positive results he reported should be evaluated with caution. DALLENBACH and VONDERLIN (1973), using new techniques, were able to demonstrate nerve fibers which extended into the endometrium to various levels, some as far as the functionalis. Where the nerve fibers ended remained unanswered since transected nerve fibrils proved to be too small to be recognized with the light-microscopic methods they used. It seems improbable that nerve fibers, which might be lost during menstruation, could regenerate and reinnervate the newly formed functionalis during the relatively short proliferative phase. We may assume therefore that the level at which we find nerve fibers in the endometrium approximates the level at which shedding occurs during menstruation.

2. Histochemical Localization of Enzymes; the Reciprocal Action Between Enzymes and Hormones

With the aid of histochemical methods, a large number of enzymes have been detected in the endometrium over the last 30 years. The activities of these enzymes are controlled in large part by hormones. On the other hand, the biological effects of the steroids depend in part on the enzyme systems of the endometrium, their "target organ" (FUHRMANN 1961). The close interaction between hormones and enzymes in the endometrium takes on clinical significance, since demonstrating the presence or absence of an enzyme may permit valuable conclusions to be drawn about the functional state of the endometrium.

Some of the methods used for detecting enzymes are technically difficult and the results obtained are often equivocal owing to diffusion-artefacts. In addition, the numerous investigators of different laboratories have employed diverse methods on dissimilar material, making it difficult to evaluate or compare their results. I shall discuss here only those enzymes that are important in the diagnosis of the functional state. We shall confine ourselves to the results of histochemical studies of the human endometrium. Biochemical studies are not included. Further details may be obtained from comprehensive reviews (BONTKE 1960; SCHMIDT-MATTHIESEN 1963).

Of all the enzymes, the activity of **alkaline phosphatase** has been studied the most. Since the results of the studies have consistently agreed, we can assume they are realiable. The activity is greatest during the proliferative phase, reaches its peak shortly before or at ovulation, then rapidly falls in the secretory phase to minimal levels (ATKINSON and ENGLE 1947; ANDRES et al. 1949; ATKINSON 1950; HALL 1950; OBER 1950; WISLOCKI et al. 1950; RUNGE and EBNER 1954; MCKAY et al. 1956; BERGER and MUMPRECHT 1959; BARBOUR 1961; FUHRMANN 1961; LEWIN 1961; MOOKERJEA 1961; BOUTSELIS et al. 1963; GROSS 1964; KUCERA 1964; SAKSENA et al. 1965; TAKI et al. 1966; FILIPE and DAWSON 1968; ELIAS et al. 1983). As judged from the precipitation reaction that takes place in the test, the enzyme is localized primarily at the apical end of the glandular epithelial cell. During glycogenolysis the cell membrane becomes more permeable (HUGHES 1976). In the stroma only the vascular endothelium gives a positive reaction. Apparently the activity of alkaline phosphatase is closely associated with the action of estrogen on the endometrium. Although biochemically different from alkaline phosphatases of other organs (WILSON 1976), it is most probably also important for protein synthesis and in the associated processes of growth and proliferation. It possibly participates in the formation of mucoids (SCHMIDT-MATTHIESEN 1963), enhancing cell membrane permeability at the time of glycogenolysis.

The large number of **lysosomal enzymes** in the endometrium increase their activities up to and during the secretory phase when the lysosomal membranes begin to become destabilized, leading to either a gradual or a drastic increase in free, non-lysosomal-bound enzymes (ROSADO et al. 1977). Apparently the important mechanism regulating the number of these lysosomal enzymes and the stability of their membranes is the appropriate equilibrium between estrogens and progesterone.

The histochemical reactions for demonstrating *acid phosphatase* are technically complicated; therefore we should expect they would occasionally yield erroneous results. According to the reports of most investigators, the activity of the acid phosphatase during the menstrual cycle is just the opposite of that of alkaline phosphatase. Its activity during the proliferative phase is very low but rises continuously after cycle day 21 to reach its peak just before menstruation (ANDRES et al. 1949; GOLDBERG and JONES 1956; MCKAY et al. 1956; FUHRMANN 1961; MOOKERJEA 1961; BOUTSELIS et al. 1963; VACEK 1965; SAWARAGI and WYNN 1969). Some investigators found the peak of activity at the time ov ovulation (BERGER and MUMPRECHT 1959; GARCIA-BUNUEL and BRANDES 1966). Others were unable to detect obvious differences between the proliferative phase and the secretory phase (WISLOCKI et al. 1950; GROSS 1964; BITENSKY and COHEN 1965; FILIPE and DAWSON 1968; BARON and ESTERLY 1975). Acid phosphatase is primarily localized in the cytoplasm of the glandular epithelium. Here it gradually migrates from its initial basal subnuclear accumulation to the apex of the cell (ELIAS et al. 1983). In addition, some stromal cells usually give a positive reaction. GOLDBERG and JONES (1956) and VACEK (1965), however, reported a premenstrual increase in the activity in cells they called "macrophages". In studies on the permeability of lysosomal membranes, BITENSKI and COHEN (1965) were able to demonstrate that acid phosphatase in the endometrium was located in the lysosomes. The reaction for the enzyme was positive only with permeable membranes. Since progesterone affects the permeability of lysosomal membranes, it is easy to understand that the activity of acid phosphatase might depend on the level of progesterone.

Glucose-6-phosphatase can be localized ultrastructurally within cisternae of the endoplasmic reticulum and in the nuclear membrane of glandular epithelial cells around the time of ovulation and during the early secretory phase (SAWARAGI and WYNN 1969). It apparently converts the large amounts of glycogen produced at that time into glucose.

Specific and non-specific *esterases* behave very much like acid phosphatase and like it are localized in lysosomes. GROSS (1964), VACEK (1965) and MANSOUR and BARADI (1967) found an increase in the activity in the secretory phase, whereas NACHLAS and SELIGMAN (1949), MCKAY et al. (1956), BOUTSELIS et al. (1963), GARCIA-BUNUEL and BRANDES (1969), and TAKI et al. (1966) were unable to detect any significant variations during the menstrual cycle. In the late secretory phase, however, these authors found a high activity of esterase in stromal "macrophages", which JIRASEK and DYKOVA (1964) were able to prove were actually endometrial granulocytes. In my own studies I have been able to confirm that endometrial granulocytes contain esterases and acid phosphatase. Since relaxin begins to exert its effect when progesterone falls, the release of relaxin seems to be closely associated with the increase in activity of the esterases and acid phosphatase, or rather, with the permeability of the lysosomal membranes (cf. p. 33).

Proteolytic enzymes also occur in the endometrium. *Aminopeptidase,* however, is the only one that has been studied histochemically (FUHRMANN 1959;

FILIPE and DAWSON 1968; BARON and ESTERLY 1975). Its activity increases during the menstrual cycle and is greater in the stromal cells than in the glandular epithelial cells.

Using biochemical methods, SCHMIDT-MATTHIESEN (1967) studied some other proteolytic enzymes (the fibrinolysokinases and tryptases), which he extracted from endometrial tissue along with such active agents as plasminogen, plasmin, and other activators of fibronolysis. He referred to the combined effects of these enzymes and agents as the "fibrinolytic activity" of the endometrium. He found that the activity reached its peak during midsecretory phase. If pregnancy ensues, then the activity falls. Just before menstruation it rises again, attaining a second peak on the 1st day of menstruation (RYBO 1968). The administration of estrogen causes the activity to increase; progesterone causes it to decrease. In contrast, intact decidua and placenta reveal no fibrinolytic activity. Attempts to localize the fibrinolytic enzymes histochemically indicate they are probably confined to the intima of small arteries, capillaries and venules, and to the stromal cells about the glands of the superficial endometrium (WEISS and BELLER 1969). Also a possible source of fibrinolytic enzymes is the endometrial granulocytes, which most likely retain the enzymes in lysosomes (HENZL et al. 1972). Some of these enzymatic activators contain lipids; accordingly, most are bound to microsomal fractions. The fibrinolytic enzymes become effective only after they are released from the cell. Their liberation appears to be induced by hormonal conditions like those that are necessary for the release of relaxin. Perhaps, however, pathological changes in hormonal balance also cause the cells to liberate their fibrinolytic activators. In contrast, the acid mucopolysaccharides that appear in the ground substance during the early proliferative and late secretory phases can act as fibrinolytic inhibitors by binding with the fibrinolytic enzymes to form complexes. From all that we have said, it appears that the fibrinolytic activity of the endometrium is closely related to the release and action of relaxin; the relationship is not only functional but morphological as well.

Some other lysosomal enzymes that have been histochemically demonstrated should be briefly mentioned. *β-glucuronidase* has its peak of activity in all probability during the secretory phase (GROSS 1964; VACEK 1965). Other authors found, however, that the enzyme showed no important fluctuations during the menstrual cycle (FUHRMANN 1961; BOUTSELIS et al. 1963; TAKI et al. 1966; FILIPE and DAWSON 1968). Although β-glucuronidase is chiefly present in the glandular epithelium, small amounts of the enzyme are also found in some stromal cells. Apparently it is important in the metabolism of carbohydrates. *Phosphoamidase* reaches its greatest activity in the glandular cells of the endometrium during the first half of the secretory phase (OEHLERT et al. 1954; GROSS 1964). BARON and ESTERLY (1975) reported that the activities of *galactosidase* and *glucosaminidase* peak in the late secretory phase.

A group of other enzymes are important in the metabolism of carbohydrates. *Glycogen-synthetase* activates the synthesis of glycogen from glucose. *Glycogen-phosphorylase* catalyzes it back to glucose. Both enzymes have their greatest activities in the secretory phase. *Glucose-6-phosphatase* shows a cyclic fluctuation with an abundant activity in the secretory phase (ELIAS et al. 1983). It can be localized electron-microscopically in the cisternae of the endoplasmic reticulum and in the nuclear membrane of glandular epithelial cells at ovulation and during the early secretory phase (SAWARAGI and WYNN 1969). It also participates in the breakdown of glycogen into glucose.

The few studies of the *dehydrogenases* indicate some of these enzymes probably fluctuate very little during the menstrual cycle (FORAKER et al. 1954; MARCUSE 1957; COHEN et al. 1964; VACEK 1965; LUH and BRANDAU 1967). Recent studies on the histochemical localization of 17β- and 3α-hydroxysteroid-dehydrogenases showed almost no activity of these enzymes during the proliferative phase of the menstrual cycle, but distinct activity during the secretory phase with a maximum around the 22nd day. The enzymes were localized mainly in the apical end of the glandular cells, and here within the outer membranes of the mitochondria and in microsomes (POLLOW et al. 1975). Stromal cells showed no activity. The prime function of these two enzymes, particularly the 17β-hydroxysteroid-dehydrogenase, seems to be to stimulate the secretory activity of the glandular cell by steroid oxidation (BRANDAU et al. 1969). *Carbonic anhydrase,* primarily localized at the base of the glandular epithelial cells during the entire cycle, appears to be important in processes of implantation (FRIEDLEY and ROSEN 1975).

3. Structural Changes Induced in the Endometrium by the Physiological Action of the Ovarian Hormones

a) Molecular Biology of Steroid Hormones

The rapid and great advances in the molecular biology of steroid hormones during the last decades have made this subspecialty a particularly exciting discipline of endocrinology. As one might guess, the wealth of new information gained virtually defies adequate summary, especially in these few paragraphs. For details I refer the interested reader to comprehensive treaties covering various aspects of the subject, many of which remain controversial or unclear (JENSEN et al. 1969; MAINWARING 1975, 1977; CHAN and O'MALLEY 1978; SCHRADER and O'MALLEY 1978; JENSEN 1979; MARKS 1979).

Since steroid hormones have molecular weights of about 300, they can readily diffuse into all cells of the body, but as we know, they trigger characteristic reactions only in cells of their target tissues. As tritiated steroids in radioautographic, affinity chromatographic, cell fractionation and gradient centrifugation studies have revealed, the high affinity of these target tissues for a steroid comes from the capacity of their cells to produce special cytoplasmic proteins, which specifically and rapidly intercept and bind the hormone as it diffuses into the cell. Because of that "welcoming" function, the cytoplasmic protein has been named a "receptor". To be able to respond to a steroid hormone, a target cell must produce receptors specific for that hormone. Consequently, receptor proteins specific for estrogens, progesterone or androgens, for glucocorticosteroids or mineralcorticosteroids have been identified.

The receptors actually have two functions (BAXTER and FUNDER 1979). The first is to recognize and select out of the hodgepodge of hormones in the fluid bathing the cell the appropriate hormone as a signal. The second is to relay that signal to the nucleus where it specifically affects the genome, bringing about definite changes in the cell. Most investigators assume that all steroid hormones act alike. GORSKI and GANNON (1976), however, present data detailing differences that exist between different steroid hormones. They explain in detail why they believe the differences should be considered. Steroids of lower biological activity, such as estrone and estriol, seem to have lower affinities for receptors (BAULIEU et al. 1980).

Because receptor proteins are difficult to purify before they become denatured, various investigators have described at least eight different subunits for the estrogen receptor. SICA and BRESCIANI (1979) have reported the molecular weight of the denatured subunit of estrogen to be close to 70000 daltons. Each subunit has one binding site for estrogen. O'MALLEY and SCHRADER (1976) estimate the molecular weight of the progesterone receptor to be about 200000. They describe it as a dimer of two unlike subunits. Each weighs about 100000 and consists of a cigar-shaped chain of aminoacids four to five times as long as it is wide, providing one binding site for progesterone. Nonetheless, as GORSKI and GANNON emphasize, depending on the techniques used to collect them from the cytosol of the target cells, complexes of steroid hormones with receptors may have a variety of forms and molecular weights. BAULIEU et al. (1980) thoroughly review the many problems associated with measuring the properties of receptors bound to radioactive hormones.

Most cells of a target organ maintain about 10000 such steroid receptors in their cytoplasm. GORSKI and GANNON (1976) estimate about 16000 receptors per cell. The number may fluctuate, however, depending on the intensity and duration of prior hormonal stimulation, on the degree of cellular differentiation, and such factors as phase of cell cycle, cell age, metabolism, genetic state (GEHRING et al. 1971; KIRKPATRICK et al. 1971; SIBLEY and TOMKINS 1974), nutrition, pharmacological pretreatment, effects of other hormones, pathological states, and so on. For example, a hormone (agonist) may depress the levels of its own receptors, a process known as "down-regulation" or "tachyphylaxis" (BAXTER and FUNDER 1979). This may explain in part why large doses of estrogen over long periods may lead to ultimate failure of its target cells to respond. According to MILGROM et al. (1973), progesterone seems to inactivate its own receptor system. On the other hand, a hormone such as estrogen is known to increase the levels of receptors for progesterone and prolactin (LEAVITT et al. 1977). In contrast, progesterone may depress the level of estrogen receptors, making the target tissue less sensitive to estrogen (MESTER et al. 1974; HSUEH et al. 1975). Whether estrogens under certain physiological conditions can bind to more than its class of receptors, as spirolactone does to androgen receptors (FUNDER et al. 1976), or whether other non-estrogenic hormones can bind readily to estrogen receptors, is not known. BAXTER and FUNDER (1979) recommend one should take such "overlap" in action into account when hormone therapy is considered, and ROCHEFORT and GARCIA (1976) reported the binding of androgens to the estrogen receptor can bring about an estrogenic effect.

Although its affinity for the estrogen receptor is relatively low, tamoxifen acts as a powerful anti-estrogen because it is metabolized so slowly and lingers at high concentrations in the cytoplasm competing with estrogens.

As several studies indicate (BAXTER and FUNDER 1979; BAULIEU 1979), when a given steroid fails to stimulate its target tissues, it is usually because the tissues lack receptors for that hormone.

The affinity of a hormone for a receptor involves electrostatic forces, whereby hydrogen bonds unite charged groups on the hormone with oppositely charged groups on the specific binding site of the receptor. These processes are dependent on temperature. All facts suggest the receptor changes its shape and its molecular weight (referred to as "conformational change") whereby it becomes activated, enabling it to slip through nuclear pores, to enter the nucleus where it signals specific changes (Fig. 11). The process of translocation from cytoplasm to nucleus proceeds quickly but apparently requires no energy. Perhaps it represents, as some suggest, nothing more than a flow initiated by gradient differences.

On arrival in the nucleus the hormone receptor complex interacts and binds with high affinity to specific acceptor sites on the chromatin, thereby inducing

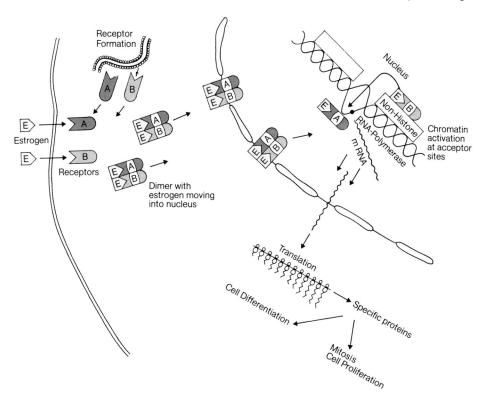

Fig. 11. Schematic portrayal of how steroid hormones (estrogen here) seem to bind to receptors at plasma membrane to be carried into nucleus where they activate specific "acceptor" sites and genes to induce transcription, then translation, with either cell differentiation or cell proliferation (for details see text)

changes in numerous gene loci (GORSKI and GANNON 1976; YAMAMOTO and ALBERTS 1976; BAULIEU 1979; BAULIEU et al. 1979). For the estrogen receptor complex there seem to be more acceptor sites than receptors, thus the nuclear binding sites never become saturated. Whether the acceptor sites for the progesterone receptor complexes also outnumber the progesterone receptors is not known but seems probable.

O'MALLEY and SCHRADER (1976) review the results of their studies with progesterone and explain how they believe the subunits A and B of the dimeric progesterone receptor bind at different but specific acceptor sites on the chromatin to activate genes. It remains to be proved whether their hypothesis applies to all steroid hormones.

As these investigators postulate, when the progesterone receptor complex enters the nucleus the B subunits bind to a specific acceptor protein on the chromatin, where a special AP_3 fraction of the non-histone chromosomal proteins is located. The other subunits A, unable to bind to intact chromatin, dissociate from the B subunits and react with specific genes situated nearby on the chain of naked DNA. The choice of specific genes is presumably determined by the B subunits as they bind with the AP_3 fraction or some protein of it. The reaction of the subunits A with the specific genes attracts a molecule of RNA polymerase to the site to initiate a locus for DNA transcription. Accordingly, strands of messenger RNA are transcribed and move off into the cytoplasm to serve as templates for protein synthesis, bringing about changes in cell structure and function we recognize histologically as characteristic of that hormone. In part this hypothesis agrees with that of YAMAMOTO and ALBERTS (1976) for estradiol. Yet attempts to purify the estrogen receptor have not led to the isolation of two binding forms as with progesterone, nor has the estrogen receptor revealed a specific binding to a single AP_3 acidic non-histone protein of chromatin.

The number of chromatin acceptor sites exceeds the number of messenger RNAs stimulated by the steroid hormone. This suggests receptor-steroid complexes may be bound to sites which serve other supportive functions of less physiological importance. Only about 1% of the messenger RNAs in the cell are regulated by the steroid hormone.

What happens to the steroid after it partakes in gene stimulation, whether it is destroyed or extruded from the cell, little is known. In vivo estradiol has a half-life of about 90 min. What the fate of the hormone receptor is remains unknown. It may be deactivated, returned to the cytoplasm for reuse, or may be destroyed by proteolysis. BAULIEU (1979) states that in humans under normal conditions, the steroid concentrations never saturate all binding sites on the cytoplasmic and nuclear receptors.

b) Endometrial Steroid Receptors

Studies to date indicate that the receptors for estrogen and progesterone in the endometrium fluctuate during the menstrual cycle and may determine when the fertilized ovum will implant (BAYARD et al. 1978; BAULIEU 1979; SOUTTER et al. 1979). LUNAN and GREEN (1975) were able to confirm earlier results showing that endometrium from various parts of the uterus yielded differences in uptake of estradiol, especially in the secretory phase, proving it is unwise to assume that all samples of endometrium taken from a single uterus will yield like values for estrogen receptors. They suggested the differences might be related to variations in vascular supply or to variations in distribution of endogenous hormones. As is to be expected, the concentrations of cytosolic estrogen and progesterone receptors are higher in the fundal region than in the middle and isthmic portion of the uterus (KAUPPILA et al. 1982).

In *the early proliferative phase,* estradiol receptors gradually increase. The progesterone receptors are only slightly fewer. In the *late proliferative phase* the concentration of total estradiol receptors increases. Those of the nucleus more than double, whereas those of the cytoplasm remain unchanged. The cytoplasmic progesterone receptors increase greatly, correlating with the surge of plasma estradiol.

After ovulation, the total estradiol receptor decreases rapidly in the early secretory phase, mostly through a fall in cytoplasmic receptors, and continues to decrease in the late secretory phase, reaching levels well below those at the onset of the cycle. The total concentration of progesterone receptors gradually falls, with a sharp decrease in cytoplasmic receptors. The nuclear receptors remain at their highest levels, correlating well with the luteal secretion of progesterone. In the late secretory phase the concentration of nuclear receptors falls to values of the early proliferative phase.

During the first trimester of pregnancy, the cytoplasmic estradiol and progesterone receptors are barely detectable whereas progesterone nuclear receptors are high, exceeding concentrations of total progesterone receptors of preovulatory endometrium. The concentrations of estradiol nuclear receptors resemble those of the early secretory phase.

Biochemical measurements of receptor concentrations in cytosol fractions are, however, of limited value, since they imply the tissue being measured is homogeneous, which it never is. With immunohistochemical methods, receptor-positive cells can be individually localized in the tissue sections. The binding of radioactively labeled hormones can only detect unoccupied receptor sites. In contrast the recent development of monoclonal antibodies against estrogen receptor proteins (estrophilin) allows the recognition of occupied as well as unoccupied antigenic sites (GREENE et al. 1980, 1984; KING et al. 1985). The positive staining with the ER-ICA assay is observed in cell nuclei only; it permits, by precise intracellular localization, an accurate quantification of receptor sites which often have a heterogenous distribution and density in the tissue (PRESS et al. 1984; CHARPIN et al. 1986; KUPRYJANCZYK et al. 1986). With this method, estrogen receptors can be detected in the nuclei of most glandular and stromal cells during the proliferative phase of the cycle, but barely in the secretory phase where the reaction is greatly decreased. The basal endometrial layers show a constantly positive receptor binding independent of the cycle phase. Hyperproliferating as well as postmenopausal endometria also show a high receptor content, whereas in endometrial carcinomas great variations can be detected depending on the degree of cellular differentiation. Although the estrogen activity is found biochemically in the cytosal, immunohistochemically the activity is localized in the cell nucleus. The discrepancy may be explained by artefacts and molecular shifts that occur with the biochemical fractionation.

c) Estrogen

In contrast to other steroid hormones, minute amounts of estrogen (17β-estradiol) are very potent, capable of producing rapid and significant changes in the target cells.

Within 15–30 min after estradiol is administered, the rate of nucleotide uptake by the endometrial cells rises and the RNA of their nuclei markedly increases (SEGAL 1967). A shift of the nucleoli to the nuclear membrane takes place (RICKERS and KRONE 1969). Between 1 and 2 h after giving estradiol the amounts of glycogen, phospholipid and fluid in the uterine cells sharply rise. Shortly thereafter the cells begin to synthesize protein, and cell growth ensues (HAMILTON 1964); at the same time the activity of alkaline phosphatase and adenosine triphosphatase increases (HENZL et al. 1968). Estradiol remains in the nuclei of "target cells" for many hours, stimulating the synthesis of DNA (KING and GORDON 1967; LEROY et al. 1967; STUMPF 1970); the result is a wave of mitoses. In the endometrium both the stromal cells and epithelial cells briskly respond. EPIFANOVA (1966), who injected mice with estrone, found the mitotic index of the uterine epithelium to be increased by a factor of 4.5

The prompt hyperemia of the endometrium, occurring within 1 min after intravenous injection of estradiol, and the subsequent rapid uptake of water were often regarded as responses to estrogen. We now realize these changes are mediated by histamine that is released locally by estrogen; how estrogen sets histamine free, however, is unknown.

In summary, estrogen regulates the amount of genetic material available for transcription and helps to control the chemical composition of the genetic material (VILLEE 1961; JENSEN 1963; KARLSON 1965, 1967; TENG and HAMILTON 1968).

Of special interest are the studies of KOHRMAN and GREENBERG (1968) who, confirming and elaborating on the results of other investigators, showed that a single injection of estradiol into neonatal mice produced changes in the vaginal epithelium that persisted long into adult life. Not only did the vaginal cells proliferate persistently and hornify, but the rates of synthesis of DNA, RNA and protein of these target cells remained permanently altered. The mice that DUNN and GREEN (1963) studied after similar neonatal injection ultimately developed cervical carcinomas.

The first morphological and histochemical effects of estrogen that we can see in the glandular and stromal cells of the human endometrium are the increase in RNA in the nuclei and nucleoli, followed by increase in cytoplasmic RNA. Thereafter, the synthesis of cytoplasmic protein accelerates, leading to growth and proliferation of the cells (DAVIDSON 1965; POTTER 1965; PODVOLL and GOODMAN 1967). At the same time we find the activity of alkaline phosphatase rises. As its cells enlarge, its glands grow longer, its stromal cells proliferate, and the endometrium increases in height. Many of the epithelial and stromal cells may be found undergoing mitosis. The more the endometrium grows, the more estrogen the ovaries secrete, adapting, it seems, to the steady increase in endometrial tissue. Finally with the secretion of progesterone, the endometrial cells cease to proliferate.

d) Progesterone

As explained above under Molecular Biology of Steroid Hormones, specific receptors for progesterone have been detected in the endometrium (EDWARDS et al. 1969; RAO and WIEST 1970; TRAMS et al. 1971; RAO et al. 1974). The progesterone binding increases quantitatively after pretreatment of castrated animals with estradiol-17β (RAO et al. 1973).

In the test named after them, HOOKER and FORBES (1947) determined the smallest dose of progesterone that corrects the changes induced in the endometrial cells of the mouse by castration: after 0.0002 µg of progesterone are injected into the uterine cavity, the nuclei of the endometrial stromal cells enlarge and become clear after 2 days. If the dose of progesterone is doubled, then the nuclei "revert to normal" within 24 h; with a four-fold dose, the reversion occurs within 6 h. The effect is specific for progesterone, and is given by no other hormone. Cytophotometric measurements have disclosed (LEROY et al. 1967) that as the nuclei enlarge the DNA increases by 20%.

In human endometrium the first evidence of a progesterone effect is detectable with the light microscope after 36 h; one sees a clearing of the nuclei of the glandular and stromal cells, and glycogen granules begin to appear at the base of the glandular epithelial cells. Before these changes can occur, however, the cells must have been stimulated by estrogen as in a normal menstrual cycle (HUGHES et al. 1969). During organ culture in media containing progesterone, the glycogen content of proliferative tissue was increased as much as 13-fold (SHAPIRO et al. 1980). In electron-microscopic studies MERKER et al. (1968) found giant mitochondria containing DNA near the glycogen granules; these investigators postulated that progesterone stimulated these mitochondria to synthesize protein. Later in the menstrual cycle, under the effects of progesterone, a nuclear channel system develops (see p. 26). Mitotic activity ceases, and the amount of alkaline phosphatase decreases; the glandular cells differentiate. In addition to glycogen, they produce and secrete neutral and acid mucopolysaccharides and lipids. In the 2nd week of the secretory phase the stromal cells differentiate either into large predecidual cells or into small endometrial granulocytes; the spiral arterioles begin to grow. The activity of acid phosphatase rises.

e) Relaxin

HISAW (1926) discovered the hormone relaxin and described its action on the symphysis pubis of the guinea pig. He defined the guinea pig unit (GPU) of relaxin as the smallest dose to cause within 6 h a widening of the symphysis pubis in 66% of castrated female guinea pigs pretreated with estrogen. In sexually mature monkeys the levels of relaxin in the blood fluctuate between 0.2 and 0.3 GPU/ml serum (HISAW and HISAW 1964). At the beginning of pregnancy women average about 0.2 GPU/ml, but at the end of pregnancy about 2 GPU/ml (ZARROW et al. 1955). Recent observations, however, showed stable concentrations (QUAGLIARELLO et al. 1979) or a slight decline in plasma concentrations toward the end of gestation (SCHWABE et al. 1978). Non-pregnant women can produce relaxin when given HCG (QUAGLIARELLO et al. 1980). Mammals with a primitive placentation produce the hormone primarily in the ovary (as in pigs), but in women (DALLENBACH and DALLENBACH-HELLWEG 1964) and in monkeys (DALLENBACH-HELLWEG et al. 1966) the hormone or its precursor seems also to be formed by the granulocytes of the endometrial stroma and by cytotrophoblastic cells in the basal plate of the human placenta. Granules resembling those of endometrial granulocytes have been found in granulosa lutein cells of porcine (BELT et al. 1971; KENDALL et al. 1978) and human (CRISP et al. 1970) ovaries. The occurrence of these granules also correlates with the production of relaxin, which could be demonstrated immunohistochemically in the human gestational corpus luteum (MATHIEU et al. 1981). The lysosomes found near the granules in the endometrial and ovarian cells suggest that enzymes may activate the precursor prorelaxin to relaxin, which then acts only at definite times in specific tissues; the stimulus inducing the release of lysosomal enzymes like ubiquitin and of relaxin is the fall of progesterone.

As recent studies have disclosed, relaxin is a polypeptide hormone of 5447 molecular weight with an A chain of 22 amino acids and a B chain of 26 amino acids connected by disulfide bridges much like insulin. Consequently, the specifity of earlier observations made with labeled antibodies directed against relatively impure relaxin should be tested and proved by using the pure relaxin now available. Recently with such specific anti-relaxin antibodies, relaxin was demonstrated immunohistochemically in human decidua and in the basal plate of the placenta at term (BIGAZZI et al. 1980; FIELDS and LARKIN 1981) and in the endometrium of the pregnant guinea pig (PARDO et al. 1980). As yet no receptor specific for relaxin has been detected.

Like other hormones, beside a distant action on target organs, relaxin has a local paracrine action at the site of its production or secretion. During the last days of the normal secretory phase, relaxin stimulates dilatation and congestion of the thin-walled capillaries located just beneath the surface epithelium (those that communicate with the anastomosing lacunae), and induces dissolution of the reticulum fibers of the endometrial stroma. That dissolution, in turn, allows the stromal cells to dissociate, facilitating menstrual shedding (Fig. 9). A similar disintegration of the connective tissue takes place at the onset of implantation, but only about the embedding blastula. The much larger amounts of relaxin released at the end of pregnancy or with an abortion stimulate profound dilatation of the thin-walled capillaries and extreme hyperplasia of their endothelial cells, as well as of those of the spiral arterioles. Further, immediately after birth relaxin produced in the basal trophoblast of the placenta causes the fibers of connective tissue that hold the placenta in place to undergo dissolution. These actions of relaxin have been confirmed in monkeys by injecting them with relaxin (DALLENBACH-HELLWEG and DALLENBACH 1966; Fig. 10). The dissolution of collagen fibers could be verified in electron-microscopic observations (CARDELL et al. 1969). In addition to these local effects of relaxin that may be brought about in part by intermediary systems of enzymes, there are the distant effects of relaxin on the cervix and symphysis pubis. These distant effects are also controlled to take place at definite times; since they are not pertinent they shall not be discussed further.

4. Changes in Structures in the Endometrium During Nidation

Although we described earlier how the various structures of the endometrium change with the advent of pregnancy, we shall review these changes here in detail. As emphasized before, virtually every structural component of the endometrium takes part in preparing for implantation. That would seem to provide multiple assurances to guarantee success of the processes involved. On the other hand, it is essential that the intricate interplay between tissue components, so carefully regulated by the delicate balance of hormones, is precisely maintained to insure a normal implantation. Knowledge of all of the tissue components and their changes gives us insight into the diversity of possible causes for infertility.

At the time of implantation on the 7th day after ovulation the endometrial glands are at the height of secretion. The endometrial stroma is maximally edematous, its fibers loosely dispersed, and its ground substance watery and richt in depolymerized substances that are more easily absorbed because of their reduced molecular sizes. The fibrinolytic activity is at its peak. The spiral arterioles proliferate and hypertrophy, finally reaching the upper compacta just beneath the surface epithelium. In women (as in other mammalian species) the blastocyst implants directly over a group of these spiral arterioles, and as it does so it apparently stimulates the adjoining endometrium to undergo profound structural changes. The group of spiral arterioles beneath the lower pole of the imbedding blastocyst responds by intense hypertrophy, and in the surrounding stroma the capillaries dilate widely and their walls become thin. Large, "true" decidual cells develop. These possess gap junctions that connect processes from the same cell but fail to show similar junctions with neighboring cells as predecidual cells do (LAWN et al. 1971). The decidual glands and stromal cells express specific carbohydrate moieties different from those in the nonpregnant endometrium, as studies with labeled fluorescein isothiocyanate-conjugated lectins have shown (LEE and DAMJANOV 1985; BYCHKOV and TOTO 1987). The granulocytes increase in number; those that have assembled about the implanting blastocyst release their relaxin, most probably owing to a local deficit of progesterone (or to an estrogen excess). The liberated relaxin causes the reticulum fibers to disintegrate locally. In addition, probably because of the same hormonal stimulus, the fibrinolytic activity reaches its peak and proteolytic enzymes are set free in the same region. Perhaps it is the hormonal activation of lysosomal enzymes that finally brings about the release of the relaxin. The blastocyst readily penetrates the region where the reticulum fibers have disintegrated, and becomes firmly imbedded after establishing contacts with the maternal blood vessels. Thereafter, the surrounding decidua develops, serving to limit further spread of the trophoblast. Over the next few days the hormones secreted by the corpus luteum of pregnancy cause the endometrium to grow even higher. The reticulum fibers become denser, the ground substance turns more viscid, and the blood vessels proliferate and dilate. The decidual cells develop a distinct pericellular basement membrane which contains laminin, type IV collagen, heparan sulfate proteoglycan, and fibronectin (WEWER et al. 1985). As a result, the decidua that surrounds the imbedding blastocyst becomes established and stable. Its granulocytes accumulate their relaxin for later use in the frequent, local processes of destruction and remodeling which characterize the fluctuating state of the decidua throughout pregnancy. Thus we see, contrary to earlier opinion, that the endometrium participates in the process of implantation, not only by providing little resistance for the blastocyst, but particularly by taking an active part in the dissolution of its reticulum fibers, as long as that is essential for implantation. In addition, through their decidualization about the blastocyst, the endometrial cells help to anchor it in place. Thereby, as electron-microscopic studies show, the contact between decidual cells and trophoblasts becomes close (TEKELIOGLU-UYSAL et al. 1975). In contrast, the decidualization of the more distant endometrium about the implantation site remains less differentiated during the entire period of gestation (ARRONET et al. 1973).

In addition to the morphological changes as sketched here, numerous biochemical alterations also take place (STRAUSS 1964; SCHMIDT-MATTHIESEN 1968; EDWARDS and SURANI 1978; LEROY 1980; BEIER 1981). In this brief review, however, it is impractical and impossible to cover all aspects of the entire, complex process of implantation. Animal experiments of the last few years have brought us some information (cf. NILSSON et al. 1978; BÖVING 1964; WYNN 1967; FRIDHANDLER 1968) but the field is still much in flux; many questions remain unanswered.

5. The Endometrium Before Puberty

In *fetal* endometrium isolated invaginations of epithelium begin to form glands by the 5th month, and the epithelial cells begin to grow taller. By the 8th months the cells are columnar, contain basal glycogen vacuoles, and discharge some secretions into the glandular lumen (KAISER 1963; HUBER et al. 1971). Although the fetal endometrium is acted upon by estrogen and progesterone from the beginning, its development is that of a pure estrogen effect. Only after reaching a certain stage of maturity in the 8th month does the endometrium respond to progesterone. The tortuosity of the glands increases until birth. The nuclei of the epithelial cells become rounded; the cytoplasm shows activity of alkaline and acid phosphatases (PRYSE-DAVIES and DEWHURST 1971). The dense stroma of small cells becomes loose, the nuclei increase in size (HIERSCHE and MEINEN 1971), and occasional predecidual cells may be seen.

Because of the hormonal effects on it during pregnancy, the endometrium of baby girls is still hyperplastic at birth. In 169 *newborns,* OBER and BERNSTEIN (1955) found that 68% had a proliferative endometrium. 27% had a secretory endometrium, and 5% had an endometrium with predecidual change or early signs of menstrual shedding. Within 14 days after birth, however, the endometrium regresses to a height of at most 0.4 mm; its short glands are sparse, embedded in a delicate stroma of spindly cells. The surface epithelium is low.

With the onset of *puberty* the endometrium begins to proliferate again. After the mucosa builds up under the influence of estrogen, cyclic changes then gradually set in. Since the hemorrhages that soon follow are anovulatory, secretory changes in the endometrium are absent for the time.

6. The Normal Menstrual Cycle and Its Possible Variations

Here we shall examine in detail the histological changes induced in the endometrium by the ovarian hormones from day to day during a normal cycle. A thorough knowledge of these changes is a prerequisite for making accurate functional diagnoses of curettings (Fig. 12).

After the first histological description of the cyclic changes of the endometrium by HITSCHMANN and ADLER (1908), numerous supplementary reports followed (SCHRÖDER 1913, 1915, 1928; O'LEARY 1929; BARTELMEZ 1933; HERRELL and BRODERS 1935; ROCK and BARTLETT 1937; FALCONER 1948; and many more). The results of these studies and the information learned about the function of hormones helped to clarify notions of the menstrual cycle. We are most indebted to NOYES et al. (1950), however, for the first detailed description on how "to date the endometrium" from histological criteria; that is, on how to diagnose how far an endometrium has developed in the menstrual cycle

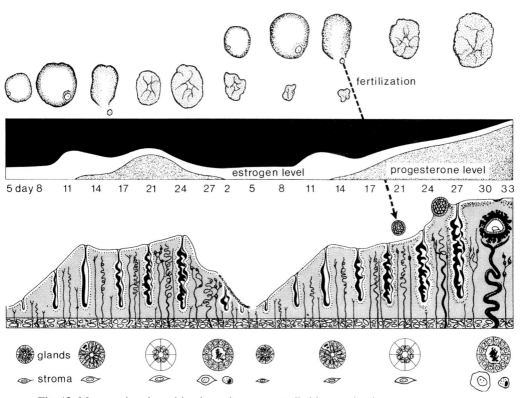

Fig. 12. Menstrual cycle and implantation as controlled by ovarian hormones

from characteristic histological changes that are known to occur at specific times (Fig. 13). MORICARD (1954) and PHILIPPE et al. (1965) confirmed the data of NOYES et al.

Recent advances in hormone therapy in gynecology have required that we attempt to learn how estrogen and progesterone act on the endometrium under

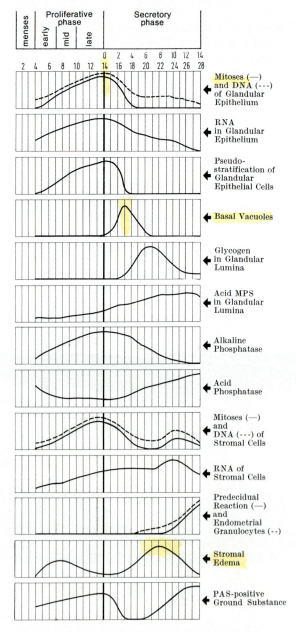

Fig. 13. Morphological criteria important in dating the endometrial cycle

normal and pathological conditions. Since hormones control the time and amount of DNA, RNA, glycogen, and mucus synthesized by endometrial cells, by determining these substances in histological sections with special stains (particularly with acridine orange fluorochromatin, the gallocyanin chromalum stain, and the PAS reaction) we can detect subtle changes in ovarian function (DALLENBACH and DALLENBACH-HELLWEG 1968). By correlating that information with corresponding changes we see in hematoxylin-eosin-stained sections prepared at the same time, we learn how to accurately evaluate the routine "H&E" sections and to determine what their limits of infallibility are. Such studies are indispensable for differentiating from the normal state the earliest variations produced by hormonal imbalance of endogenous or exogenous origin, and are of utmost importance for diagnosing functional changes. Although electron-microscopic studies may disclose finer details of hormonal action, they are of no help in recognizing functional disturbances. For that, a light microscope is needed, because the cyclic changes develop at somewhat different times from region to region or from cell to cell. To ascertain the extent of these differences, in order to date the endometrium accurately, we must examine all parts of the curettings carefully. Only the light microscope affords us such a thorough examination.

Although some investigators have elected to divide the menstrual cycle into three functional phases (FORBES and HEINZ 1953; BARTELMEZ 1957; STRAUSS 1962; THEMANN and SCHÜNKE 1963), I prefer to retain the customary division into the proliferative phase and the secretory phase. My reasons are: first, ovulation logically sets the two phases apart. Second, the differences in the amounts of the two ovarian hormones secreted during the cycle favors its divisions into two halves. Estrogen predominates in the proliferative phase, the progesterone effect prevails in the secretory phase. That the secretion of the hormones overlaps in both directions is well-known and to be expected in such a biological reaction.

a) The Normal Proliferative Phase

This phase generally lasts 2 weeks but under physiological conditions may fluctuate between 10 and 20 days. Consequently, it is impossible to determine each day of the cycle during the proliferative phase. Therefore, we subdivide it only into the early, middle and late stages. The classification suffices since the important functional changes first become evident in the secretory phase. The proliferative phase is under the control of the growth-stimulating hormone estrogen. Only at the end of the phase do criteria appear, as revealed by special stains, that indicate ovulation is imminent. These criteria are of value in distinguishing a normal cycle from the anovulatory cycle.

The early proliferative stage (4th–7th day of a 28-day cycle) is characterized by a low endometrium and represents essentially a freshly epithelialized basalis. Its glands are sparse, narrow, and straight, embedded in a loose stroma of spindly cells. The regenerating superficial epithelium remains flat. The epithelial cells of the glands are low columnar; their cytoplasm contains little RNA.

Their nuclei appear small, oval and the chromatin is dense. Nucleoli are inapparent. The spindle-shaped stromal cells are all alike, poorly differentiated and well anchored in the reticulum network. The chromatin of their nuclei is dense, surrounded by scanty cytoplasm (Fig. 14).

As the effect of estrogen steadily intensifies, the endometrium gradually changes; a state is finally reached that we recognize as the *midproliferative stage* (8th–10th day of a 28-day cycle). The prime change characterizing this stage is the great increase in the height of the endometrium resulting from generalized stromal edema induced by estrogen. The glands not only keep pace with that increase by rapidly growing longer but even exceed it, as their beginning tortuosity indicates. Their epithelial cells become compressed and tall columnar. Although the chromatin of their large, oval nuclei is still dense, nucleoli soon become apparent. In general, the nuclear content of DNA increases, as measurements have shown (Harkin 1956); many of the cells may be in mitosis. Usually, the cytoplasm of the epithelial cells now contains only a small amount of RNA. With appropriate histochemical methods we can demonstrate poorly polymerized acid mucopolysaccharides at the apical ends of the cells (Strauss 1962). The epithelial cells of the endometrial surface also are of the tall columnar type. The spindle-shaped stromal cells, separated by the interstitial edema, lie attached to the reticulum network. Their cytoplasm is scanty; their fusiform nuclei are enlarged. Stromal cells in mitosis generally abound (Fig. 15).

The transition to the *late proliferative stage* (11th–14th day of a 28-day cycle) is marked by the regression of the edema. As that abates, the endometrium temporarily shrinks and as a result the glands, which continue to grow, become more tortuous. Although their epithelial cells continue to proliferate, increasing the tortuosity of the glands, the length to which they can grow is limited. Consequently, the epithelial cells lining them begin to pile up against one another with their nuclei at different levels, producing a pseudostratified appearance. Since all the cells maintain contact with the basement membrane, in some instances only by a thin cytoplasmic extension, the apparent multilayered epithelium is in fact just a single layer. The apical edges of the cells are now so sharp and smooth it appears as if the lumina of the glands had been punched out (Fig. 16). As the cytoplasm of the epithelial cells increases and RNA accumulates, the nuclear-cytoplasmic ratio shifts gradually in favor of the cytoplasm. The nuclei, though enlarged, remain fusiform. They now contain several to many small nucleoli, which become especially prominent with acridine orange fluorochromation. Also at this time we will find tiny green granules of glycogen at the basal parts of the cells if we stain frozen sections with acridine orange and examine them under UV light. With the PAS reaction the granules are red (Color Plate I a). Their appearance before ovulation indicates that the ovary has already begun to secrete progesterone. Minute amounts of progesterone have been detected in the blood of patients at this time (Hoffmann 1948; Edgar 1952; Forbes 1953; Zander 1954). From the results of studies in animals it seems most likely that the progesterone is secreted by the theca interna of the mature Graafian follicle (McKay and Robinson 1947). The lumina of the glands are either empty or contain at most scanty, ill-defined substance composed in part of proteins and mucopolysaccharides shed by the cells (Strauss

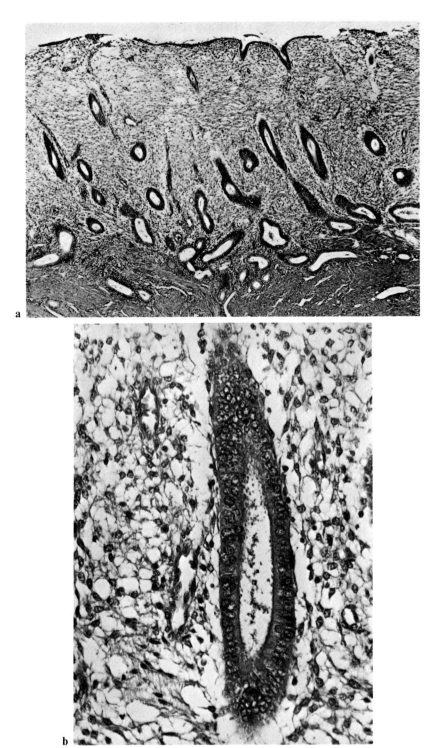

Fig. 14a, b. Early proliferative phase. Narrow, straight glands surrounded by a loose stroma of spindle-shaped cells. a Low magnification; b higher magnification

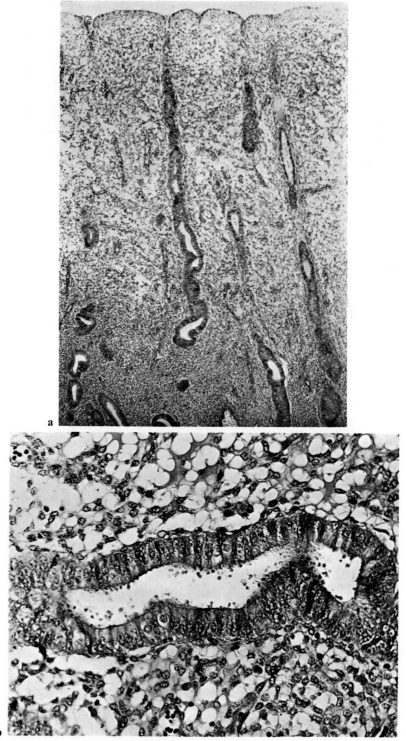

Fig. 15a, b. Midproliferative phase. Slight tortuosity of glands, stromal edema. **a** Low magnification; **b** higher magnification

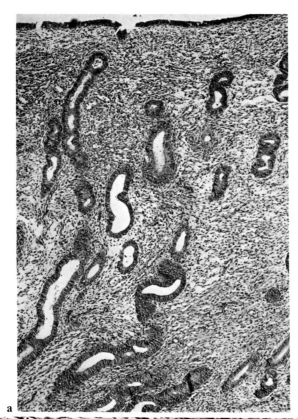
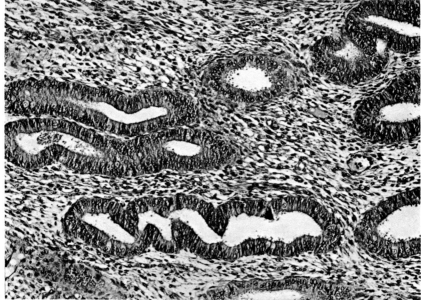

Fig. 16a–c. Late proliferative phase. Glands are more tortuous, the epithelium pseudostratified, the stromal edema has subsided. **a** Low magnification; **b** higher magnification; **c** (see p. 62) high magnification

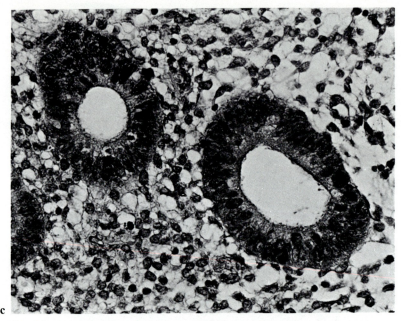

Fig. 16c. Legend see p. 61

1962; SCHMIDT-MATTHIESEN 1963). The stromal cells, again compact because the edema has subsided, have in the meantime enlarged and proliferated; their nuclei bear prominent nucleoli. The stromal cells in the upper half of the functionalis have especially abundant RNA in their enlarged cytoplasm, whereas the stromal cells of the lower half contain only sparse amounts. We can clearly dinstinguish these two layers, which correspond later to the compacta and spongiosa, with acridine orange fluorochromation since the more the RNA, the redder the cells fluorescence. With hematoxylin-eosin-stained sections, however, RNA fails to stain specifically, thus the differences in the two layers go undetected.

The estrogen effect, optimal when it lasts 2 weeks, leads to the build-up of the functionalis through growth and proliferation of the glands and stromal cells. With their high content of RNA, the cells of the superficial stroma and glands are ideally primed by the time ovulation occurs and are receptive to progesterone and the differentiation it induces.

Color Plate I

a Endometrium at the end of the proliferative phase. Beginning secretion of glycogen as droplets in the basal cytoplasm of the glandular epithelium. Unfixed cryostat section. Stain: PAS

b 7 days after ovulation. The dilated glandular lumen is filled with green-staining glycogen, the apical ends of the glandular cells are frayed. Unfixed cryostat section. Acridine orange fluorochromation

c Same endometrium as in **b**. The glycogen in the lumen is red. Unfixed cryostat section. Stain: PAS

The Normal Proliferative Phase 63

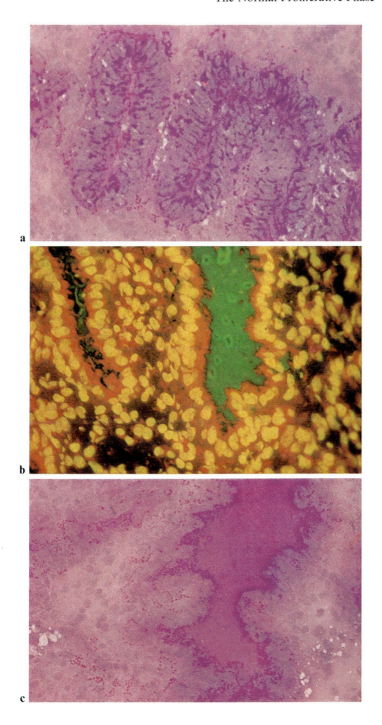

Color Plate I

b) The Normal Secretory Phase

After ovulation the normal corpus luteum develops and involutes at a definite rhythm in a precise sequence, causing changes in the endometrium to take place at the same rate. Consequently, the normal secretory phase, also called "luteal phase", of most cycles lasts 14 days (± 1) (ROCK and HERTIG 1944; ZUCKERMAN 1949). If that limit is decreased (or exceeded) by more than 2 days, then we should diagnose a pathological shortening (or lengthening) of the secretory phase. In order to evaluate such fluctuations precisely, the clinician must determine the time of ovulation just as accurately as we define the morphological changes and criteria that occur in the endometrium. The peak of LH signalizes ovulation more precisely than does the measurement of the basal temperature (KONINCKX et al. 1977). The greater fluctuations in the length of the secretory phase occasionally observed (variations between 9 and 16 days) most probably cause the infertile cycles that occur sporadically in healthy, sexually mature women. Such deviations are most frequent at the beginning and end of the childbearing period (SCHRÖDER 1913, 1928; VOLLMAN 1967; TRELOAR et al. 1967). Since the corpus luteum develops and involutes at a definite rate and rhythm, the associated changes regularly induced in the endometrium enable us to date the endometrium (to diagnose the day of the cycle). Histological changes in the endometrium serve as our criteria. Whereas the changes in the glandular epithelium during the 1st week of the secretory phase are more striking and easier to detect, during the 2nd week we base our histological dating chiefly on the daily changes that take place in the stromal cells. The histological and cytological changes induced in the endometrium by the sex hormones are never uniform. Some cells in some regions always reveal greater differentiation than cells in other parts although adjacent. Such differences are related to many variable factors, such as differences in local blood supply, in amounts of hormones reaching the target cells, and in cellular nutrition and metabolism. We should therefore never expect the endometrium to present the same picture in all equivalent parts. In dating the endometrium we should be guided by those regions showing the most advanced changes or by the appearance of the majority of the cells.

The *1st day after ovulation* (15th day of an ideal cycle) is morphologically "mute" because it takes 36–48 h before the initial progesterone secreted by the corpus luteum produces enough change to be detected in hematoxylin-eosin-stained sections. Since sporadic vacuoles appear in some of the glandular epithelial cells in the first hours after ovulation and since deposits of glycogen, as revealed by special stains, may occasionally form just before ovulation, these vacuoles and deposits are unreliable as definite signs that ovulation has taken place. The earliest that ovulation can be detected with certainty is 36 h later; that is, on the *2nd day* (16th day of the cycle) when numerous basal vacuoles appear in the glandular epithelium. The endometrium should not be dated as the 16th day, however, unless at least 50% of the glands have basal vacuoles. In hematoxylin-eosin sections the vacuoles are produced by the dissolving away of glycogen that formed basally and pushed the nucleus towards the lumen. By this 2nd day the epithelial cells again form a single row. The glands continue

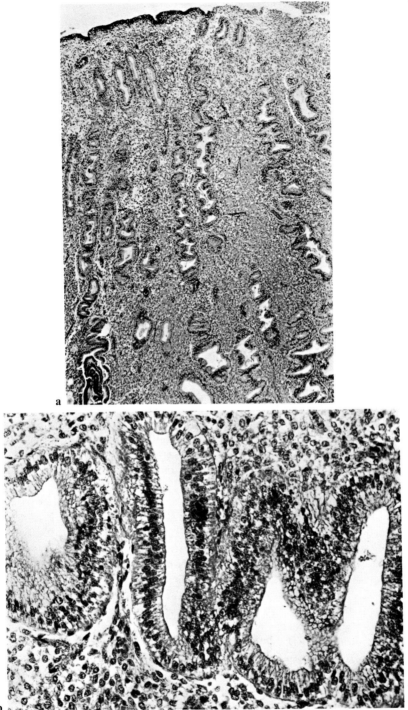

Fig. 17a, b. The 2nd day after ovulation. Prominent tortuosity of glands; basal vacuoles begin to appear in the glandular epithelial cells. **a** Low magnification; **b** higher magnification

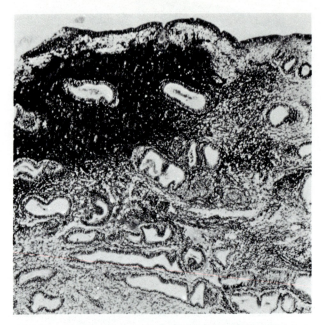

Fig. 18. Ovulatory bleeding: focal extravasation of blood in the superficial stroma

to grow longer and become increasingly more corkscrew-shaped (Fig. 17). As a consequence, the entire surface of the epithelium greatly increases, a change that promotes the secretion soon to occur from the surface into the glandular lumen. At this time fairly brisk hemorrhages may develop in the stroma ("physiological ovulatory bleeding"; Fig. 18), if the transient fall of estrogen at ovulation is great or if the capillaries prove to be unusually sensitive to that decrease in estrogen.

Whereas most of the glandular epithelial cells on the 2nd day after ovulation disclose basal vacuoles, by the *3rd day* these vacuoles have enlarged to push all nuclei toward the apical end of the cell where they form a uniform row around the lumen (Fig. 19). Few mitoses are to be found since the epithelial cells generally lose their ability to divide with the onset of this specific differentiation brought on by progesterone. The nuclear-cytoplasm ratio now is clearly in favor of the cytoplasm (1:3.6) (STURGIS and MEIGS 1936). The cytoplasm still contains abundant RNA. As histochemical studies disclose, acid mucopolysaccharides begin to accumulate at the apical rim of the cell.

On the *4th day* after ovulation some of the nuclei return to the base of the cell (Fig. 20), while the glycogen on both sides of the nucleus moves towards the lumen, a shift that is particularly easy to follow with the PAS reaction.

On the *5th day* after ovulation most of the nuclei have returned to the base of the cell. The accumulated glycogen now located above the nucleus is secreted at the free margin as a globular cap, which bulges into the lumen (Fig. 21). The cytoplasm is still rich in RNA. The nuclei are round, vesicular and unusually clear or pale staining, making it easy to distinguish them from

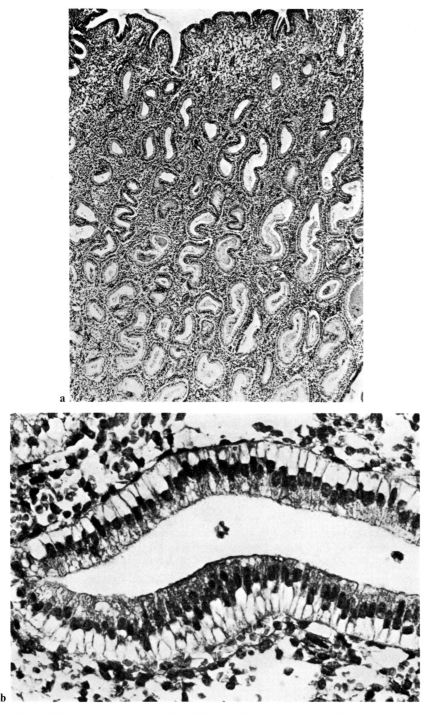

Fig. 19a, b. The 3rd day after ovulation. Dinstinct basal vacuoles in all glandular epithelial cells. The nuclei generally still elongated. **a** Low magnification; **b** higher magnification

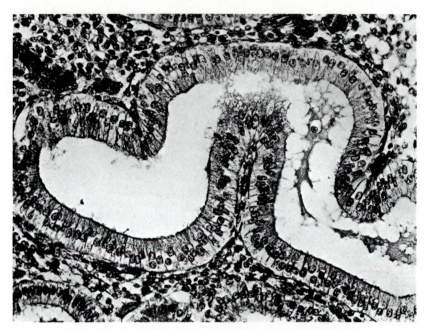

Fig. 20. The 4th day after ovulation. Basal vacuoles are still readily visible. The nuclei are more rounded

the dense, elongated nuclei that were basal just before the glycogen vacuoles appeared. The nucleoli by now have greatly enlarged.

The *6th day* after ovulation is characterized by a dilatation of the glandular lumina produced by the continued secretion of glycogen (Fig. 22). The apical ends of the low glandular cells appear shredded with hazy margins owing to the apocrine secretion. Since the RNA content of the cytoplasm gradually falls but the nucleoli remain large, it seems probable that the nuclear RNA ceases to be discharged into the cytoplasm.

In the ensuing days of the cycle, which are diagnosed primarily from the changes taking place in the stroma, the secretion distending the glandular lumina becomes thicker (Color Plate I b and c), now intermixed with acid and neutral mucopolysaccharides, and through polymerization becomes stringy and metachromatic; gradually it disappears. Although we find glycogen in the glandular lumen only until the 7th day after ovulation, remnants of acid and especially neutral mucopolysaccharides remain at the apical end of the cell and in the glandular lumen until shortly before menstruation. The glandular cells become more cuboidal and their stores of RNA continue to decrease; a few days before menstruation starts their RNA is depleted.

Fig. 21 a, b. The 5th day after ovulation. The basal vacuoles are fading away and the nuclei are returning to the base of the cell; beginning secretion of glycogen. Slight stromal edema. **a** Low magnification; **b** higher magnification

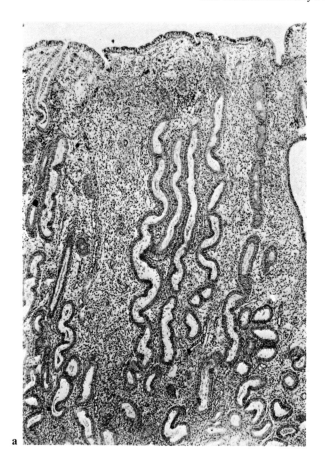
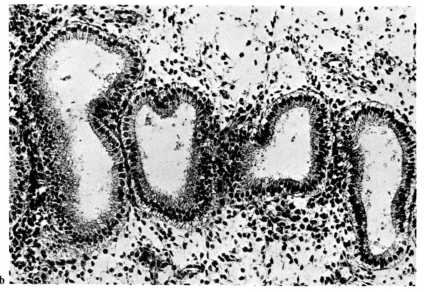

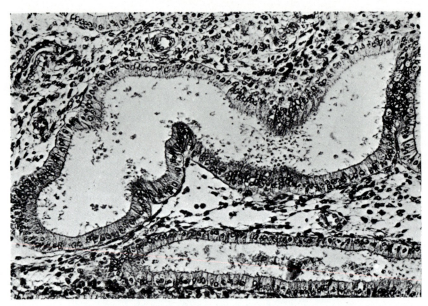

Fig. 22. The 6th day after ovulation. The nuclei are now almost entirely basal. The glandular lumen begins to dilate with fine droplets of glycogen

During the 1st week of the secretory phase little happens to the endometrial stroma, as compared with the drastic changes that take place in the glandular epithelium. During the 2nd week, however, changes in the stroma make it possible to readily subdivide the functionalis into the compacta and the spongiosa. On the 7th day after ovulation stromal edema develops again (Fig. 23), reaching its maximum on the 8th day (Fig. 24) when the secretion of estrogen during the secretory phase is also at its highest. Although the stromal cells are now somewhat larger, they are still spindle-shaped; the edema fluid causes them to become widely separated. Mitoses cease to appear.

As the edema subsides on the 9th day after ovulation, groups of spiral arterioles become prominent (Fig. 25). During the proliferative phase these vessels have a straight course, but in the secretory phase, owing to the effects of progesterone, they grow much longer, thicker, and become spirally twisted. Although the volume of the endometrium doubles in the secretory phase, the volume of the arterioles enlarges three-fold (MASSHOFF and KRAUS 1955) and their length increases five-fold (MARKEE 1950). It is obvious that the growth of these vessels exceeds that needed for mere nutrition of the endometrium. The stromal cells surrounding these spiral arterioles grow larger, become rounded and their content of RNA increases markedly.

On the 10th day these periarteriolar stromal cells turn into predecidual cells, forming prominent, broad mantles about the vessels. The nuclei of the cells are large, round, and clear (Fig. 26; Color Plate II a). Among the predecidual cells, and almost as numerous as they, are small endometrial granulocytes with lobated, chromatin-rich nuclei and characteristic phloxinophilic granules in their cytoplasm, which also contains abundant RNA (HAMPERL 1954; HELLWEG

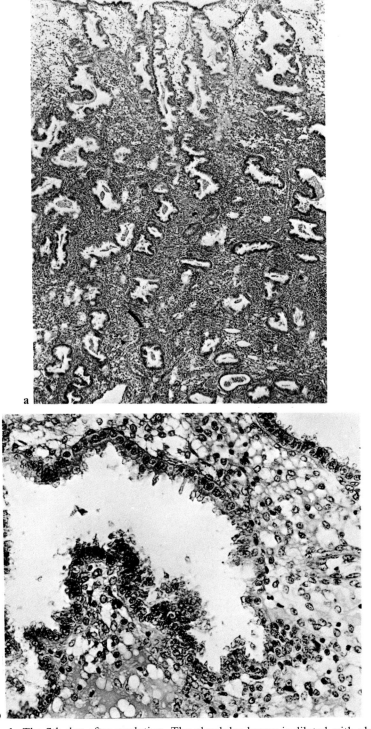

Fig. 23a, b. The 7th day after ovulation. The glandular lumen is dilated with abundant glycogen. The border of glandular epithelium appears shredded owing to intense secretion. a Low magnification; b higher magnification

72   The Normal Histology of the Endometrium

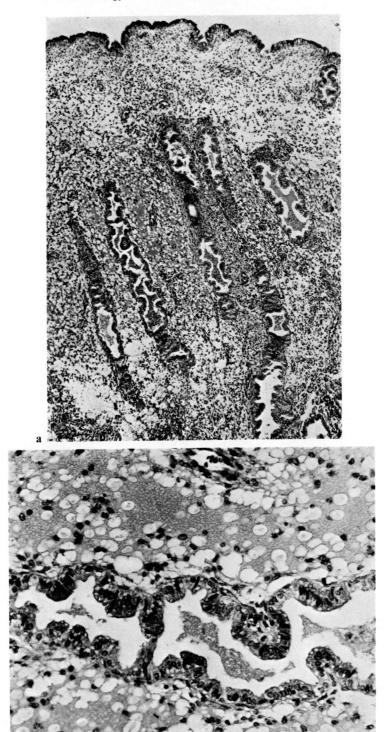

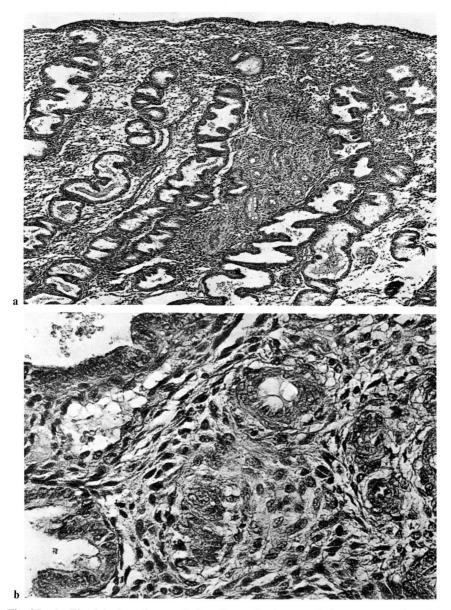

Fig. 25a, b. The 9th day after ovulation. Stromal edema and glycogen secretion abate, first evidence of predecidual reaction around spiral arterioles. **a** Low magnification; **b** higher magnification

---

Fig. 24a, b. The 8th day after ovulation. Glandular lumina still contain traces of glycogen, intermixed with mucopolysaccharides. Greatest stromal edema during secretory phase. **a** Low magnification; **b** higher magnification

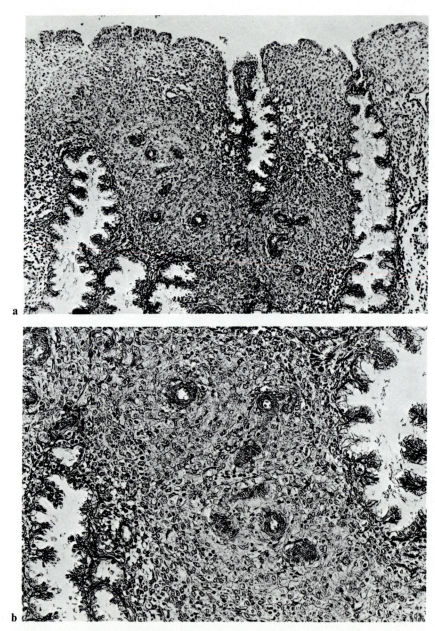

Fig. 26a–c. The 10th day after ovulation. Almost sheet-like predecidual reaction around the spiral arterioles and beneath the superficial epithelium. **a** Low magnification; **b** higher magnification. **c** The glandular epithelium in the spongiosa is prominently dentated. Residual secretion in the glandular lumen

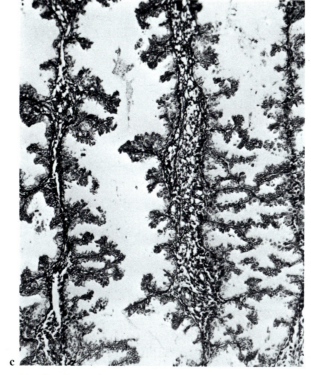

Fig. 26 c. Legend see opposite page

1954). Thus, as one might expect, the first stromal cells to undergo differentiation by rounding up to become predecidual cells or by freeing themselves from the reticulum network to turn into small granulocytes are those nearest the arterial blood supply; that is, those first affected by progesterone.

By the *11th day* after ovulation the stromal cells of the upper compacta located close to the superficial epithelium differentiate into predecidual cells and granulocytes (Fig. 27); by the *12th day* the entire compacta discloses that transformation. Numerous lacunae of dilated capillaries appear close to the surface. When the corpus luteum begins to regress (4 days before menstruation sets in, since pregnancy has failed to take place), we begin to see the first signs of endometrial involution with incipient shrinkage (Fig. 28).

On the *13th day* after ovulation the endometrium greatly contracts because of the fall in both progesterone and estrogen. The glands collapse, assuming a saw-toothed appearance (Fig. 29), and the predecidual stroma becomes very dense.

On the *14th day* the Golgi apparatus of the stromal and glandular cells involutes and the remaining RNA in these cells disappears. As the reticulum network disintegrates the stromal cells dissociate (Fig. 30). Occasionally one can find nuclear debris in the glandular cells, corresponding no doubt to the hematoxylin-positive granules described by SCHRÖDER (1914). By now the endometrial granulocytes have given off their phloxinophilic granules and can at

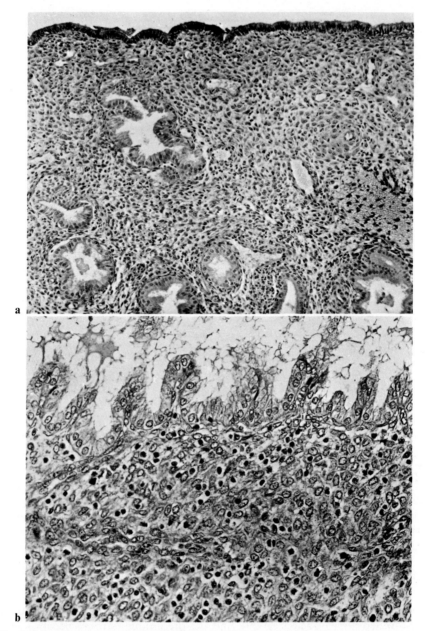

Fig. 27a, b. The 11th day after ovulation. Predecidual transformation of the entire compacta, numerous endometrial granulocytes. **a** Low magnification; **b** higher magnification

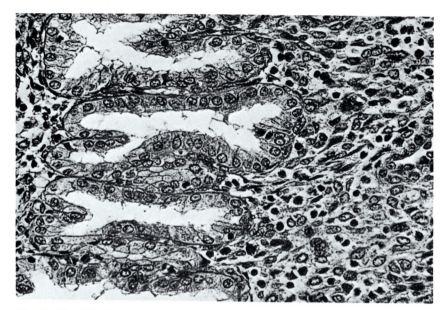

Fig. 28. The 12th day after ovulation. The glands are beginning to collapse

times be recognized only by their characteristic lobated nuclei and their vacuolated cytoplasm.

c) Menstruation

The *1st day* of menstruation is characterized by hemorrhage in the superficial stroma, whose dissociated cells still show their predecidual change (Fig. 31). From the remaining evidence of that change and from the occasional persisting signs of previous secretion in the epithelium of the collapsed glands, it is possible after the onset of menstruation to still diagnose that ovulation had taken place.

On the *2nd day* of menstruation one normally finds only scattered stromal cells and remnants of glandular epithelium liberated from their cellular connections, lying amid fresh blood and aggregates of polymorphonuclear leukocytes (Fig. 32). Contrary to earlier opinions, polymorphonuclear leukocytes are not found in a healthy endometrium before menstruation starts. The investigators who thought so mistook endometrial granulocytes for leukocytes.

The much-discussed question about the *cause of menstruation* remains incompletely understood even today, as the many theories that have been proposed for it testify; they all lack sufficient experimental confirmation. The most fundamental experiments carried out until now were made in monkeys. From the results we may assume the following is probably true: with the premenstrual fall of both hormones, especially estrogen, the endometrium loses water and greatly shrinks. According to some authors (MARKEE 1940, 1950; WITT 1963) the shrinkage is 20% of the original height, but BARTELMEZ (1931, 1941, 1957) estimates it to be as much as 40%. Such a 40% shrinkage has been observed

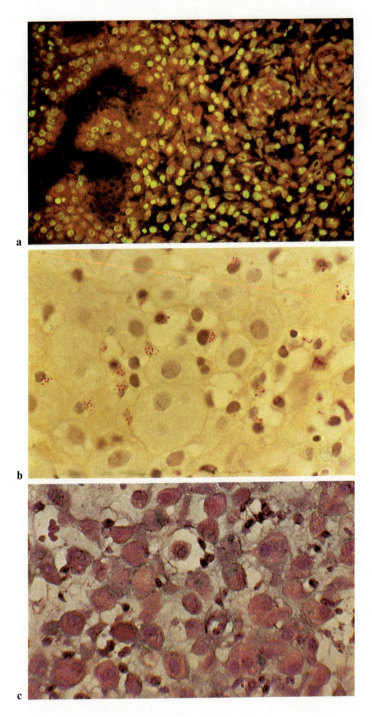

Color Plate II

to occur in an endometriosis of the vagina (HOFFMANN et al. 1953). In rare instances nothing more takes place at menstruation than the loss of water and the shrinkage of the endometrium; a real menstrual flow may fail to develop (BENGTSSON and INGEMANNSSON 1959; PHILIPPE et al. 1966). As the shrinkage progresses the spiral arterioles (DARON 1936) and veins (DARON 1937) collapse and kink, leading to ischemia and impairment of cellular respiration (BURGER 1958). With the collapse of the arterioles, further factors act to aggravate the ischemia, such as a contraction of the smooth muscle cells of the media (BARTELMEZ) and a development in the arterioles of hyaline degeneration with loss of elastic fibers (KELLER 1911). The capillaries also become more fragile. In addition, the fall in the progesterone activates fibrinolytic enzymes and induces the release of relaxin from the endometrial granulocytes, which in turn brings about dissolution of the stromal fibers (DALLENBACH and DALLENBACH-HELLWEG 1964). That dissolution must take place before the stromal cells can dissociate and the functionalis can break down to be discharged as menstruating endometrium. Some authors maintain that a part of the spongiosa normally remains and partakes in the regeneration of the next cycle (SEKIGA 1924; BARTELMEZ 1933, 1941; ROCKENSCHAUB 1960; MCLENNAN and RYDELL 1965; SENGEL and STOEBNER 1970). Contrarily, BOHNEN (1927) always observed a complete shedding of the spongiosa followed by epithelialization of the basalis. Most probably the extent to which the endometrium is desquamated depends on individual variations.

In general, the endometrium is discharged at those levels where it contains enough granulocytes to induce dissolution of the reticulum fibers. Normally, these cells pervade the compacta and part of the spongiosa, becoming increasingly sparse towards the basalis. During menstruation regressive changes begin in the parts of the endometrium not shed, which enable the glandular and stromal cells here to survive and restore themselves, in order to participate in the physiological build-up of the next cycle. When bleeding commences, the epithelial and stromal cells engage in processes of "cellular and tissue self-cleaning and rejuvenation". These processes can best be followed with histochemical and electron-microscopic methods and are seen as: autophagocytosis regulated by the cell's own lysosomes, heterophagocytosis performed by wandering macrophages, and discharge of cellular debris (FLOWERS and WILBORN 1978) through intercellular spaces (DAVIE et al. 1977) or through epithelial cells for

Color Plate II

a The 10th day after ovulation. Stromal cells show predecidual change, especially about the spiral arterioles (*upper right*), and abundant intracytoplasmic RNA (fluorescing red). The condensed nuclei of endometrial granulocytes stain intensely for DNA (fluorescing bright yellow). Unfixed cryostat section. Acridine orange fluorochromation
b Young decidua of 2nd month of pregnancy. Numerous small endometrial granulocytes with paranuclear phloxinophilic granules between large decidual cells. Paraffin section. Stain: phloxine-tartrazine
c Involuting decidua after abortion in 3rd month. Blue-staining "collagen inclusions" in the shrinking and dissociating cells. Paraffin section. Trichrome stain after MASSON

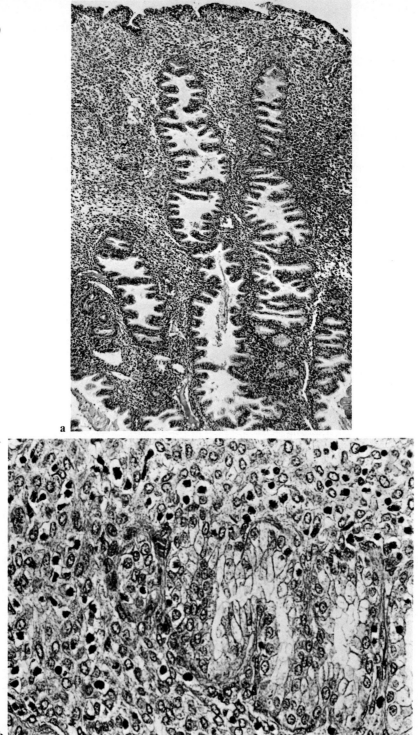

Fig. 29a, b. The 13th day after ovulation. Pronounced shrinkage of the glands and stroma with saw-toothed appearance of the glands; the endometrial granulocytes are still numerous. **a** Low magnification; **b** higher magnification

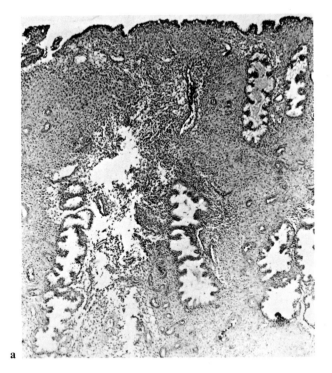

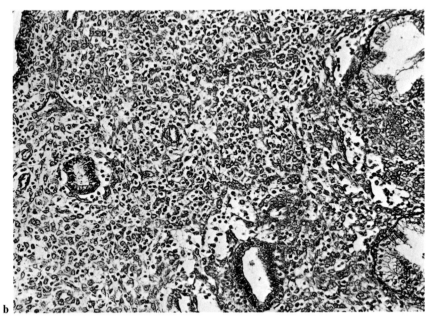

Fig. 30a, b. The 14th day after ovulation. Though the tissue in general is intact, dissociation is beginning in the compacta. Onset of relaxin release from the endometrial granulocytes with dissolution of stromal fibers. Some of the glandular epithelium is markedly shrunken. **a** Low magnification; **b** higher magnification

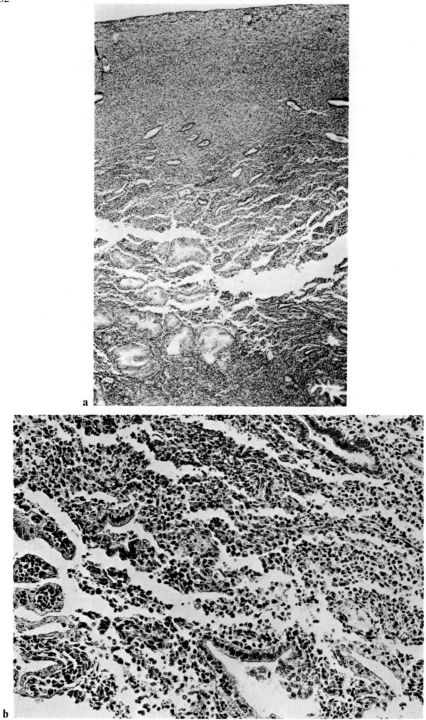

Fig. 31a, b. First day of menstruation. The compacta separates from the spongiosa. Glands and stroma dissociate. **a** Low magnification; **b** higher magnification

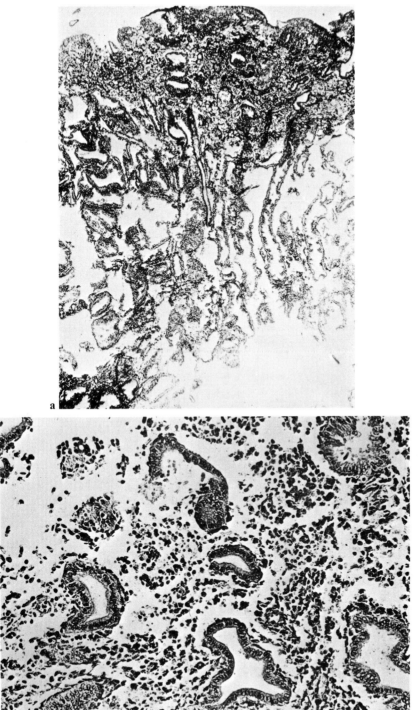

Fig. 32a, b. Second day of menstruation. The disintegration of the tissue is advanced, remnants of collapsed endometrial glands separate from the tissue. **a** Low magnification; **b** higher magnification

elimination into glandular lumina and the uterine cavity. The remaining cells rejuvenate. Consequently, menstruation represents two main processes: first, the loss of tissue, the amount of which varies from patient to patient; second, a complicated interplay of cellular regression, restoration and renewal in the parts of the functionalis that remain and are needed for the next cycle. For menstruation to take place in a regular manner, the fall of estrogen and progesterone is essential (ZUCKERMAN 1949). If their fall is disturbed by any of several possible mechanisms, then menstrual shedding may be accordingly either prolonged or incomplete.

Hemostasis is enhanced by endothelial changes, such as swelling or proliferation caused by the release of relaxin (see p. 52), and the ensuing formation of platelet thrombi in the vascular lumina. These mechanisms seem to account for hemostasis during the first 20 h of menstruation and are followed by vasoconstriction of the remaining vessels during the next days (CHRISTIAENS et al. 1980).

d) Regeneration

Immediately after menstrual shedding ceases and before proliferation begins a **regenerative phase** sets in lasting 1–2 days, during which the denuded endometrium becomes epithelialized (Fig. 33). The regeneration of the surface epithelium can be readily followed by studies with the scanning electron microscope (FERENCZY 1976; LUDWIG and METZGER 1976). It proceeds on the one hand from the stumps of glands in the basalis or lower functionalis. From these the epithelial cells form collar-like aggregates that spread out in all directions. On the other hand, the epithelium remaining in the tubal recesses and isthmus grows out over the adjacent defects. Stromal cells do not take part in the regeneration. Since the newly formed epithelial cells fail to show mitoses, although the synthesis of nuclear DNA and cytoplasmic RNA is increased, cellular proliferation is thought to come about partly by endomitotic processes (FERENCZY 1976). On the other hand, endometrial healing involves both migration and replication of surface cells, factors that may explain the relative paucity of mitoses despite rapid restoration of the surface epithelium (FERENCZY et al. 1979). Generally, re-epithelization is completed by the 5th day of the cycle, independent of hormonal stimuli. When estrogen stimulation is increased, however, as for example with glandular-cystic hyperplasia, the regeneration is accelerated. As one might expect, the onset, progress, and duration of regeneration vary from patient to patient, just as do the manner and extent to which the endometrium is shed during menstruation (NOGALES et al. 1969, 1978).

e) Possible Variations in the Endometrium During the Normal Cycle

The sequence of changes just described that take place in the endometrium from day to day occasionally fail to develop uniformly in all parts. If extreme differences are evident with variations exceeding 2 days, then the changes are clearly not normal and a functional disturbance exists. Such endometria are impossible to date accurately.

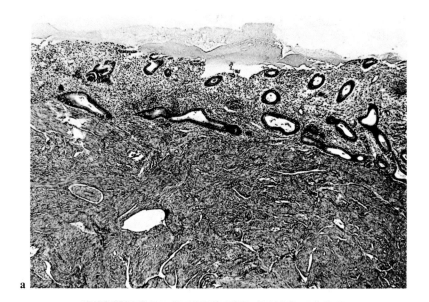

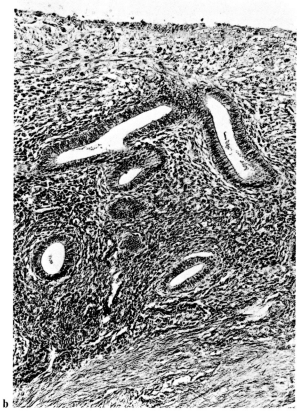

Fig. 33. a Onset of regenerative phase after menstruation ceases (low magnification). **b** High magnification: beginning local regeneration of surface epithelium

Here we are primarily interested in the possible deviations that may take place in the height of normal endometrium, in the abundance of its glands, and in the shape of its glands (BEHRENS 1953; WINTER 1955). Fully developed and normal secretory endometrium may vary from 1 to 10 mm in *height,* depending primarily on the amount of fluid in the stroma. The height of the basalis or the number of glands in it that fail to participate in the cyclic changes may likewise show great differences from patient to patient, or may vary from one part of the endometrium to another, particularly when focal hyperplasia develops in the basalis. Further, although still within normal limits, the boundary between the basalis and the myometrium may be very irregular, simulating at times adenomatous hyperplasia. In like manner, the surface of the endometrium may be wavy, nodular or folded owing to local variations in the content of fluid or glands but without an overgrowth of glands or collagenous fibers that characterizes polyps. A circumscribed or generalized *paucity of glands* in the functionalis may arise from a comparable scarcity in the basalis. Both deficiencies should be regarded as variations within the range of normal, although the glands that are present may overproliferate, dilate, and grow irregularly. In addition, a localized or generalized *excess of glands* may also develop, even though the glands are normal. *Cystic dilatation* of an occasional gland is not necessarily a sign of focal hyperplasia (WILSON and KURZROK 1938). When the surrounding stroma is unusually loose or when the flow of glandular secretions becomes obstructed, the glands may enlarge; the change, however, should not be misinterpreted as a functional deviation. The distinction can easily be made if the glandular epithelium fails to show the changes characteristic of a functional disturbance (Fig. 34a, 35). *Sporadic glands without secretory activity* may occasionally be found at the height or end of the secretory phase, located incongruously among the otherwise homogeneous, actively secreting glands; such inactive glands apparently represent local unresponsiveness to hormonal stimuli, a variation belonging within the range of the biological norm. It is of no pathological importance (Fig. 34b).

7. The Endometrium in the Climacterium and After the Menopause

An increasing frequency or persistence of irregular cycles portends the approaching end of the reproductive period. Slight irregularities in the hormonal balance, indicating ovarian function is waning because of age, may still be within the range of normal yet cause the endometrial glands to proliferate irregularly. At times an insufficient corpus luteum results in imperfectly developed secretory changes. Ovulation may recur sporadically, even years after a menopause; the associated corpus luteum is insufficient (NOVAK 1970). In addition, a local alteration of endometrial reactivity to estrogen or gestagen may develop owing to climacteric ageing of the endometrium. The arrangement of the glands, their spacing and growth pattern, the width of their lumina, and the height and maturity of their lining epithelium may all vary markedly without these changes implying that a functional disturbance, such as a circumscribed of diffuse glan-

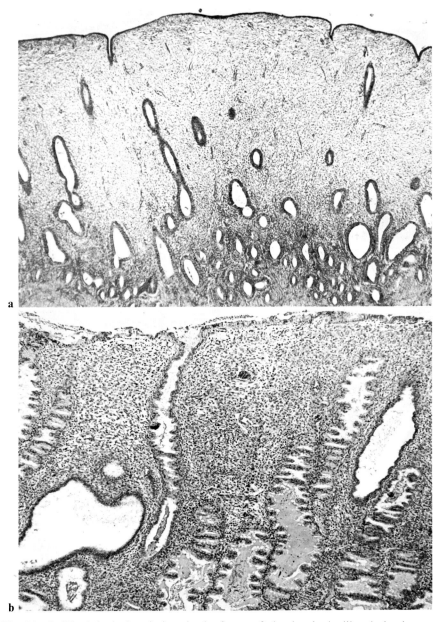

Fig. 34a, b. Physiological variations in the forms of glands; single dilated glands among those of normal size. **a** Early proliferative phase; **b** late secretory phase

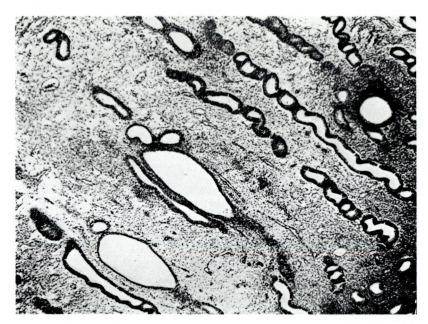

Fig. 35. Elliptical dilatation of the midportion of a gland as a physiological variation, midproliferative phase

dular-cystic hyperplasia or adenomatous hyperplasia, is present (Fig. 36). We refer to endometria with these changes, therefore, as the preclimacteric or *climacteric transitional type*; we find it occurs in almost 50% of all endometria studied in the climacteric age group. Some patients with endometria of this type will already have anovulatory cycles when first seen (BEHRENS 1956). Anovulation can be easily diagnosed, even in the first half of the cycle, if the endometrium is examined with the acridine orange fluorochromation method. Such studies will show that the cytoplasm of the superficial stromal cells fails to fluoresce red, as it should in a normal cycle. Consequently, there is no distinction into two layers (superficial red staining stromal cells rich in RNA; poorly stained stromal cells of the lower half of the functionalis deficient in RNA) characteristically seen at this time in a normal menstrual cycle of the reproductive period. We can also detect an anovulatory cycle or an irregular proliferative phase of the preclimacterium by the absence of the glycogen granules, which normally appear just before ovulation in the basal parts of the glandular epithelium. For such studies we recommend frozen sections prepared with the cryostat and stained with either acridine orange or the PAS reaction.

After the physiological decline of ovarian function and the sharp fall in the secretion of both progesterone and estrogen, the resting, afunctional endometrium that evolves after the menopause[1] ends as an atrophic endometrium

---

[1] The term "menopause" means etymologically: time of the last bleeding. We prefer to hold to that definition and will refer to the period after the last menstrual period as the "postmenopause", often incorrectly designated the menopause.

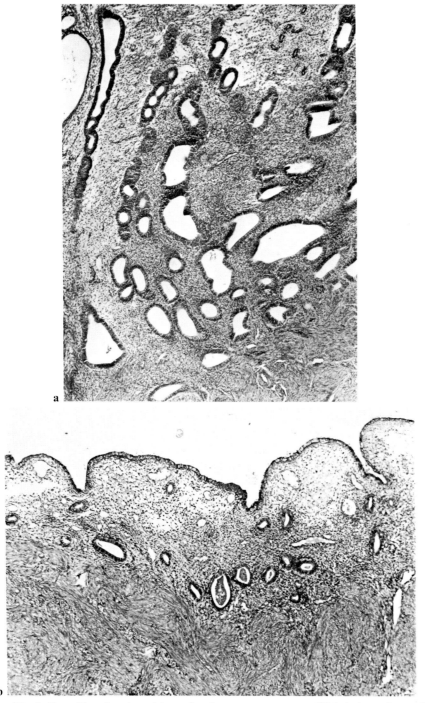

Fig. 36a, b. Transitional endometrium of early postmenopause. a Slightly irregular proliferative phase with variation in width of glands, in height of glandular epithelium, and in the density of the stroma. b Additional variation in the total height of the endometrium

Table 5. The preclimacteric and postclimacteric endometrium

	Preclimacterium – climacterium		Postmenopause
Last ovulatory cycle	Physiological waning of the secretion of hormones	→ Resting endometrium	→ Atrophic endometrium
	Preclimacteric hormonal dysfunction (ovary-hypophysis)	→ Climacteric transitional endometrium with irregular secretion; some glands well developed (secretory hypertrophy, "glandular hyperplasia")	→ Atrophic endometrium
	Anovulatory cycles	→ Climacteric transitional endometrium with irregularly proliferating glands, some cystically dilated	→ Cystic atrophy endometrium
	Persistent follicle	→ Glandular-cystic hyperplasia	→ Cessation of hormonal section → Regressive hyperplasia → Persistent secretion of estrogen → Adenomatous hyperplasia

after a few years (see Table 5). Since that atrophic state represents, so to speak, the preserved or "petrified" cycle that existed when the menopause set in, it may have many forms. If the last cycle is ovulatory and ends with a regular menstruation, then a *simple atrophy* will develop with sparse remnants of narrow glands lined by a low epithelium with small inactive nuclei and supported by a dense, fibrous stroma of spindly cells (Fig. 37a). Spiral arterioles will be lacking. The functionalis cannot be separated from the basalis. The amount of RNA and the activities of enzymes are either very low or absent (GOLDBERG and JONES 1956; GROSS 1964; personal studies). In contrast, if the last cycle or cycles were anovulatory, or if the proliferative phases were irregular, then what we should find after the menopause sets in is the "petrified" state of that last proliferative phase. Because some glands may be cystically dilated, the histological picture found may be misdiagnosed as a glandular-cystic hyperplasia (Fig. 37b). That a *cystic atrophy* is present, however, is evident from the inactive, flattened glandular epithelium that contains no enzymes (MANSOUR and BARADI 1967) and no RNA (MCKAY et al. 1956), as we could show with acridine orange fluorochromation (DALLENBACH and DALLENBACH-HELLWEG 1968). The stroma is dense, composed of spindly cells devoid of most RNA. The only morphological difference between simple atrophy and cystic atrophy is the diameter of the glandular lumen, but that difference is of no clinical

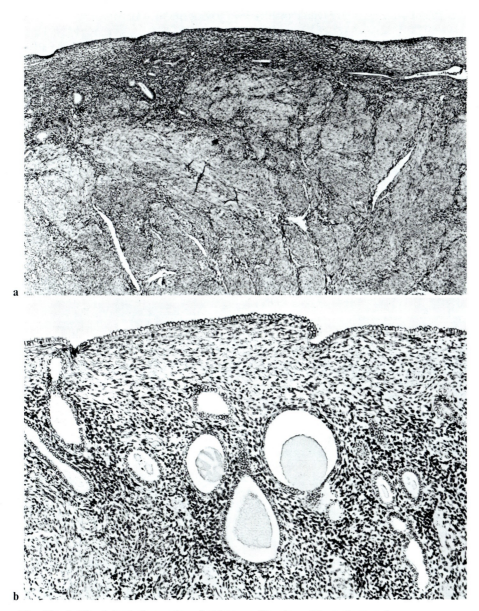

Fig. 37 a, b. Physiological atrophy of old age. **a** Simple and **b** cystic atrophy

importance. Both conditions are to be regarded as physiological forms of regression (KELLER and ADRIAN 1939; SPEERT 1949; TOTH and GIMES 1964), of which the cystic atrophy is seen most commonly. According to NOER (1961) it occurs in 76% of all cases, as compared with 7.8% for simple atrophy. In contrast, all other endometrial conditions encountered after the menopause (16.2%) are caused either by an abnormal persistence in the production of estrogen or by treatment with estrogen (Breipohl 1935; Novak and Richardson 1941; Husslein 1948; Dhom 1952; Novak 1953; McBride 1954; Parks et al. 1958). Thus, the proliferation produced should be regarded as pathological; it usually causes bleeding.

Endometrial atrophy is the most frequent cause of postmenopausal bleeding (Choo et al. 1985), which develops because of sclerotic degeneration of the endometrial vessels (Meyer et al. 1971), local or systemic hypertension as in apoplexia uteri (see p. 97), or senile endometritis.

C. The Histopathology of the Endometrium

Almost all hormonal dysregulations (that is, endocrinopathies) and organic diseases of the endometrium produce atypical uterine bleeding. Clinically, the cause of the bleeding often remains unclear. Therefore, the attending gynecologist

Table 6. Causes of atypical uterine bleeding

A. *Systemic diseases:*

> Cardiac and circulatory failure
> Hypertension
> Blood dyscrasia with thrombocytopenia
> Hemophilia, avitaminosis, intoxications, infectious diseases

B. *Functional disturbances:*

> Dysfunction of the ovaries,
>   pituitary, diencephalon,
>   thyroid, or adrenal glands
> Death of extrauterine pregnancy
> Hormone-producing ovarian tumors
> Exogenous administration of hormones

C. *Local anatomic disturbances:*

> Endometrium: Endometritis
>   Abortion or retained products of conception
>   Foreign bodies (talcum powder, intrauterine device)
>   Polyps, Hyperplasia
>   Neoplasms

Myometrium: Vascular anomalies (aneurysms)
            Myometritis

>   Fibromyoma-submucous, intramural, subserous

            Adenomyosis
            Neoplasms

> Portio and cervix: Cervicitis
>   Polyps, Hyperplasia
>   Glandular-papillary ectropium
>   Neoplasms

Structural changes of the vagina, vulva, parametrium
Anomalous positions of the uterus with circulatory disturbances (hemostasis)

☐ Can usually be diagnosed by histological study of curettings.

☐ Can be diagnosed only at times.

will attempt to establish a diagnosis in all his patients with unexplained bleeding by submitting curettings for histological study. Most causes of atypical uterine bleeding can be revealed histologically. The percentage of patients whose endometrial curettings fail to disclose pathological changes is small, varying from 3.6% to 18%, depending upon the investigator who makes the examination (LAU and STOLL 1963; also for further literature). The cause of the bleeding in that small percentage of women is either morphologically extrauterine or functionally extraovarian (see Table 6).

By carefully correlating the histological study of the endometrium with the patient's anamnesis and the results of clinical tests, and by using special stains and eventually histochemical reactions, it is often possible to diagnose conditions that are unclear in sections prepared by routine methods. At least a presumptive diagnosis can be made at times. For example, a stretched and compressed endometrium may suggest a submucosal leiomyoma, or microaneurysms of the endometrium may mean thrombocytopenic purpura.

In evaluating pathological changes of the endometrium one should consider all the causes for the disturbance that led to curettage. These causes may be divided into three main groups, as shown in Table 6. In the following chapters we shall examine as precisely as possible how each condition of these groups varies histologically from the norm, enabling us then to differentiate the causative disturbances from one another and to reach a definitive diagnosis.

1. Morphological Effects of Circulatory and Coagulation Disturbances

a) Edema

The vascular system of the endometrium is unusually sensitive to fluctuations in levels of the sex hormones and reacts to such variations by promptly dilating; that leads to hyperemia, slowing of the blood flow, and edema. Similar changes also take place at specific times during a normal menstrual cycle (see Fig. 12). Thus, before one diagnoses a pathological edema of the endometrium one must determine the phase of the cycle. In our differential diagnosis it is necessary to exclude the physiological edema that develops when the levels of estrogen in the blood are highest; namely, in the middle of the proliferative phase and around the 21st–24th day of the cycle.

Pathological edema of the endometrium may be traced back to a circulatory disturbance that can be caused either by venous or lymphatic obstruction (increased hydrostatic pressure) or like physiological edema, by hormones (functional abnormality) (DERICHSWEILER 1934; CRAMER 1952).

Often in *ovarian dysfunction* only estrogen is secreted; its unopposed action induces focal or diffuse hyperplasia of the endometrium and polyp formation. The stroma of the proliferated regions frequently is extremely edematous; the glands are pushed apart and the reticulum network pulled apart (Fig. 38). Occasionally small lakes of edema fluid form, as serous exudates seep from the greatly distended vessels, their walls often swollen with hyaline material. Not

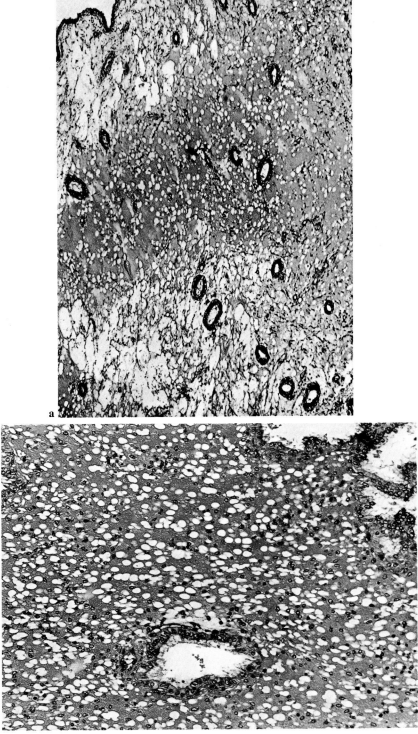

Fig. 38a, b. Pathological edema of the stroma; the stromal cells are pushed widely apart and the reticulum fibers are sparse. **a** Low magnification; **b** higher magnification

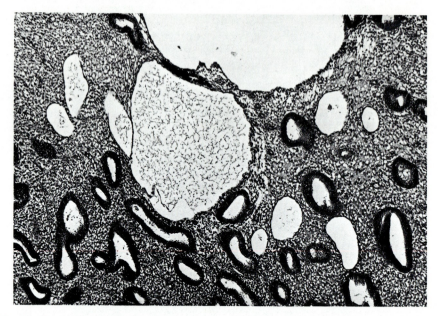

Fig. 39. Cystic lymphatic channels of various sizes in the lower functionalis. Their flattened endothelial lining can be readily distinguished from glandular epithelium

infrequently we find a distinctly patchy edema of the endometrial stroma of women who are taking oral contraceptive agents (see p. 170). Its uneven character is comparable to the diversity of changes we see in the neighboring glands and stromal cells, which disclose marked disparity in their development. We must assume that in these women the changes also represent intense, local variations in the effect of estrogen.

Among the *mechanical causes of increased hydrostatic pressure* are: changes in the position of the uterus, leiomyomata, and polyps. In a retroflexio uteri the pressure in the capillaries may simply be increased by venous or lymphatic obstruction. Submucous myomata may lead to local disturbances of the circulation by stretching or compressing endometrial vessels (HEINICKE 1959). During hysterectomy ligation of the blood vessels may obstruct lymphatic channels. Depending on how long the operation lasts, the blocked endometrial lymphatics dilate, and in extreme cases form cysts which may be mistaken for dilated endometrial glands. The cystic lymphatics can be distinguished by their lining of flattened endothelial cells (Fig. 39).

b) Chronic Passive Hyperemia; Hemorrhage Caused by Extragenital Diseases

The causes that induce a pathological edema may also give rise to chronic passive congestion. If blood flow in the vessels stops (stasis), then the walls of the vessels become injured, and as injury progresses the walls may leak not only edema fluid but blood cells as well. Mild but protracted bleeding follows. Chronic passive hyperemia with hemorrhages in an otherwise normal endometrium may be a sign of cardiac failure. In contrast, a hemorrhagic infarct of the endometrium from venous thromboses is extremely rare.

The term *apoplexia uteri* refers to a diffuse hemorrhage of the endometrium caused by chronic passive hyperemia. We see it most often in old women afflicted with sclerosis of the uterine arteries and generalized arteriosclerosis. Most of the patients have either an organic or functional disturbance of the heart and circulatory system (DALY and BALOGH 1968). Some facts suggest, however, that apoplexia uteri is nothing more than an agonal hemorrhage after inadequate circulation in a vascular system already impaired by arteriosclerosis (TERASAKI 1928). It is usually encountered incidentally at autopsy. We also see it occasionally in the uteri of older women that were removed by vaginal operation. In these instances, besides the vascular disease, the operative trauma is important in causing the endometrial hemorrhage. Grossly, the hemorrhage confines itself to the endometrium and ends sharply at the internal uterine os. Histologically, the striking feature is the widespread extravasation of blood throughout the superficial endometrial stroma (Fig. 40). One occasionally finds small aggregates of polymorphonuclear leukocytes about scattered focal necroses. Hemosiderin-filled macrophages are absent; therefore, the hemorrhage has not been present long. In this context it is important to recall that postmenopausal bleeding may be associated with, and is frequently even caused by, endometrial atrophy (see p. 100f.; MEYER et al. 1971; CHOO et al. 1985).

Menorrhagia due to extragenital disease may occasionally develop in severe infections, poisonings, avitaminoses, or in blood dyscrasias that are associated with disturbances of coagulation owing to decreased numbers of platelets, partic-

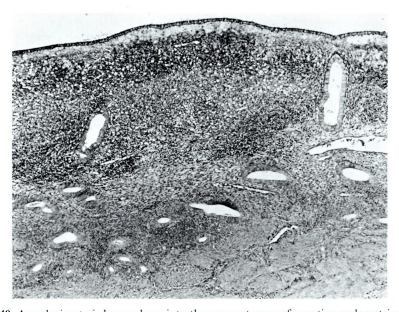

Fig. 40. Apoplexia uteri: hemorrhage into the upper stroma of a resting endometrium

ularly as in *thrombocytopenia* (HALBAN 1922; GOECKE 1932; GREMME 1932). A thrombotic thrombocytopenic purpura may lead to a severe menorrhagia (SYMMERS 1959; "thrombotic microangiopathia"). Histologically, the involved vessels are dilated; some reveal microaneurysms; others are partially occluded by a thrombus covered with endothelial cells. In our differential diagnosis we must differentiate this condition from the much more common thrombosis of vessels associated with tissue necrosis that develops in a glandular-cystic hyperplasia or after estrogen therapy.

Occasionally we observe a *pseudomelanosis* of the endometrium that closely resembles intestinal pseudomelanosis. Histologically, the glandular lumina to the level of the spongiosa are filled with old blood, which in the central parts has been converted into hemosiderin. Most of these patients had been taking oral contraceptive agents; these, it seems, had brought about persistent withdrawal bleeding without dissolution or shedding of the endometrium. Blood had simply seeped into the glandular lumina (Fig. 41).

No matter what their etiology may be, if hemorrhages occur when the isthmus, cervical canal, or cervical os are stenosed, then a *hematometra* develops, and the superficial layers of the endometrium imbibe blood (ARRATA and ZAROU 1963). If the hematometra persists then the resulting pressure and distention may cause the endometrium to atrophy.

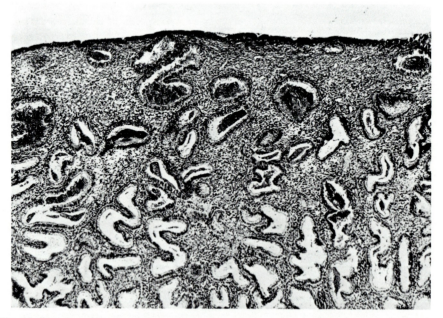

Fig. 41. Pseudomelanosis of the endometrium. The portions of glands near the surface are distended and filled with old blood

2. Functional Endogenous (Hormonal) Disturbances

Of the several target organs for the ovarian hormones, the endometrium, without doubt, is the most sensitive indicator of ovarian function. It responds promptly to every disturbance in ovarian hormonal balance that may develop from either absent, deficient, or excessive functions of the ovarian cells which secrete the hormones. The morphological changes produced in the endometrium will vary greatly, depending on the stage of maturation in which a follicle becomes injured. In the following we want to review what happens in the endometrium when the follicle becomes arrested at various stages of its maturation.

a) Atrophic Endometrium from Non-Functioning Ovaries

If in the childbearing age both ovaries are excised or functionally eradicated (for example, by X-irradiation, by chemical toxins, or by damage of the controlling centers in the hypothalamic-pituitary system), then the endometrium receives no hormonal stimulus and remains in a functionless, resting phase. If that resting phase persists, the stroma and glands continue to atrophy and disappear since as non-functioning components of tissue they are gradually absorbed. Histologically and histochemically the atrophic endometrium of castration resembles the physiological atrophy of the endometrium seen before puberty or after the menopause. Its narrow glands are extremely sparse and lined by low cuboidal epithelial cells with small, round nuclei of dense chromatin. Their cytoplasm is scanty (Fig. 42b). Mitoses are lacking. The stroma consists of small, densely packed, spindly cells. The entire height of the atrophic endometrium is equivalent to but a fraction of the original basalis, which now cannot be recognized. In extreme instances no glands remain, and the flat epithe-

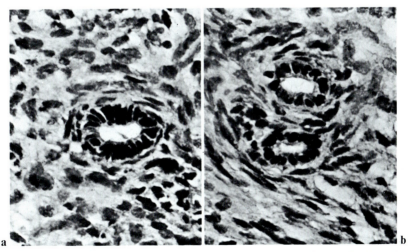

Fig. 42a, b. Endometrium from a patient without ovarian function. **a** Resting glands, **b** atrophic glands

lium of the surface is separated from the myometrium by a stromal layer just a few cells thick. The spiral arteries are undeveloped. The glandular and stromal cells contain little RNA, alkaline or acid phosphatase. Glycogen and glycoproteins are nowhere to be found (GOLDBERG and JONES 1956; MCKAY et al. 1956; LEWIN 1961; GROSS 1964).

In rare instances we see atrophic endometrium associated with normal ovarian function and a regular biphasic menstrual cycle (PLOTZ 1950; EUFINGER 1952; STIEVE 1952). In these instances the ovarian hormones, although secreted, fail to stimulate the endometrium, apparently because it is refractive to them ("silent ovulation" of STIEVE). Perhaps the endometrial cells are unable to produce estrogen receptors. Immunocytochemically, with the ER-ICA assay no estrogen receptors can be detected in the nuclei of glandular epithelial or stromal cells. Instead of menstruation, vicarious bleeding may develop in the adnexae or myometrium.

Independent of the levels of the ovarian hormones, a localized atrophy of the endometrium may be produced by mechanical causes, as for example, by the compressing and stretching from a large submucosal leiomyoma. We refer to this type of atrophy as *pressure atrophy* (Fig. 43), realizing, however, that the cellular changes are not to be distinguished from those seen in atrophy due to lack of hormones. As pressure atrophy is always focal and usually surrounded by rather hyperplastic glands, the coexistence of atrophic and hyperplastic or irregular portions of endometrium in the same curettings may be an aid in diagnosing a submucosal leiomyoma (DELIGDISH and LOEWENTHAL 1970). Abnormal bleeding in these cases may be due either to pressure necrosis

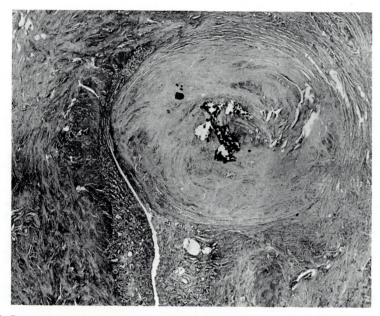

Fig. 43. Pressure atrophy of the endometrium overlying a submucosal leiomyoma. The endometrium of the opposite side also reveals pressure atrophy

or to mechanical obstruction which causes congestion and dilatation of the overlying venules (FARRER-BROWN et al. 1971).

b) Resting Endometrium Resulting from Inadequate Ovarian Function (Ovarian Insufficiency, Hypofolliculinism)

Clinically, we expect to find a resting endometrium when the ovaries are underdeveloped (hypoplastic, rarely polycystic), and when the hormones they produce are insufficient for the endometrial build-up and differentiation of a normal cycle. Another cause for a resting endometrium is a recent but complete arrest of ovarian function. If the ovaries remain inactive, then the resting phase regresses further into an atrophy. Hence, the resting endometrium may represent on the one hand a transitional stage; on the other hand, it may indicate ovarian insufficiency with hypofolliculinism (hypoestrogenism).

Histologically, the resting endometrium has more glands than the atrophic endometrium, a characteristic we use to differentiate the two conditions. The glands are narrow, lined by a single row of columnar epithelial cells (they rarely are stratified) with chromatin-rich, oval nuclei that lie close together in scanty cytoplasm (Fig. 42a). The cells of the stroma are spindly and in general densely packed but may at times be dispersed by edema fluid. Mitoses are very rare. Both glandular and stromal cells contain little RNA; their enzyme activities also generally are low. The height of the resting endometrium may vary but its maximum is 3 mm. Because the subthreshold amounts of estrogen remain inadequate for inducing a regular proliferation, the processes of regression soon counterbalance those of growth.

Clinically, an *amenorrhea* or *hypomenorrhea* almost always accompanies an atrophic or resting endometrium. An exception is the endometrial bleeding in senile atrophy that may develop secondarily to apoplexia uteri associated with hypertension (STOLL and BACH 1954), myometrial arteriolosclerosis (MEYER et al. 1971) or mechanical vascular obstruction by submucosal leiomyoma or uterine prolapse. On the other hand, the question whether we will find an atrophic or resting endometrium with every amenorrhea or hypomenorrhea should be answered with a no (see Table 7). Some women experience no menstruation though their ovaries function normally, and their endometrium develops a secretory phase like that of a normal cycle (TEN BERGE 1936; LAUTERWEIN 1941; PLOTZ 1950; HOFFMANN 1951; BENGTSSON and INGEMANSSON 1959; PHI-

Table 7. Histological and clinical results in the various types of amenorrhea

Ovary	Endometrium	Menstruation	Basal temperature	Infertility
❙ Atrophic	Atrophic	None	Monophasic	Yes
Normal	❙ Atrophic	None	Biphasic	Yes
Normal	Biphasic	❙ None	Biphasic	No

❙ Stimulating effect of hormone blocked.

LIPPE et al. 1966). In primary[1] or secondary[2] amenorrhea all that happens at the end of the menstrual cycle is the functionalis contracts intensely. Histologically LAUTERWEIN found a secretory endometrium in 13.7% of his patients with amenorrhea; PLOTZ reported a secretory phase in 15% of his amenorrheic patients. In the histological and histochemical studies of the endometrium from 221 women with oligoamenorrhea, MYRHE (1966) diagnosed an atrophic endometrium 47 times, a resting endometrium 26 times, and a hyperplastic endometrium five times; 52 of the women histologically were in the early proliferative phase, 24 in the late proliferative phase, and 19 in the secretory phase. In 48 instances the biopsy specimen was inadequate for histological diagnosis. The greater the endometrial atrophy the lower the levels of estrogen in the urine. In a histological study of a large group of women with functional amenorrhea, WALLAU (1948) found an atrophic endometrium in only 6.4%. Occasionally a persistent corpus luteum may cause secondary amenorrhea, since with the greatly retarded fall in progesterone the decidualized endometrium undergoes functional hypertrophy (so-called pseudopregnancy).

Histological studies of endometrial biopsies (single stroke, strip specimens) from patients with hypomenorrhea often disclosed a normal endometrium. In 75% of such patients (PLOTZ 1950), however, only the superficial endometrium desquamated, the remaining endometrium merely contracted (HOFFMANN 1947). This histological appearance of these endometria may so closely resemble irregular shedding of the endometrium of quite a different cause (persistent corpus luteum, see p. 143) that the two conditions may be confused with one another. Here the pathologist is dependent on exact clinical information before he can make a correct functional diagnosis. Since high doses of estrogen fail to provoke withdrawal bleeding in these hypomenorrheas or amenorrheas of similar cause (HOFFMANN 1951), we must assume that because the endometrium lacks certain factors it is unable to shed properly. In spite of persistent primary amenorrhea, this type of cycle need not be infertile (secretory changes to develop) and pregnancy may take place; the correct diagnosis is therefore of great prognostic importance for the patient. Consequently, in all patients with amenorrhea of unclear etiology an attempt should be made to explain the amenorrhea by histological studies. Because the subject is so complicated I must refrain from discussing the clinical problems and various forms of primary and secondary amenorrhea or their etiological mechanisms. I refer the interested reader to standard texts of clinical gynecology and gynecological endocrinology.

c) The Endometrium Associated with a Persistent Follicle

If LH fails to rise after the leading follicle has normally matured, or if with abnormal oocytes or insufficient FSH stimulation no leading follicle has been selected, then ovulation does not take place. Furthermore, a hypersecretion

---

[1] In primary amenorrhea – the patient has never menstruated.
[2] In secondary amenorrhea – the patient ceases to menstruate after having had menstrual bleeding, which may have been either regular or sporadic.

of prolactin may inhibit ovulation or block the effects of FSH or LH on the ovary. The unruptured follicle may either become atretic forthwith (insufficient follicle) or regress slowly (persistent follicle). As the estrogen gradually decreases, withdrawal bleeding sets in about 14 days later when menstruation would normally start, and the anovulatory cycle ends. With the maturation of a new follicle, ovulation may take place, followed by a regular menstruation. If anovulation occurs again, then with every subsequent persistence of a follicle a chain of anovulatory cycles may develop. With a prolonged persistence of a follicle, however, the sustained secretion of estrogen from the persisting follicle and from any newly ripening follicles may induce the endometrium to undergo a glandular-cystic hyperplasia.

α) The Anovulatory Cycle

Described by MAZER and ZISERMAN in 1932, and NOVAK in 1933, the anovulatory cycle occurs predominantly at the beginning and end of the childbearing age (DÖRING 1963). It is the second most common cause of infertility, accounting for 6.9% (DÖRING 1968) –13.6% (OVERSTREET 1948). Beside the afore-mentioned causes, the polycystic ovary syndrome is the most important, being responsible for infertility in 75% of the women with anovulation. In this syndrome, an elevated LH/FSH ratio results in increased androgen production by the follicle, caused by lack of follicular maturation and resulting follicular atresia. Instead, the androgen is metabolized in the fatty tissue to estrogen which is the source of the hyperestrogenism in these patients. Less frequently responsible for anovulation are the luteinized unruptured follicle (LUF) syndrome (MARK and HULKA 1978; KONINCKX and BROSENS 1982), gonadal dysgenesis, autoimmune antibody reactions against granulosa cells or oocytes and demonstrable by immunoperoxidase staining (DAMEWOOD et al. 1986), deficiency of FSH receptors resulting in a gonadotropin-resistant ovary syndrome (KONINCKX and BROSENS 1977; DALEMANS et al. 1979), enzyme deficiencies, or neoplasms.

HAMMERSTEIN (1965) distinguished three types of anovulatory cycle based on how high and how long the secretion of estrogen persists. In the first type A, the follicle continues to secrete for about 7–10 days (persistent follicle resulting in irregular proliferation, see p. 106). In the second type B, an additional secretion of gonadotropin (LH) takes place with little luteinization of the follicle (resulting in abortive secretion). In the third type C, the follicle becomes insufficient early and the estrogen levels remain low (insufficient follicle resulting in deficient proliferation). The duration of the anovulatory cycle may vary, depending on whether the atresia of the follicle begins early or late. At times the interval between the withdrawal bleedings is shorter than between the menstruations of normal cycles. Often the interval is longer. In general, the follicles that persist for a short time are more common than those that undergo premature atresia. Usually the concentrations of receptors for estrogen and progesterone correspond to those of the late proliferative phase. Only the concentration of the intranuclear progesterone receptor, however, is lower than that of the preovulatory endometrium, a finding which correlates with the very low levels of plasma progesterone.

As we should expect, commensurate with the waxing and waning of the hormone levels, the histological picture of the endometrium also fluctuates: all histological stages may be found, from atrophy to hyperplasia (NOVAK 1940). The most important criterion for making the diagnosis from curettings is the absence of secretory changes in the second half of the cycle. In contrast, the first half of the cycle differs little from the proliferative phase of a normal cycle. Consequently, if an anovulatory cycle is suspected, then the curettage should be performed during the second half of the cycle, and when possible, just before the onset of the expected bleeding or at its onset. Absence of secretory changes in the 3rd week, however, may also result from a prolonged proliferative phase and subsequent delay in ovulation. If during the last days of the cycle or at the onset of bleeding one finds a proliferating endometrium that resembles either the early, middle or late proliferative phase, then with corroborating clinical data (known day of the cycle, monophasic curve of basal temperatures) and with convincing results of cytological studies (estrogen smear) one can diagnose an anovulatory cycle. SEDLIS and KIM (1971) described a band of collagen beneath the surface epithelium in 17% of their infertility cases. The band was associated only with anovulation; its diagnostic significance, however, has been questioned in further investigations (AGRAWAL and FOX 1972). In contrast to a normal proliferative phase and a glandular-cystic hyperplasia, the endometrium of the 4th week of an anovulatory cycle shows no alkaline phosphatase activity (ATKINSON 1950), since the level of estrogen has already decreased. From the degree of proliferation, however, it is possible to infer how high the level of estrogen still is. If it has fallen, then we often find focal

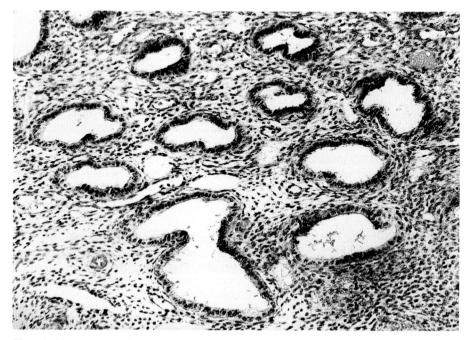

Fig. 44. Abortive secretion

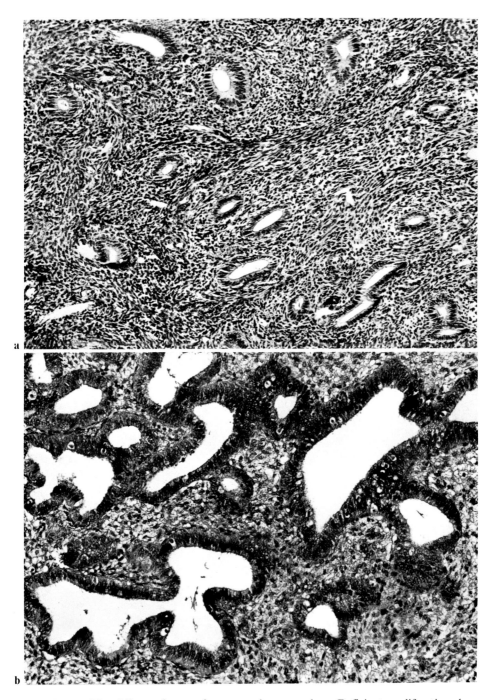

Fig. 45a, b. The different forms of an anovulatory cycle. **a** Deficient proliferation due to follicular insufficiency. The glands are sparse, narrow, their proliferation retarded. **b** Irregular proliferation due to a persistent follicle: glands variably dilated, convoluted, their proliferation pronounced. Magnifications in **a** and **b** are the same!

hemorrhagic necroses or fresh hemorrhages in the stroma without dissolution of the reticulum fibers or dissociation of the stromal cells. On the other hand, if a follicle persists for a short time and continues to secrete estrogen, then occasional glands scattered among the normal proliferating glands undergo cystic dilatation. At times *abortive secretion* with small amounts of glycogen becomes evident in the glandular epithelium leading to focal abortive secretion among the proliferating glands (Fig. 44). These deposits indicate that the persistent follicle underwent a limited and deficient luteinization due to an insufficient secretion of LH without a peak and therefore incapable of inducing ovulation. These unusual endometria prompted PLOTZ (1950) to distinguish them as an "intermediate type" within the spectrum of the anovulatory cycle.

Because of the practical and therapeutic advantages attained, the anovulatory cycle has been divided into two histological patterns readily distinguished from one another: (a) the deficient proliferation; (b) the irregular proliferation.

Compared with those of the normal proliferative phase, the glands and stroma in the **deficient proliferation** remain clearly retarded. The glands are slender and straight. The height of the endometrium is only moderate (Fig. 45a). The cause of the anovulation if follicular insufficiency.

In **irregular proliferation** (previously called "glandular hyperplasia", see LETTERER and MASSHOFF 1941) the growth of the glands and stroma clearly exceeds that of the normal proliferative phase. The glands vary in their distribution, lying either closely packed or widely dispersed, and their diameters differ consid-

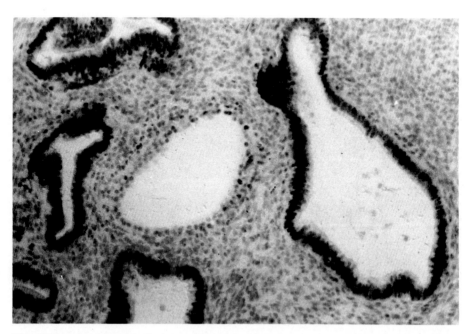

Fig. 46. Immunohistochemical demonstration of estrogen receptor sites in the nuclei of proliferating glandular epithelial cells in irregular proliferation of the endometrium. Note weak to negative reaction of gland in the center lined by flat, non-proliferating epithelium. ER-ICA assay.

erably. Some may be lined by a pseudostratified epithelium, others by a proliferated epithelium that forms several layers. The cellular stroma is composed of spindly cells and is irregularly edematous. Although the height of the endometrium varies considerably, it can often be extreme (Fig. 45b). Here, the cause of the anovulatory cycle is a persistent follicle that secretes either excessive estrogen or androgen, which is then metabolized to estrogen in the fat tissue. On immunohistochemical examination, the nuclei of the proliferating glandular epithelial cells show strong staining for estrogen receptors (Fig. 46). We may regard the irregular proliferation as a direct precursor of glandular-cystic hyperplasia. It is often the first sign that estrogen levels are remaining elevated.

The *withdrawal bleeding* that sets in at the end of an anovulatory cycle must develop differently from a normal menstrual bleeding, since the fall of progesterone, so necessary for a normal menstruation, cannot take place. The withdrawal bleeding, therefore, represents bleeding due to cessation of estrogen secretion alone. Numerous theories have been postulated to explain how the bleeding is brought about. Initially the abnormal hormonel stimulation probably induces increased vascular fragility with changes in the ground substance and in the activities of enzymes and other substances (SCHMIDT-MATTHIESEN 1965). Then as the levels of estrogen fall, additional circulatory disturbances are most likely provoked. With the loss of fluid the endometrium contracts, the vessels become compressed, and stasis follows, giving rise subsequently to thrombosis, hemorrhagic infarction and necrosis (MARKEE 1950; CRAMER 1952; HIN 1957). Accordingly, dissolution of the reticulum fibers is not brought about by the action of relaxin and associated enzymatic proteolysis, as in a normal menstrua-

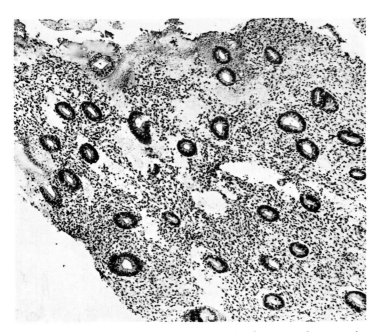

Fig. 47. Withdrawal bleeding in the 4th week of an anovulatory cycle

tion, but rather by necrosis. Hence, bleeding is often prolonged. At times when the estrogen decreases slowly the bleeding becomes unusually protracted. The regressive changes in the glandular and stromal cells, such as nuclear shrinkage and karyolysis, are more pronounced than in normal menstrual shedding (VASEK 1947). Large fragments of tissue with intact reticulum fibers may be discharged (TERASAKI 1928) (Fig. 47).

On the other hand, if the bleeding after an anovulatory cycle is of short duration, then it probably was not proceeded by a persistent follicle. Instead, we may assume that the endometrium is inadequately developed and involuting, chiefly by shrinkage as in hypomenorrhea.

β) Glandular-Cystic Hyperplasia

Glandular-cystic hyperplasia of the endometrium usually is the morphological consequence of either: (a) a persistent follicle that has maintained high levels of estrogen over a long period (SCHRÖDER 1915); (b) repeated anovulatory cycles with limited persistence of follicles, as in polycystic ovarian disease; (c) repeated follicular atresia with hyperplasia of estrogen-secreting theca cells; or occasionally (d) the recurrent development of severe luteal insufficiency or follicular deficiency with androgen production may also result in endometrial hyperplasia. Other causes for the hyperplasia may be exogenous sources (prolonged therapy with estrogens ZONDEK 1940; SCHRÖDER 1954; BLOOMFIELD 1957) or endogenous pathological conditions that produce excessive estrogen, such as stromal hyperplasia (NOVAK et al. 1965; BILDE 1967) or reactive forms found about ovarian tumors, which themselves secrete no estrogens (MACDONALD et al. 1976), hilarcell hyperplasia (HUSSLEIN 1948; DHOM 1952), thecomas and granulosa-cell tumors (LIMBURG 1947; FIENBERG 1958; KOTTMEIER 1959). Here the height of the estrogen is less important than the duration of its unopposed (by gestagens) effect. Glandular-cystic hyperplasia is most common between the ages of 41 and 50 years, a period when ovarian function is in transition, as evidenced by pronounced fluctuation in estrogen production (GRUNER 1942; SCHRÖDER 1954). The condition is comparatively rare in adolescent girls (FRASER and BAIRD 1972). It has been known for many years that glandular-cystic hyperplasia can be produced in animals by excessive estrogen (for review of literature see TAYLOR 1938; MEISSNER et al. 1957), in organ cultures of human endometrium when estradiol is added to the medium (DEMERS et al. 1970), and in women by immoderate therapy with estrogen (SCHRÖDER 1954; BLOOMFIELD 1957). FASSKE et al. (1965) have confirmed these observations with electron-microscopic studies. Depending on the duration and constancy of the hyperestrogenism and on the individual sensitivity to the hormone, the endometrium responds by various changes, all of which may be seen in glandular-cystic hyperplasia. The most common is the *homologous hyperplasia,* in which the glands and stroma proliferate concurrently (LETTERER 1948) (in about 65% of the cases of STOLL 1949). The *heterologous hyperplasia* may be subdivided into the *interstitial* type, in which the stromal proliferation predominates (in about 25% of STOLL's cases, 1949) and into the *glandular* type, in which hyperplasia of the glands prevails (in about 10% of the cases). Perhaps the kind of estrogen compound that stimulates the endometrium is also important in regulating the type of changes produced. Estradiol induces generalized proliferation of the glands. Estriol, however, is thought to cause primarily a proliferation of the basalis (PUCK et al. 1957).

Grossly the endometrium is almost always tall, varying from 3 to 12 mm in height and in extreme cases may measure up to 20 mm. Its surface may be either smooth or irregular with polyps. The surface of these polyps is shiny and sleek, in contrast to that of a papillary carcinoma. In general, the hyperplastic endometrium is edematous and glassy. Occasionally some of the greatly dilated, cystic glands can be seen with the naked eye (Fig. 48).

Histologically, it becomes impossible to distinguish the three layers of the endometrium; they are obliterated by the marked proliferative changes. In the homologous type of glandular-cystic hyperplasia the intense mitotic activity of the glandular and stromal cells leads to an expansion in the volume of the stroma and an extension in the surface area of the glands. This increase in the glandular epithelium comes about in three ways (LETTERER and MASSHOFF 1941): by cystic dilatation, which is most common, by an abnormal enhancement of glandular tortuosity, and by the protrusion of epithelial papillae into the lumen. In the most common type of glandular-cystic hyperplasia the glands, although not increased in number, proliferate intensely and undergo cystic dilatation, producing in the endometrium the characteristic "Swiss cheese" appearance (Fig. 49). In reconstruction of serial sections it could be shown, that in addition to the intense proliferation of the glandular epithelium, the cystic dilatation is due to a constriction of the gland in the narrow neck part near the

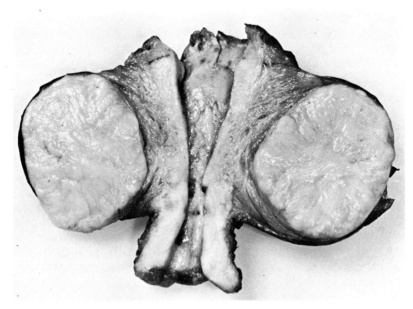

Fig. 48. Uterus from total hysterectomy, laid open to show hyperplastic endometrium and an intramural leiomyoma

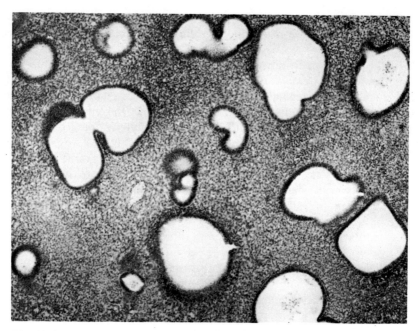

Fig. 49. Pronounced glandular-cystic hyperplasia ("Swiss cheese-like pattern")

surface (RATZENHOFER and SCHMID 1954) caused by pressure from the growing stroma or by unequal epithelial proliferation.

The luminal margin of the *glandular epithelial cells* is sharp, as is that of the superficial epithelium. The cells are uniformly tall and, depending on the degree of hyperplasia, may be pseudostratified (Figs. 50 and 51). Their nuclei are elongated, the chromatin dense; their cytoplasm, although sparse, contains abundant RNA; consequently it stains blue. Several large nucleoli with dense ultrastructures may be seen in the nuclei. Many of the cells may be undergoing mitosis. Not only are the mitoses increased in number but are often blocked in prophase or metaphase by the excessive estrogenic stimulation (PICARD 1949). Such a disturbance of mitosis could explain the frequent occurrence of "clear cells" in the glandular epithelium, which FUCHS (1959) held as forerunners of mitosis. SARBACH (1955) found many "swollen cells" in the hyperplastic glandular epithelium and regarded them as pathological mitoses that had failed to reach completion. The synthesis of DNA in the epithelium in the actively proliferating and less cystically dilated glands is greatly intensified (FETTIG 1965). As measurements have proven, the nuclei are enlarged (PICARD 1950). The more the glandular epithelial cells proliferate, the greater their RNA content becomes (ATKINSON et al. 1949; REMOTTI 1956; MOOKERJEA 1961). In the extremely dilated, cystic glands the RNA may decrease again (BREMER et al. 1951). Droplets of glycogen can always be demonstrated (ATKINSON et al. 1952; CRAMER and KLÖSS 1955; BUSANNI-CASPARI and UNDEUTSCH 1956; RUNGE et al. 1956; ARRONET and LATOUR 1957; LEWIN 1961; STRAUSS 1963). The number of small droplets found is comparable to that of the midproliferative phase (FASSKE

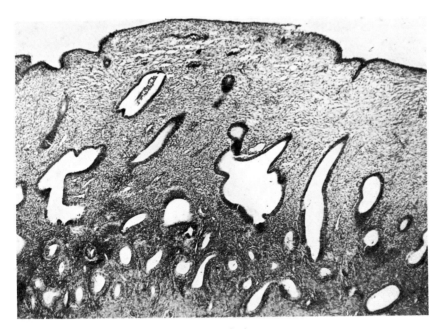

Fig. 50. Beginning glandular-cystic hyperplasia

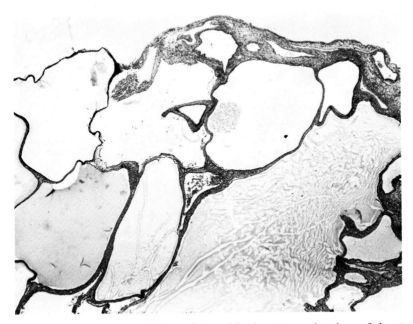

Fig. 51. Extreme glandular-cystic hyperplasia with almost complete loss of the stroma between the greatly dilated cysts lined by flattened epithelial cells

et al. 1965). Granules of lipid are increased (CRAIG and DANZIGER 1965). The glands contain more mucus than normal (SALM 1962); especially the acid mucoids accumulate at the apical margin of the cell. The increase in the activity of alkaline phosphatase is directly proportional to the level of estrogen (ATKINSON and GUSBERG 1948; HALL 1950; MCKAY et al. 1956; LEWIN 1961; MOOKERJEA 1961; KUCERA 1964; FILIPPE and DAWSON 1968). The activities of acid phosphatase and esterase are decreased (GOLDBERG and JONES 1956; MCKAY et al. 1956). HUGHES (1976) suggests that faulty hormonal control of endometrial metabolism may lead to the increased activities of TPN-isocitric dehydrogenase and glucose-6-phosphate dehydrogenase found in hyperplastic and cancerous endometria. He postulates the increased activities of these enzymes may be the basis for further altered cellular metabolism and ultimate transformation to uncontrolled cell growth.

Electron-microscopically, several types of glandular cells may be distinguished in glandular-cystic hyperplasia (WESSEL 1961). The first type resembles the epithelial cell of the proliferative phase but has shorter microvilli and its cytoplasm contains numerous granules of lipid and a widely distributed Golgi apparatus. The second type of cell is dark with cytoplasmic processes, numerous ribosomes, osmiophilic granules and a nucleus rich in DNA. The third type is the clear cell, some of which are ciliated (HAMPERL 1950); others represent degenerating cells after interrupted mitoses (SARBACH 1955; FUCHS 1959).

In the *stroma* the characteristic signs of differentiation induced by progesterone fail to develop. The stroma consists of cells with scanty cytoplasm and no glycogen. Many of the nuclei are small, rich in chromatin and densely spaced. Others, however, are large, have little chromatin, are widely dispersed, and show minimal proliferative activity (FETTIG 1965). Granulocytes are not evident. Mast cells may be adundant (RUNGE et al. 1956). Although the reticulum fibers become increased in number and thickness (WERMBTER 1924; TIETZE 1934; CENTARO and SERRA 1949; ECKERT 1955) their distribution varies, and in many places they are pulled apart by focal edema. Typical collagen fibers are lacking (in contrast to atrophic endometrium). The ground substance varies as well. Where the stroma is dense it contains abundant mucopolysaccharides and protein. In the edematous regions the stroma is partly depolymerized and often contains fibrin-like exudates, apparently the result of increased vascular permeability (SCHMIDT-MATTHIESEN 1965). The fibrinolytic activity is high. The spiral arteries and arterioles are poorly developed and run a straight course (SCHRÖDER 1954; BEILBY et al. 1971); that is, since progesterone is necessary for their proliferation, none takes place, hence the vessels merely suffice to nourish the tissue (MASSHOFF and KRAUS 1955). In contrast, the superficial capillaries and venules are very numerous, dilated and often congested. Some may contain hyaline thrombi that occlude part or all of the vessel lumen (Fig. 52a). One may find many similar hyaline deposits lying in the stroma; most probably these represent thrombi extruded from ruptured vessels (MASSHOFF 1941). Eventually these hyaline deposits become organized. In addition, there are often localized fresh and old hemorrhages in which focal hemorrhagic necroses may develop (Fig. 52b).

Like the bleeding at the end of an anovulatory cycle, the shedding of a glandular-cystic hyperplasia is clinically characterized by a protracted bleeding

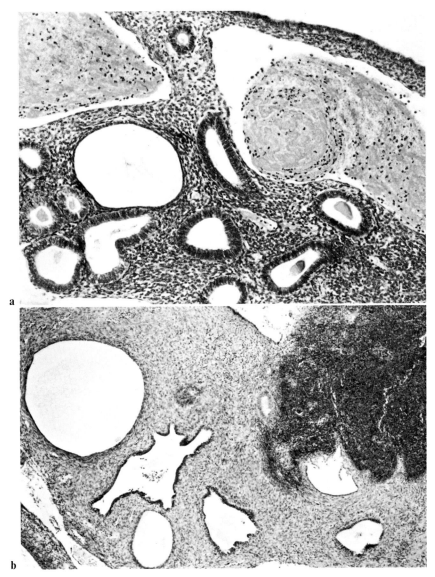

Fig. 52 a, b. Hyaline thrombi **a** and focal hemorrhagic necroses **b** in a glandular-cystic hyperplasia

after a long interval; that is, after about 3 months – the time required for a relative deficiency of estrogen to develop. It also represents a pathological *withdrawal bleeding* caused by estrogen deficit. The deficiency may be brought about in various ways: 1. Under constantly rising levels of estrogen the endometrium grows higher and higher until one day the concentration of estrogen becomes insufficient to sustain the voluminous tissue. By means of this relative estrogen deficiency the endometrial tissue then degenerates ("breakthrough bleeding"), although the level of estrogen in the blood remains stable (LETTERER 1948). 2. Through feedback mechanisms the level of estrogen may be depressed by the pituitary, perhaps even quite early; the decrease in estrogen will, however, lead to the same effect of breakthrough bleeding. As in the anovulatory cycle, the relative or absolute decrease of estrogen is only the last factor in a long sequence that induces the breakthrough bleeding. The protracted bleeding from the non-dissociated mucosa (for dissociated mucosa, see Menstruation, p. 77) comes about in the following manner. Owing to the abnormally developed vascular bed and the aberrant composition of the stroma and ground substance, the circulation in the endometrium becomes slowed and inadequate. Thrombi form. The vessels soon rupture, hemorrhage occurs, deposits of hyaline thrombotic material are extruded into the stroma, and necroses develop. Shedding often proceeds with a brisk and unremitting menorrhagia, not only because the lack of relaxin prevents the mucosa from disintegrating but also because the further secretion of estrogen stimulates the remaining mucosa to proliferate. In addition, proteolytic enzymes become activated, inhibiting coagulation in the endometrium while it is slowly shed. On the other hand, estrogen causes the fibrinolytic activity to rise (SCHMIDT-MATTHIESEN 1965, 1967). Perhaps the many hyaline (fibrinoid) deposits so characteristic of glandular-cystic hyperplasia represent products of partial fibrinolysis that, for reasons of local deficiencies in enzyme activities, are left behind in the tissue to organize.

After a prolonged menorrhagia the major part of the hyperplastic endometrium may eventually be discharged. A curettage carried out at this time yields only sparse, hemorrhagic remnants with shrunken stroma and collapsed glands, whose circumferences perhaps suggest they had originally been cystic (Fig. 53). Our diagnosis in such instances is *discharged glandular-cystic hyperplasia*. In extreme cases, when almost all endometrial tissue has been shed, that diagnosis cannot be made histologically. Since glandular-cystic hyperplasia tends to recur (Fig. 54) (according to TIETZE 1934, in 67.2% of young women and in 36.3% of older women) a repeat curettage after a long interval and at the onset of a renewed, extended bleeding usually leads to the diagnosis.

Secretory changes occasionally occur in a glandular-cystic hyperplasia without hormonal treatment (according to GRUNER 1942, in 6.2%; according to BEHRENS 1954, in 3% of the cases). Glycogen may accumulate in some epithelial cells as solitary basal vacuoles. We surmise these accumulations are stimulated by small amounts of progesterone secreted either by the ripe follicle, as at the end of the proliferative phase, or by the temporarily luteinized cells in the persisting follicle (BUSANNI-CASPARI and UNDEUTSCH 1956; HINZ 1957). At times even sporadic stromal cells differentiate. Further spontaneous (unprovoked) changes of differentiation, however, are rare. In contrast, with progestational therapy or with clomiphene the cystically dilated glands may undergo secretory change (Fig. 55) and the fibrinolytic activity of the stroma may disappear. Depending upon the type of gestagen administered, predecidual or decidual changes may also develop (KISTNER et al. 1966). Occasionally such therapy induces the endometrium to regress to a normal state or even to atrophy (WENTZ 1966).

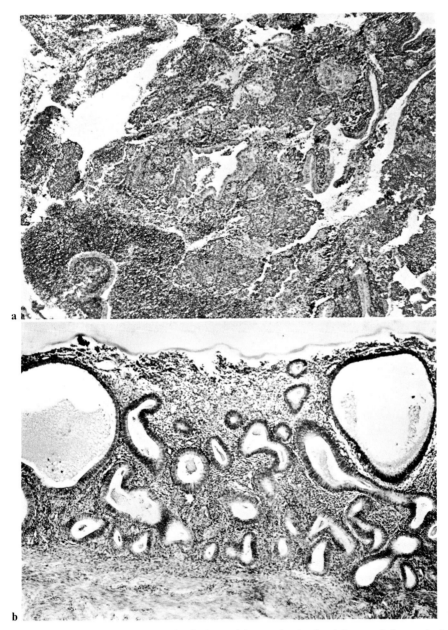

Fig. 53a, b. Remnants of a partially discharged hemorrhagic glandular-cystic hyperplasia. **a** Remnants obtained by curettage after several weeks of bleeding; cysts are collapsed and the stroma shows complete hemorrhagic necrosis. **b** Cystically dilated glands remaining in the basalis of an extirpated uterus

Small nodules of *squamous epithelium* ("morules") sometimes arise from the glandular epithelium of the hyperplastic endometrium (HUNZIKER 1911; according to KUTLIK 1962, in 2.5% of all endometria examined). Most probably

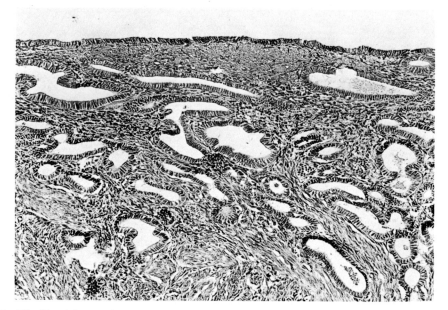

Fig. 54. Glandular-cystic hyperplasia developing again at site where it was previously shed

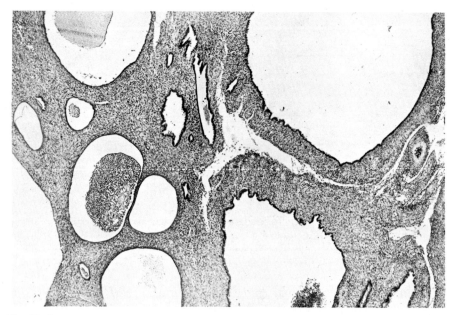

Fig. 55. Secretory transformation of some of the glands of a glandular-cystic hyperplasia

these nodules represent squamous metaplasia of columnar epithelial cells, or perhaps of pluripotential cells of the Müllerian epithelium (MEYER 1922; HINTZE 1928; FLUHMANN 1928, 1953, 1954; BRUNTSCH 1950). The assumption of STRAUSS and HIERSCHE (1963) that these nodules arise from "dedifferentiated descendants of the endometrial epithelium" seems less plausible. The cells making up the nodules have histological characteristics that are typical of squamous epithelium. They may cornify centrally as the phloxine-tartrazine stain clearly shows. A basement membrane can often be made out delimiting these morules from the surrounding stroma (see Fig. 56). Merely because the cells lack intercellular bridges does not mean they are not of squamous epithelial origin. Frequently the morules protrude into the glandular lumen and may even fill it. At other times they grow outwards, bulging into the stroma. We regard the appearance of the nodules of squamous epithelium merely as an individual variation in the reaction of the endometrium to elevated levels of estrogen. Among other observations supporting our view is the long-term prospective follow up of patients who were observed to pass through all stages of hyperplasia, ending with a carcinoma. As these observations disclosed, if nodules of squamous epithelium were demonstrable in the glandular-cystic hyperplasia then they were also found in the subsequent adenomatous hyperplasia, and the carcinoma ultimately developing from that proved to be an adenoacanthoma since it also contained nodules of squamous epithelium. The appearance of the squamous epithelium in the glandular-cystic hyperplasia, however, in no way predisposes to the development of a carcinoma. Their differentiation from adenoacanthoma may be of considerable clinical importance, particularly in the young patient (BLAUSTEIN 1982). The morules in the adenoacanthoma usually represent remnants of metaplastic squamous epithelium that arose in the pre-existing benign hyperplasia. They commonly appear after years of estrogen therapy (see Fig. 57; cf. SIEGERT 1938; GOSCH 1949). Similar changes have been produced in animals with estrogen (GUMBRECHT 1936).

The duration of the hyperestrogenism determines what happens to the glandular-cystic hyperplasia. If the levels of estrogen fall with the onset of menopause, then regressive changes may appear. If the hyperestrogenism persists, either because of abnormal endogenous production or because of continued therapy with estrogen, then glandular-cystic hyperplasia progresses to an adenomatous hyperplasia (see Table 5). Whereas glandular-cystic hyperplasia develops most commonly at the beginning and end of the reproductive years because these periods of adaptation predispose to anovulation and persistent follicles, after the menopause the histological picture of hyperplasia changes.

As ovarian function wanes, the secretion of estrogen gradually subsides, finally falling to such levels that endometrial proliferation ceases and no withdrawal bleeding occurs. Mitoses become rare; the glandular epithelial cells become more cuboidal. This histological picture of *resting glandular-cystic hyperplasia,* although fully developed in all other respects, can still be distinguished from the *active* form (KAISER and SCHNEIDER 1968). During subsequent years or decades, as atrophy increases, the resting form slowly transforms into *regressive hyperplasia* (Fig. 58). The glandular epithelium becomes a single row again, which flattens out more and more with time. The cells lose RNA and cytoplasmic

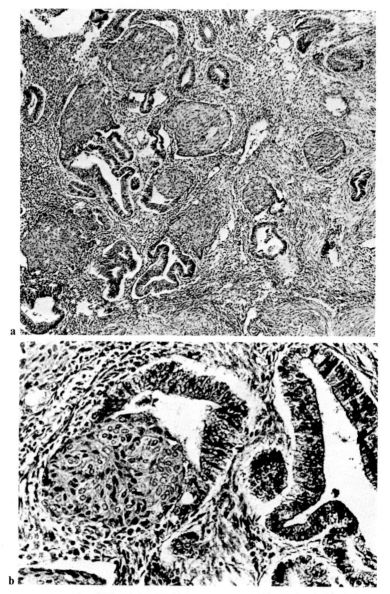

Fig. 56a, b. Nests of squamous epithelial cells ("morules") in glandular epithelium of a glandular-cystic hyperplasia. **a** Low magnification; **b** higher magnification

organelles, and their nuclei become rounded, small and hyperchromatic. The stromal cells shrink and become more closely packed. During this process of involution we have never observed the atypical proliferations of glandular cells that RATZENHOFER and SCHMID (1954) described. We believe such atypical proliferations rather indicate an aberrant hormonal stimulation (see p. 177). The glands do not collapse but instead remain cystic well into old age. Thus we

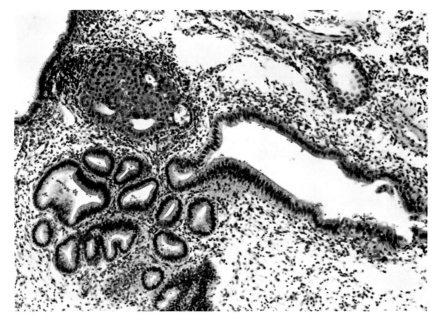

Fig. 57. Glandular-cystic hyperplasia with squamous metaplasia and beginning adenomatous proliferation after years of estrogen therapy during the postmenopause

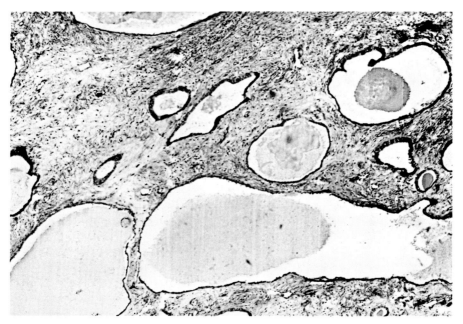

Fig. 58. Regressive hyperplasia with flat, in part endothelial-like glandular epithelium and stroma poor in cells

see a "petrified" state of the hyperplasia that had developed just before menopause set in when no withdrawal bleeding occurred because the estrogen levels had decreased so slowly. Regressive hyperplasia differs from the cystic, atrophic endometrium of the postmenopausal period (cf. p. 91; Fig. 37b) merely by its greater number of cystically dilated glands.

γ) Adenomatous Hyperplasia

If the secretion of progesterone ceases at menopause but that of estrogen continues at high or moderately high levels then we speak of "an unopposed estrogenism". That stimulates the glandular-cystic hyperplasia to further sustained growth, leading to the development of an **adenomatous hyperplasia.** The proliferation, until now principally characterized by cystically dilated glands, sharply accelerates. The glandular epithelium begins to bud, sending forth offshoots; the *new glands* that form are in part quite small and of the branched alveolar type (Figs. 59, 60). The larger glands are lined by tall columnar, stratified epithelium from which epithelial papillae develop to protrude into the lumen. The elongated, chromatin-rich nuclei of the epithelial cells begin to show abnormalities; their synthesis of DNA greatly increases (FETTIG 1965). Their cytoplasm remains sparse but basophilic owing to abundant RNA. Cytoplasmic structures indicative of differentiation (progesterone effect) are absent. The histochemical reactions essentially resemble those of glandular-cystic hyperplasia (McKay et al. 1956).

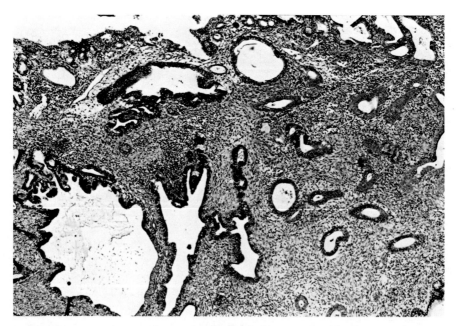

Fig. 59. Beginning adenomatous proliferation that has developed in a glandular-cystic hyperplasia by excessive epithelial proliferation, appearing here mainly as intraluminal (epithelial) papillae

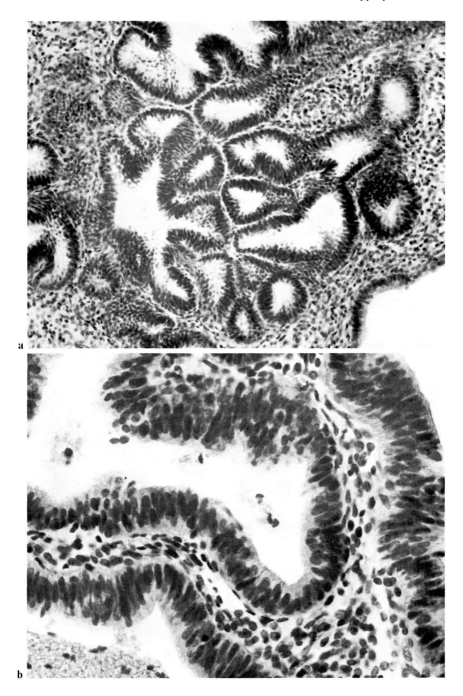

Fig. 60a, b. Adenomatous hyperplasia grade 1 with extreme atrophy of the stroma and some alveolar branching of glands. The epithelium is pseudostratified or stratified. **a** Low magnification; **b** higher magnification

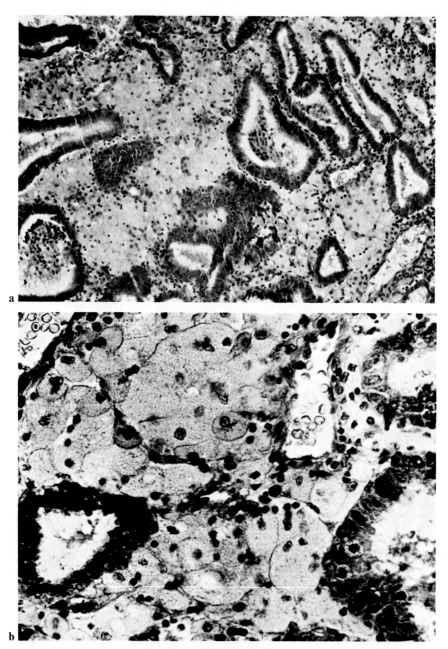

Fig. 61a, b. Transformation of stromal cells into foam cells in adenomatous hyperplasia. **a** Low magnification; **b** higher magnification

As the glands proliferate and grow they push the stroma lying between them together. It is gradually adsorbed, so that ultimately the basement membranes of some of the glands come to touch one another (back-to-back position of the glands). In the remaining gusset-like patches of stroma, groups of *foam cells* may be found in over 50% of the adenomatous hyperplasias (Figs. 61, 63). They contain lipids that have a green autofluorescence. From histochemical reactions (DALLENBACH-HELLWEG 1964) it seems these lipids are most probably either cholesterol esters or estrogen derivatives. The foam cells show no relationship to inflammatory processes, either etiologically or anatomically. They are,

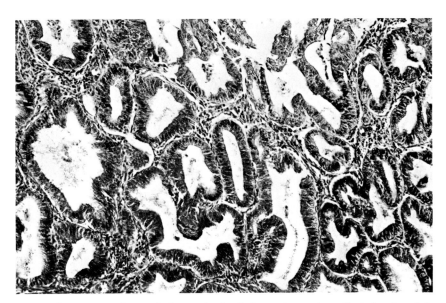

Fig. 62. Adenomatous hyperplasia grade 2 of the endometrium that developed in a 37-year-old woman after many years of estrogen therapy

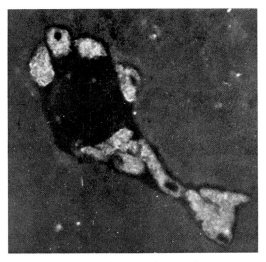

Fig. 63. Autofluorescence of foam cells

like decidual cells, transformed stromal cells and always associated with a hyperestrogenism, at times even with that resulting from estrogen therapy. Their stromal origin could be confirmed ultrastructurally by FECHNER et al. (1979) who also found intermediate stages between normal stromal cells and foam cells. They can be differentiated from the histiocytic-inflammatory-type foam cell by a hemosiderin stain, since the stromal foam cells do not contain hemosiderin (ASHKENAZY et al. 1983). Endometrial foam cells serve as reliable indicators that the levels of estrogen have remained elevated; they are especially useful in evaluating the prognosis of adenomatous hyperplasias. In general, the more numerous the foam cells the sooner an adenomatous hyperplasia progresses to a carcinoma. About 30% of all glandular-cystic hyperplasias contain some foam cells in the stroma. It was in the stroma of such hyperplasias that first SCHILLER (1927) and later VON NUMERS and NIEMINEN (1961) discovered foam cells; SALM (1962) also found them in the stroma of polyps. The results of experimental studies refute the notion that the endometrium is able to produce and secrete estrogenic substances (DALLENBACH and RUDOLPH 1974). Mos likely a derivative of estrogen is stored in the cytoplasm of the foam cells, when the endometrial tissues are flooded by excessive estrogen they cannot properly metabolize. Cells morphologically identical to those in the endometrium appear in prostatic carcinomas after estrogen therapy (EPSTEIN 1976).

Adenomatous hyperplasia develops under the influence of unopposed estrogen, consequently almost exclusively after the menopause. During the reproductive years it is seen only with persistent anovulation (as with the Stein-Leventhal syndrome), or following prolonged estrogen treatment (Fig. 62). Whether it regresses, remains, or progresses further depends on the secretion of estrogen. If the levels of estrogen fall or if gestagens are given as therapy, then adenomatous hyperplasia may regress. If the levels of estrogen remain elevated, however, as they often do after the menopause, then after various periods of time, if the patient has a predisposing constitution, the adenomatous hyperplasia through progressive overgrowth of its glands may develop into an adenocarcinoma (see p. 255f.; cf. Fig. 119).

Recent experience has convinced us that a division into three histological grades has proved worthwhile for evaluating prognosis and choice of therapy:

Grade 1: mild adenomatous hyperplasia is characterized by mild diffuse or marked focal glandular crowding and pseudostratification of epithelium with beginning intraluminal infolding and budding (Fig. 60).

Grade 2: moderate adenomatous hyperplasia (or complex hyperplasia) shows marked diffuse glandular crowding with reduced intervening stroma approaching a back-to-back position of glands and focal microalveolar formation, and with increased pseudostratification and intraluminal budding exhibiting structural complexity (Fig. 62).

Grade 3: marked adenomatous hyperplasia (or atypical hyperplasia): in addition to the criteria of grade 2 there are foci with atypical epithelium showing depolarized nuclei of various shapes and chromatin density and with several enlarged nucleoli in a pale, eosinophilic cytoplasm. Consequently, grade 3 represents cytological atypias in addition to architectural glandular changes. Such foci may develop in only one part of an adenomatous hyperplasia or also multicentrically (BUEHL et al. 1964), but generally in the basalis. The cells of these atypical glands are often distinct, for their pale cytoplasm contains only small amounts of RNA (McKAY et al. 1956). Their nuclei are large, round or polygonal and

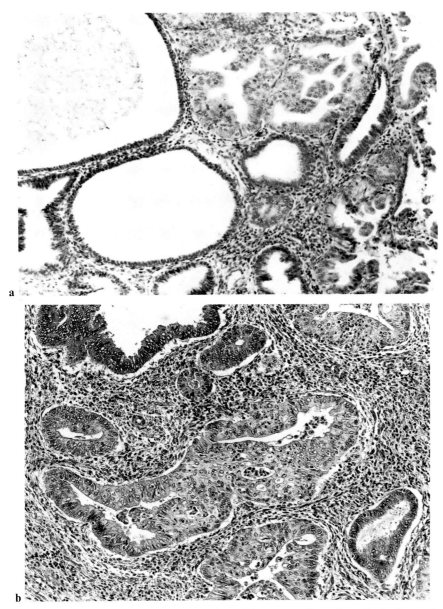

Fig. 64a, b. Adenomatous hyperplasia grade 3 with structurally and cytologically atypical glands

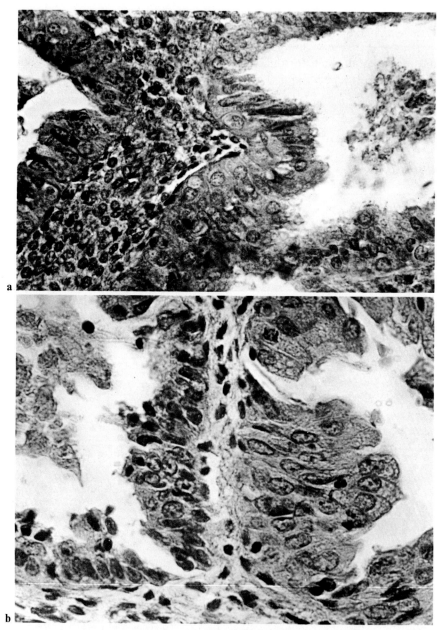

Fig. 65a, b. Adenomatous hyperplasia grade 3. **a** Basally located round nuclei push away the overlying elongated nuclei. **b** The nuclei of the atypical gland *on the right* are aneuploid

unevenly distributed (Figs. 64–66). Cytophotometric studies of these nuclei reveal an aneuploidy like that found in invasive carcinoma; in contrast, the glandular-cystic hyperplasia and most of the adenomatous hyperplasias without atypias (grades 1 and 2) show unequivocal diploid values for DNA (WAGNER

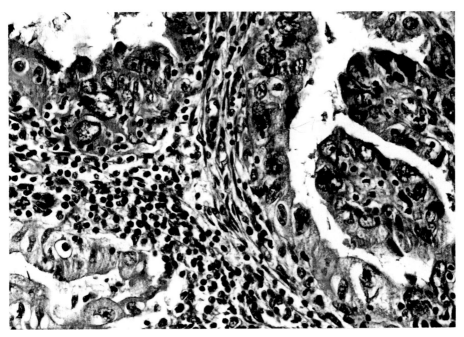

Fig. 66. Adenomatous glands with cytological atypia surrounded by lymphocytic infiltrates within an adenomatous hyperplasia grade 3 (atypical hyperplasia)

et al. 1967). The chromatin is clumped, and the nucleoli are enlarged. Profound changes occur in the histochemical reactions but thereafter remain constant in the carcinoma. Immunohistochemically, the nuclear estrogen receptor content is very high in the glands of grade 1 and 2 adenomatous hyperplasias, but decreases in the atypical nuclei of grade 3 hyperplasia. Parallel observations have been made with biochemical measurements of the progesterone receptor (ROBBOY and BRADLEY 1979). There is also a switch in activity of the phosphatases during the transition: alkaline phosphatase decreases, whereas acid phosphatase rises. Because it resembles a secretory endometrium, focal cytologic atypia often goes unrecognized, or it may mislead one into believing that an adenomatous hyperplasia is undergoing secretory changes. The PAS stain readily decides the issue: the atypical glands are free from glycogen. The focal excessive proliferation associated with the adenomatous hyperplasia paves the way, so to speak, for the transformation into carcinoma. The change is like that occurring in a carcinoma in situ of the cervix which causes it to invade. CULLEN (1900), R. MEYER (1923) and LAHM (1928) were the first to describe these changes as direct precursors of cancer. HERTIG et al. (1949) suggested they be called "carcinoma in situ". Follow-up studies of patients with foci of such changes, however, prove they really are immediate precursors of early endometrial adenocarcinoma (DALLENBACH-HELLWEG 1979; cf. p. 255f.).

Because the distinction between adenomatous hyperplasia and early adenocarcinoma may be problematic for the examining pathologist, an extensive search for foci of cytological atypias and their differentiation from benign me-

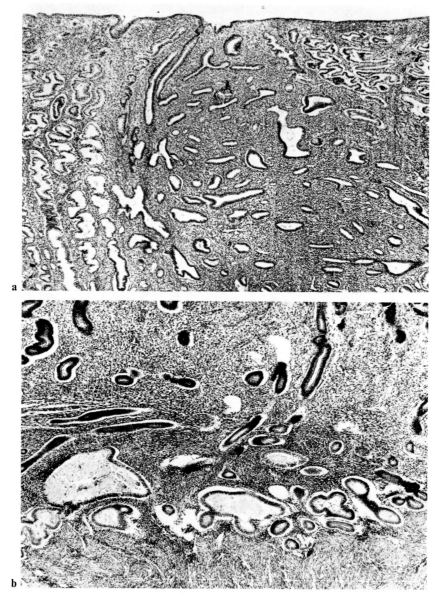

Fig. 67. a Focal hyperplasia, pushing normal secretory glands aside. **b** Hyperplasia of the basalis. Basal glands are cystically enlarged; the glands of the functionalis are proliferating normally

taplasia on the one hand (cf. p. 214 ff.) and from early carcinoma on the other (cf. p. 230 ff.) is of paramount importance.

Statistical and epidemiological studies have helped to clarify the dignity of the adenomatous hyperplasia: grades 1 and 2 may still reverse since progression to carcinoma at these stages is hormone dependent. Grade 3, on the other hand, has to be regarded as irreversible precancerosis, if left untreated and the patient lives long enough, because of its nuclear atypias with aneuploidy. According to recent data collected by KURMAN et al. (1985) the *practical* likelihood of progression to carcinoma is about 1% for simple (glandular cystic) hyperplasia, 3% for complex (adenomatous hyperplasia grades 1 and 2), and 29% for atypical (adenomatous hyperplasia grade 3).

SHERMAN and BROWN (1979) observed that carcinomas developed in 22% of their patients with adenomatous hyperplasia without atypia (grades 1 and 2), and in 57% of their patients with atypical adenomatous hyperplasia (grade 3). The lower rates published by KURMAN et al. (1985) may be because many of their patients in all groups were premenopausal or had taken estrogens, which were discontinued after the diagnosis of hyperplasia.

δ) Special Forms of Hyperplasia
(Focal Hyperplasia, Polyps, Glandular, and Stromal Hyperplasias)

The entire endometrium is not always stimulated uniformly by estrogen. Sometimes only certain regions react to the hormone. When the stimulation persists these regions may undergo *focal hyperplasia*, from which polyps may develop or even at times carcinomas, although the remaining endometrium may show regular secretory changes. The focal hyperplasias differ from the diffuse form only in their limitation to a circumscribed region (Fig. 67a).

Hyperplasia of the basalis is not rare. In that condition the cystically dilated and excessively proliferated glands of the basalis push the normal endometrium upward and away (Fig. 67b). Consequently, many cycles may elapse before the hyperplasia makes itself clinically evident (WINTER 1955). Histologically, the dilated glands are hardly distinguishable from those of the glandular-cystic hyperplasia. In curettings hyperplasia of the basalis can be recognized by its stroma, which is usually irregularly interwoven with bundles of smooth muscle cells but for the basalis still characteristically dense with collagenous fibers. Under appropriate stimulation hyperplasia of the basalis may progress to adenomatous hyperplasia and even to carcinoma. In addition to diffuse hyperplasia of the basalis there are the focal hyperplasias. These may give rise to the formation of so-called endometrial hummocks that may continue to grow, eventually becoming tall polyps.

The polypoid, glandular-cystic hyperplasia is characterized by focal, polypoid growths within the hyperplasia. Some of the glands in these growths dilate cystically and become surrounded by a stroma that is rich in fibers but poor in cells and occasionally very edematous. These polypoid outgrowths are readily recognized by their shape and by the characteristic red of their stroma with the van Gieson stain, owing to the abundance of collagenous fibers. At times the glands within the polyps undergo excessive hyperplasia, a change less disquieting as a precancerous condition than a similar hyperplasia elsewhere in the endometrium. Nevertheless, in a rare polyp extreme glandular hyperplasia may undergo carcinomatous transformation.

At this point in our review we should discuss the **polyps of the endometrium**, which commonly develop from a non-diffuse hyperplasia of the endometrium.

These polypoid outgrowths are not neoplasias but rather only focal hyperplasias of the mucosa that develop in circumscribed regions in response to hormonal stimuli. Often they arise from focal hyperplasias of the basalis whence they slowly grow upward to reach the surface of the endometrium (SCHRÖDER 1954). At first they have broad bases but with time these become slim stalks, since the normal endometrium about them is shed away during menstruation. Their site of predilection is the endometrium of the fundus and tubal recesses. Based on their histology we distinguish four types of polyps: the glandular, the glandular-cystic, the adenomatous, and the fibrous. For each type there is an equivalent generalized change (that is, type of hyperplasia) that may involve the endometrium diffusely.

The *glandular* polyps resemble the normal endometrium. They are recognized by their loose yet fibrous stroma (seen best with the van Gieson stain) and by their usual refractoriness to cyclic changes. Their glands, having sprouted from the basalis, are clearly proliferating: therefore in a secretory endometrium they will be especially conspicuous and easy to recognize. Often their stroma supports bundles of thick-walled vessels stemming from the basalis. If a polyp remains intact during the curettage then its shape in the sections, with three sides covered by epithelium, will prove diagnostic (Fig. 68). The *glandular-cystic* polyps differ from glandular-cystic hyperplasia only by their more fibrous stroma; the glandular changes in both conditions are alike in all respects. A comparable relationship exists between the *adenomatous* polyps and adenomatous hyperplasia. Yet, these last two conditions do differ biologically. Adenomatous hyperplasia in a single polyp usually has a good prognosis and causes little concern, whereas diffuse adenomatous hyperplasia has a dubious prognosis, consequently it must be taken seriously. A polyp with a long stalk usually either pulls loose, or twists and constricts, or undergoes regressive changes. Only when the atypical hyperplastic glands overgrow the stalk does the prognosis become a matter of concern. On the other hand, a carcinoma may certainly arise in a polyp although probably only rarely. It is much more common to find polyps associated with an endometrial carcinoma (according to PETERSON and NOVAK 1956, in 2.7% of all endometria with polyps and in 15.5% of postmenopausal endometria with polyps). The *fibrous* polyps usually represent regressive forms of the glandular polyps. Consequently we find them most commonly in old women; fibrous polyps are comparable to atrophic endometrium (Fig. 69). In general they have few glands, which may be either cystic or atrophic. The stroma usually consists of parallel bundles of densely packed collagenous fibers, which stain bright red with the van Gieson method. The stroma of the polyps may also contain smooth muscle cells (*adenomyomatous* polyps), indicating that these polyps arose from a focal hyperplasia of the basalis. Some polyps are especially well vascularized (*teleangiectatic* polyps). Their vessels may be either thin-walled capillaries like those of the superficial endometrium, or thick-walled arterioles with narrow lumina like the spiral arterioles.

Theoretically these various polyps may develop at any age. The youngest patient in the series of 1314 polyps described by LAU and STOLL (1962) was 12 years old. The polyps are most common at 50 years of age. After the menopause both the hormonally sensitive adenomatous polyps and the hormonally

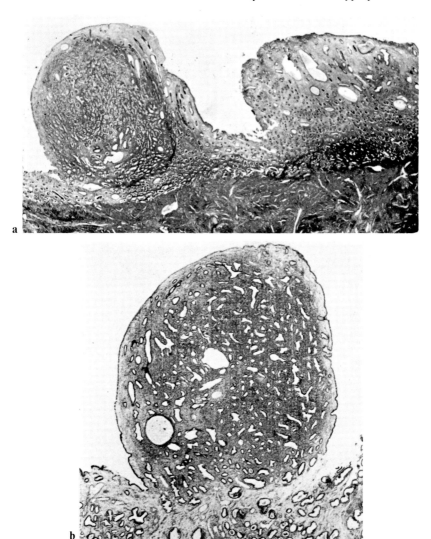

Fig. 68. a A large adenomatous polyp arising in a glandular-cystic hyperplasia. **b** A tall, glandular polyp of the corpus endometrium

insensitive "petrified" glandular-cystic polyps (counterparts of regressive hyperplasia) increase in frequency. The latter have flattened epithelial cells and often a hyalinized stroma.

A special form of polyp found in the postmenopausal period was referred to as the "matron's adenoma" or "matron's polyp". Since that term originated clinically and was applied loosely, depending on clinical manifestations, opinions about its histology have varied. Moreover, various investigators have used that name for all polyps occurring after the menopause. In 1922 MENGE classified the matron's adenoma as an actively growing, true neoplasm and separated it from the polyps. Influenced by MENGE's report, BRAITENBERG (1941) described

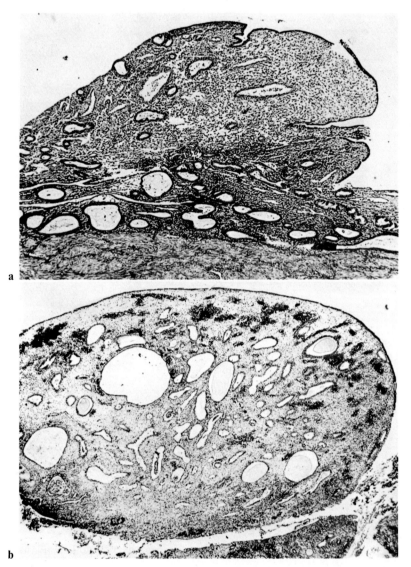

Fig. 69. **a** A broad-based senile polyp with regressive hyperplasia and **b** a fibrocystic senile polyp that has already been shed

an obvious adenocarcinoma under the expression "proliferating matron's adenoma". Although the prevailing view of ASCHOFF and SCHRÖDER was that all polyps were adenomata, ADLER (1926) pointed to the frequency of polyps in glandular-cystic hyperplasia and suggested that the two conditions had a common etiology. On the other hand, R. MEYER (1923) regarded polyps as circumscribed hyperplasia of the basalis. According to our present concepts the polypoid growths of the endometrium represent local hyperplasias induced by hormones or possibly also by trauma. Therefore, we should like to discard

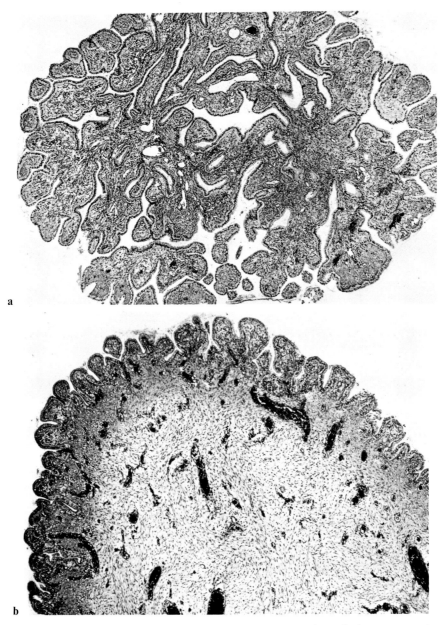

Fig. 70. a A papillary polyp and **b** a vascular polyp of the endocervical mucosa

the term "adenoma" and to refer to all benign, localized hyperplasias of the endometrium as "polyps". Since the designation "matron's adenoma" appears to be inappropriate for several reasons we prefer to forget it. We suggest instead that all polyps in the postmenopausal period be classified according to their histology into: the adenomatous, the cystic-atrophic, and the fibrous polyps of old age. That classification includes an interpretation about the prognosis, which provides the gynecologist with important information for the therapeutic measures he plans.

Since polyps are not usually discharged during menstruation and may occasionally elude the surgeon's curette, with time they may grow so large as to fill the uterine cavity. Because they are soft and pliable, they generally assume the shape of the cavity. The most important clinical symptoms that polyps produce are interval bleeding, premenstrual and postmenstrual bleeding, and occasionally labor-like pains. Through tension, stretching and pressure, *secondary changes* may develop in polyps, leading to hemorrhage and inflammation, and ultimately to extensive necrosis or diffuse endometritis. At times when the glandular-cystic polyps are traumatized cysts may burst; the mucus extruded into the stroma often provokes a granulomatous inflammation (mucus granuloma) (SALM 1962). Because they tend to persist for long periods, compared with the surrounding endometrium discharged during menstruation, the polyps may become foci of chronic inflammation such as tuberculosis or foreign body granulomata.

Curettings of the endometrial cavity may contain not only parts of endometrial polyps but often fragments of polyps from the endocervix and transitional mucosa. These fragments may be readily differentiated from the endometrial polyps by the structure of their glands and by the character of their superficial epithelium. The **polyps of the endocervical mucosa** are papillary and covered by a tall, cylindrical, mucus-secreting epithelium (Fig. 70). A similar epithelium lines their glands, which resemble normal glands of the endocervix. Three main types of cervical polyps can be distinguished: the fibrous, the glandular, and the vascular (teleangiectatic). The stromal cells of cervical polyps may undergo decidual change during pregnancy. At times such a change may be the first morphological indication that the patient is pregnant. HARRIS (1958) observed numerous foam cells in the stroma of polyps after prolonged therapy with estrogens. A special type of polyp unusually rich in cellular stroma may develop in girls. Referred to as a "juvenile cervical polyp", it must be distinguished from the sarcoma botryoides (TERRUHN 1977). The glandular and surface epithelium of cervical polyps tends to undergo reserve cell hyperplasia or squamous metaplasia, which by definition is always benign. During a pregnancy (MEINRENKEN 1956), but chiefly during exogenous gestagen therapy, and then often to an extreme degree (cf. p. 186) new glands develop which show a charateristic microalveolar proliferation. When polyps of the cervical mucosa protrude from the cervical os they become either partially or completely covered with metaplastic, squamous epithelium. They are then referred to as *polyps of the portio vaginalis*. The *polyps of the transitional epithelium* present a mixed picture, containing glands not only of the endometrial type but also of the sort found in the endocervical mucosa. Although these polyps are less common than the other types they grow to resemble the others grossly (Fig. 71).

The true or genuine **stromal hyperplasia** of the endometrium is a rare variant of the glandular-cystic hyperplasia and may be regarded as a potential precursor of endometrial sarcoma (HANSON 1959). The hyperplasia of the stromal cells predominates. These cells have large, often pleomorphic nuclei haphazardly located within sparse cytoplasm. The reticulum fibers between the cells are

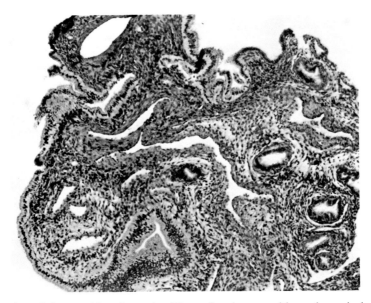

Fig. 71. Polyp of the transitional mucosa. The surface is covered by endocervical epithelium; the glands within the polyp are endometrial

abundant. The glands become widely separated, are small and narrow, and lined by a single row of epithelial cells (Fig. 72). – A moderate form of stromal hyperplasia with a striking predecidual change of the stromal cells occasionally develops after the treatment of a glandular-cystic hyperplasia with gestagens (see p. 114), or after the use of oral contraceptives (see p. 178), especially those with derivatives of 19-nortestosterone. The sarcoma-like change induced by these hormones may alarm us; however, as of now the change should not be considered as a potential precursor of endometrial sarcoma and should not therefore be confused with true stromal hyperplasia. These interesting experiences with unnatural stimulation of the endometrium with hormones may indicate that a specific (androgenic?) and protracted endogenous disturbance of hormonal balance is responsible for inducing stromal hyperplasia of the endometrium. A pseudosarcomatous stromal reaction combined with an endometrial adenocarcinoma has been described in a 75-year-old woman with ovarian hyperthecosis (RAVINSKY 1984). Since that patient had not received hormone therapy, the progestogenic stimulus must have arisen from the hyperthecosis. Because the enzymatic metabolism of androgens, estrogens and progestogens is closely related, a *combined adenomatous and stromal hyperplasia,* as occasionally seen, may be induced by a common hormonal stimulus produced in an ovarian stromal hyperplasia or hyperthecosis. – From the stromal hyperplasia we should furthermore distinguish a common type of hyperplasia with stromal cells arranged in whorls and bound by thickened reticulum fibers. LOHMEYER and VELTEN (1957) found such a hyperplasia in 92% of all uteri with leiomyomata; they believed that when found in curettings it indicated the presence of a submucosal leiomyoma.

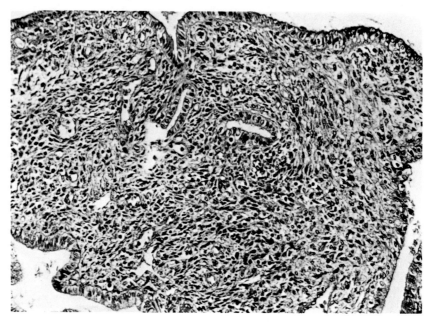

Fig. 72. Stromal hyperplasia of the endometrium. The stromal cells have large polygonal nuclei. The glands are sparse

d) The Deficient Secretory Phase Associated with Deficiency or Premature Regression of the Corpus Luteum

If the corpus luteum fails to develop normally after ovulation or regresses too quickly, then the stimulatory effect of progesterone on the endometrium becomes deficient. The hormonal balance then shifts in favor of estrogen; consequently, a normal secretory phase cannot evolve. In like manner, any disturbance resulting in decreased progesterone action on the endometrium as the end organ may cause a deficient secretory phase. The progesterone deficiency may be absolute or relative. An absolute deficiency may have various causes: (a) a primary ovarian defect with lack of enzymes or with abnormal oocytes incapable of organizing granulosa cells into mature follicles and programmed to respond to gonadotropic stimulation; (b) a central defect with insufficient FSH or LH stimulation (formation or release) for follicular growth or postovulatory luteinization, respectively. Following inadequate FSH stimulation in the proliferative phase, even a normal LH surge will result in deficient and too short progesterone synthesis and vice versa (JONES 1973). Furthermore, hypersecretion of prolactin may suppress progesterone secretion by the corpus luteum and shorten the luteal phase (DEL POZO et al. 1979). A relative progesterone deficiency may follow a preceding follicular persistency with delayed ovulation or repeated anovulatory cycles as in polycystic ovary syndrome. Here the FSH/LH ratio is low due to hypersecretion of LH with excessive androgen production which is metabolized to estrogen in the fat tissue, resulting in hyperestrogenism. The associated secretory phase is of normal length or may show an early breakdown. In rare instances, a defect of progesterone receptors in the endometrium may cause a relative progesterone deficiency in the presence of a normally functioning corpus luteum ("pseudo-corpus luteum insufficiency", KELLER et al. 1979; LAATIKAINEN et al. 1983; SPIRTOS et al. 1985).

Just as the type and cause of disturbance or interference in the function of the corpus luteum may vary, so may the histological picture of the resultant deficient secretory phase fluctuate. One has the best chance of diagnosing the changes that occur by examining tissue taken at the end of the secretory phase. The specimen obtained should be from the uterine fundus, since the cyclic changes in the endometrium near the uterine isthmus may be delayed or imperfectly developed, even normally. Because the degree of secretory differentiation may vary greatly from one cycle to the next, depending on the variable insuffi-

Table 8. Functional disturbances of the endometrium in infertility

Causes	Serum levels	Morphology of endometrium at end of cycle	Therapy
Ovarian defect			
Gonadal dysgenesis			Estrogen priming + clomiphene (+ progesterone)
Deficient enzymes or abnormal oocytes: →deficient follicle		Atrophy or deficient proliferation	
Receptor defect: →gonadotropin-resistant ovary syndrome	FSH ↑ LH ↑ E ↓		
Luteinized unruptured follicle (LUF)syndrome		Normal secretory phase	
Central defect			
Normal FSH + elevated LH (↓FSH/LH ratio):			
Polycystic ovary syndrome	LH ↑ E ↑	Irregular proliferation or abortive secretion	Clomiphene
Persistent follicle + delayed ovulation		Deficient luteal phase with coordinated apparent delay	
Inadequate FSH + normal LH	FSH ↓	Deficient luteal phase with coordinated true delay	FSH in first half of cycle followed by HCG (+ progesterone)
Normal FSH + inadequate LH	LH ↓	Deficient luteal phase with dissociated delay (slight)	
Inadequate FSH and inadequate LH	FSH ↓ LH ↓	Deficient luteal phase with dissociated delay (severe)	
Hyperprolactinemia →inadequate LH	LH ↓	Short luteal phase with early breakdown	Antiprolactin
Endometrial receptor defect (pseudo-corpus luteum deficiency)			
Estrogen receptor defect		Atrophy or deficient proliferation	Estrogen or Tamoxifen
Progesterone receptor defect		Irregular proliferation	

ciency of each corpus luteum developing, proper evaluation of the patient requires biopsy material from at least two cycles. Although histological sections stained with hematoxylin-eosin prove adequate for revealing many of the changes, other changes can be detected only with histochemical methods. When we apply strict criteria, we find that a deficient secretory phase due to endogenous disturbances is more common than previously assumed; although ISRAEL (1959) reported it in only 3.5% of his sterility patients, we found it in 20% of our sterility patients (SILLO-SEIDL and DALLENBACH-HELLWEG 1974).

By carefully correlating clinical and histological findings it is possible to divide the deficient secretory phase into three types of different causes (GIGON et al. 1970; DALLENBACH-HELLWEG 1984; see Table 8). The *deficient secretory phase with dissociated delay* is the variety most frequently encountered. The endometrium shows widely spaced, poorly convoluted glands, a variation in the development of glands and stroma from region to region, and a dissociation of development between glands and their surrounding stroma (they are "out of phase" or discordant). Adjacent to normal secretory *glands* that correspond with the proper day of the cycle one may see other glands that are poorly developed or deficient, with basal vacuoles and small rounded nuclei in low, functionally inactive epithelial cells (Figs. 73, 74). Other glands, however, may be in the proliferative phase and contain elongated nuclei with dense chromatin in a non-functioning, hormonally non-responsive epithelium. The variation in glandular differentiation results from decreased progesterone levels. Only those portions close to the blood supply (spiral arterioles) receive enough progesterone to react properly. In contrast, when levels of progesterone are normal, all parts

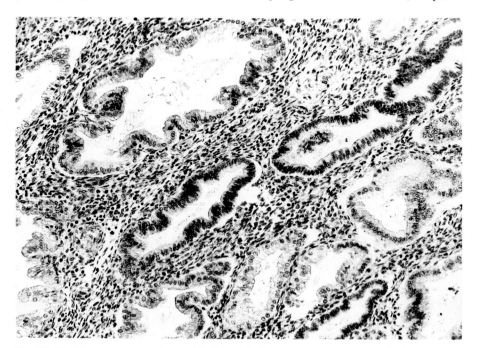

Fig. 73. Deficient secretory phase with dissociated delay of maturation, 26th day

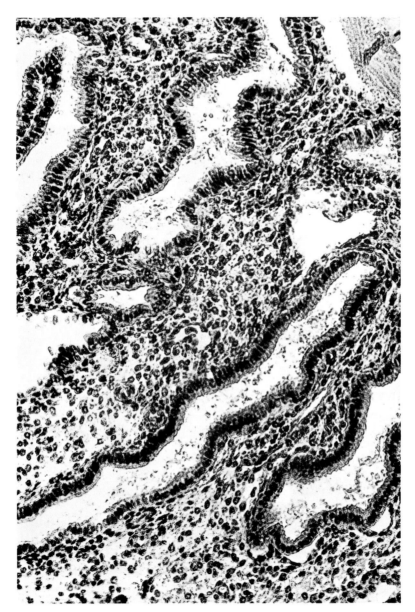

Fig. 74. Deficient secretory phase on the 26th day of the menstrual cycle, with severe dissociated delay in maturation. The glands are only slightly tortuous and lined with low epithelial cells that have round to elongated, dense nuclei. The stroma is loose and poorly differentiated

of the endometrium, including those more remote from the arterioles, are stimulated (ULM 1970). Accordingly, with deficient levels of progesterone, the epithelium of the glands will contain variable though diminished amounts of glycogen, mucopolysaccharides, proteins and acid phosphatase. The activity of the alkaline phosphatase is often increased (Noyes 1959; Schmidt-Matthiesen 1965; further literature op. cit.). Electron-microscopically the granules of glycogen, the mitochondria, and the intranucleolar channel system of the glandular cells are clearly reduced in size and number (Ancla et al. 1967; Gore and Gordon 1974). The concentrations of estrogen receptors in the nucleus and cytoplasm are lower than in the normal secretory phase. The concentrations of progesterone receptors correspond with the low values of the late secretory phase.

The *stroma* may be either poorly differentiated, arrested at about the grade of maturity of the early proliferative phase, or it may be edematous, as it is premenstrually, but reveal no predecidual change. On the other hand, it may be flecked with focal regions of predecidual change, localized edema, and small hemorrhages. At times the stroma contains large amounts of glycogen prematurely, or accumulates acid mucopolysaccharides focally. The ground substance, which normally undergoes two major transformations during the menstrual cycle, may fail to change or may remain depolymerized during the entire secretory phase. That depolymerized state is apparently associated with the focal accumulation of glycogen in the stroma (Schmidt-Matthiesen 1965). Occasionally a widespread pathological edema develops. The spiral arterioles remain small and underdeveloped.

In the *deficient secretory phase with coordinated delay* this delay in maturation may be the only histological criterion for distinguishing it from a normal luteal phase. To find an early secretory phase at the end of the cycle is characteristic for this entity, which is often caused by delayed ovulation. In consequence, the maturation of glands and stroma is only *apparently delayed*. When this type of deficient secretory phase is preceded by a persistent follicle with irregular proliferation, some of the glands characteristically retain their dilated lumina. The stromal cells are fairly large and spaced by edema (Fig. 75).

If, on the other hand, the preceding proliferation was insufficient or shortened, then the glands are small and narrow, the basal glycogen vacuoles hardly reach their normal size, and the stromal cells remain small and undifferentiated. In these rare instances, we have a *truly delayed* coordinated maturation of glands and stroma (Fig. 76).

The dissociated delay is most often the result of a true progesterone deficiency due to suppression of its production or secretion. The coordinated delay, on the other hand, is most often associated with normal secretion of progesterone which is counteracted by too much estrogen, as from a preceding persistent follicle; or the progesterone cannot act fully because of a preceding deficient proliferation with underdevelopment of glands and stroma, or of endometrial progesterone receptor defects.

Twenty-five percent of all deficient secretory phases are abnormally short. At times they last only 8 days (Buxton 1950), as concurrent studies of the ovaries have shown. The shedding of the endometrium takes place prematurely because the levels of progesterone decline before they should owing to the abnormal corpus luteum. Menstrual shedding with correct dissolution of stromal and glandular elements can take place only when progesterone has acted on the endometrium for at least 10 days. The deficient secretory phase may also terminate in pathological bleeding due to estrogen withdrawal (fall in estrogen levels); such bleeding occasionally develops late but is usually prolonged.

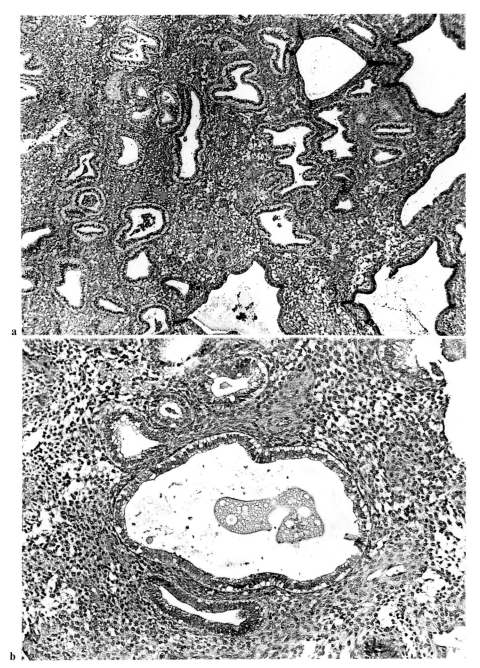

Fig. 75a, b. Deficient secretory phase with coordinated apparent delay of maturation. a Low magnification; b high magnification

The therapy of the deficient secretory phase should depend upon its specific etiology and should consist of hormone substitution. In general, good therapeutic results may be obtained by administering natural progesterone during the

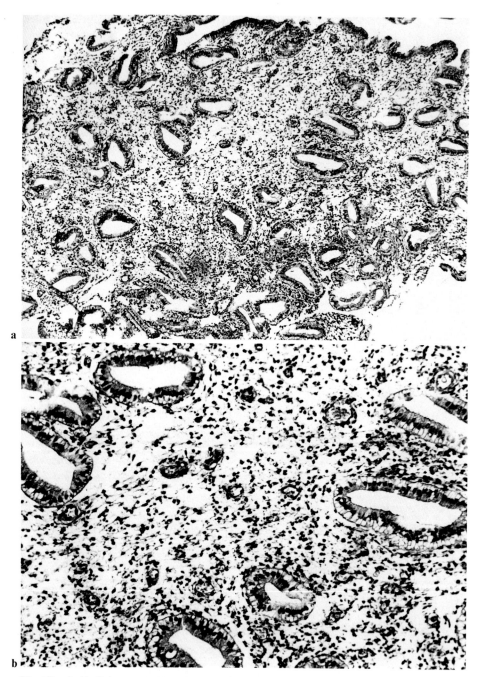

Fig. 76a, b. Deficient secretory phase with coordinated true delay of maturation. **a** Low magnification; **b** high magnification

last week or 10 days of the menstrual cycle (MOSZKOWSKI et al. 1962; JONES 1973). That is best given parenterally or as vaginal suppositories, 25 mg twice daily since synthetic gestagens taken orally depress the production of endogenous progesterones (SOULES et al. 1977). Such a treatment has led to a pregnancy rate of 50% after an average of five menstrual cycles. If the cause of the deficient secretory phase is central with inadequate FSH and/or LH secretion, then FSH during the proliferative phase (HUANG et al. 1984) or chorionic gonadotropin may prove beneficial (see Table 8) as it stimulates endogenous progesterone secretion, and may be added to the progesterone substitution therapy. Hypergonadotropic dysfunction, on the other hand, as in Stein-Leventhal syndrome, will require clomiphene therapy. Furthermore, a primary ovarian defect with abnormal corpora lutea will not respond to HCG but requires treatment with clomiphene which acts locally on the granulosa cells (see p. 188). In pseudocorpus luteum insufficiency, on the other hand, clomiphene is contraindicated, because it has been shown to reduce the number of cytosolic estrogen and progesterone receptors by inhibition of steroid receptor replenishment. In these rare instances estrogen or tamoxifen should be administered, both of which will stimulate the production of progesterone receptors.

e) The Endometrium Associated with Persistent Corpus Luteum

α) Irregular Shedding

If a corpus luteum develops normally after ovulation but fails to regress later at the proper time because of disturbances of the hormonal mechanisms controlling it, then it continues to secrete progesterone. As a consequence, the changes normally brought about in the endometrium by the decline in progesterone shortly before menstruation fail to develop or do so late; "irregular shedding" of the endometrium results. The menstrual bleeding may start at the proper time or may be delayed. In any case, it is prolonged and usually excessive. Persistence of the corpus luteum may be induced by hyperstimulation either from hypophyseal gonadotropin or from placental gonadotropin; that is, by an intrauterine or extrauterine pregnancy with increased secretion of gonadotropin. In extreme cases, a hydatidiform mole may cause several corpora lutea to become cystic. MCKELVEY and SAMUELS (1947) commonly observed irregular shedding during the first post partum menstruation, perhaps because the hypophysis then failed to function properly. Similar endometrial changes may be induced by spontaneous polyovulation (PEPLER and FOUCHE 1968) or by therapy with gestagens, as HOLMSTROM and MCLENNAN (1947) were able to demonstrate by injecting progesterone during the menses, and as results with some of the oral contraceptives have proved. It is logical, therefore, that an irregular shedding may be prevented by giving estrogen 2 days before the onset of menstruation (WEBER 1954). After the diagnosis of irregular shedding is verified histologically, if its cause remains clinically obscure, then all the various etiological possibilities just reviewed should be considered.

Irregular shedding was recognized by DRIESSEN in 1914 and described thoroughly by PANKOW in 1924 and by BANIECKI in 1928. The condition develops only during the reproductive years, predominately between the ages of 25 and

50 years (MCKELVEY 1942; 30–50 years; STADTMÜLLER 1950: 25–30 years and 40–50 years; THIERY 1955; 24–40 years). Irregular shedding occurs either at every menstrual period or only once, as for example, after a stillbirth or after a clinically unrecognized abortion of a blighted ovum. BANIECKI observed irregular shedding 61 times among 465 curettings.

The *histological recognition* of irregular shedding is not easy for the inexperienced since the histological changes are confusing. It is exactly that confusion of the histological picture, however, that should make us think of irregular shedding. Characteristic of the condition is the diverse admixture of endometrial fragments in various stages of regression and dissociation still evident several days after menstruation started. The changes cannot be diagnosed in the intervals between bleeding or just after its onset. Since the levels of progesterone do not fall, the premenstrual release of relaxin and proteolytic enzymes is prevented, and consequently the reticulum network fails to undergo dissolution (DALLENBACH-HELLWEG and BORNEBUSCH 1970). The normally developed endometrium cannot disintegrate; it merely shrinks owing to the loss of water induced by the decrease in estrogen. Since the shedding is greatly prolonged, the regressive changes in the glands and stroma become more intense. Then too, because the resulting changes lag in time, they appear much more striking than those normally seen before or during a regular menstruation.

The most characteristic sign of irregular shedding, readily seen under low magnification, is the narrow, star-shaped appearance of the *glandular* lumina Figs. 77 and 78a). The cytoplasm of many of the glandular cells is clear and often contains abundant glycogen, thus contrasting sharply with the surrounding small stromal cells that have scanty, dark cytoplasm and densely packed nuclei rich in chromatin. Often the nuclei of the glandular cells are equally shrunken with dense chromatin, but owing to the excessive hormonal stimulation they may also be enlarged, grotesquely shaped, and suspended haphazardly within a swollen, clear cytoplasm (see Fig. 154b). Such a phenomenon, first described by ARIAS-STELLA in 1954, is associated with an abnormally high level of gonadotropin and is, therefore, a sign of a dead fetus with continued production of the hormone by a trophoblast that remains viable (see p. 304). A positive Arias-Stella phenomenon, consequently, is to be expected in only some of the cases of irregular shedding of the endometrium. If the phenomenon is found, then the irregular shedding may be related to death of a fetus even though trophoblasts or decidual cells are histologically lacking (see also OVERBECK 1959).

The dense *stroma* of these portions of endometrium is composed initially of large, compact cells and many granulocytes. Later, after shrinkage takes place, the granulocytes appear more numerous than in a premenstrual stroma or in an intact decidua. Most of the granulocytes are laden with granules that are never discharged. Silver impregnation reveals an intact, tightly knit meshwork of reticulum fibers woven about the stromal cells and glands, holding them firmly in place. The spiral arterioles slowly undergo retrograde changes after the elastic fibers in their walls gradually degenerate (THIERY 1955). In the endometrium of young women with irregular shedding, BANIECKI (1928) observed that the dilated and tortuous spiral arterioles were often thrombosed because of the slow involution and prolonged bleeding; in contrast, he found that in patients in the preclimacterium the arterioles were generally narrow.

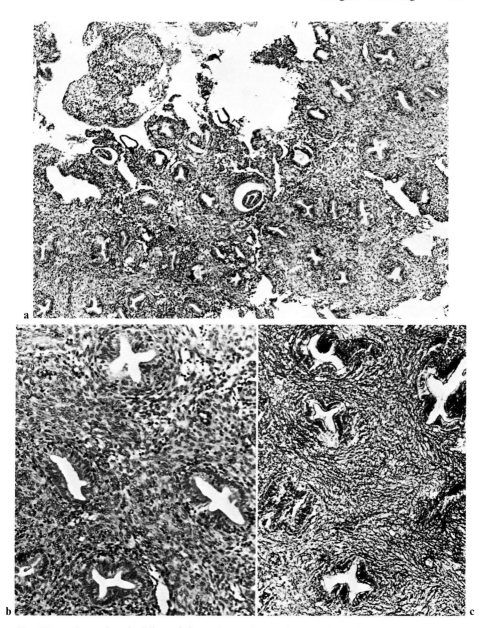

Fig. 77 a–c. Irregular shedding of the endometrium. **a** Survey view of the usual disordered appearance of focal dissolution and desquamation. **b** Higher magnification: the star-shaped glands are embedded in a stroma of large cells. **c** The network of reticulum fibers is intact and dense (silver impregnation after GOMORI)

The stromal cells about the arterioles remain intact the longest. Otherwise, the stromal cells undergo retrograde changes and shrinkage before the epithelial cells of the glands do. In brief, the sequence in the protracted involution is as follows: first stromal cells, then glandular epithelial cells, then blood vessels.

Besides these characteristic changes in some parts of the endometrium, other regions may be found that have already undergone extensive dissolution and hemorrhage. It is possible that in these regions the shrinkage of the endometrium had produced local ischemia, cutting off the supply of progesterone. Thus the granulocytes are induced to release their granules of relaxin and the reticulum fibers in these regions disintegrate, as in a normal menstruating endometrium. Between these two extremes – the intensely shrunken but intact endometrium and the normally menstruating endometrium – all transitions may be found. Further, when the bleeding is particularly protracted, other regions of the endometrium may already have begun to regenerate and may show early proliferative changes of the next menstrual cycle. These parts are recognized by the loose, edematous stroma composed of poorly differentiated spindly cells and a reticulum network of sparse, delicate fibers. The glands are narrow, straight and lined by a uniform row of inactive-appearing epithelial cells. At times the parts of endometrium undergoing the protracted irregular shedding cover in cap-like fashion the regions of regenerating endometrium (Fig. 78b). In rare instances the degenerating parts fuse with the regenerating tissue and become organized. The regressing glands in these regions are transformed and incorporated into the next cycle. Regeneration of the superficial epithelium takes place only after complete detachment of the menstruating endometrium; consequently, the regeneration is greatly prolonged.

Depending upon the intensity and quality of the hormonal stimulus still persisting or upon the speed with which it abates, the regressive and progressive changes just described may accordingly vary in extent and kind. One of the components of the endometrium may change more than the others. Borderline cases may show changes that merge gradually with those of a normal menstruation. In differentiating irregular shedding from protracted bleeding due to other causes, it is important to demonstrate that the glandular *and* stromal cells clearly show secretory (progestational) effect.

It may be possible histologically to draw conclusions about the *etiology* of irregular shedding by disclosing endometritis, hyalinized arterioles, and necrotic or degenerated remnants of decidua, placental villi, trophoblasts or an Arias-Stella phenomenon. Some of the degenerating glands may dilate cystically after the fetus dies, whereas the regressing glands of irregular shedding due to other causes usually remain small. In curettings it may be exceedingly difficult to differentiate the cystic, degenerative changes occurring post abortum from those of a hemorrhagic, glandular-cystic hyperplasia in secretory transformation. Accurate clinical information is extremely helpful here. Occasionally the use of oral contraceptives may lead to irregular shedding of the endometrium, since they may induce a deficiency in progesterone resulting in an insufficiency of endometrial granulocytes and consequently of relaxin. The reticulum fibers therefore fail to undergo dissolution. If, however, such histological clues are lacking, then the genesis of the irregular shedding must be explained clinically. Precise clinical data are exceedingly valuable in the accurate interpretation of regressive changes of the endometrium. Without knowledge of the menstrual cycle it may be impossible to differentiate a prolonged menstruation from the terminal, late discharge of a decidualized endometrium associated with an extrauterine pregnancy (HINZ 1954). The cause of the irregular shedding can be

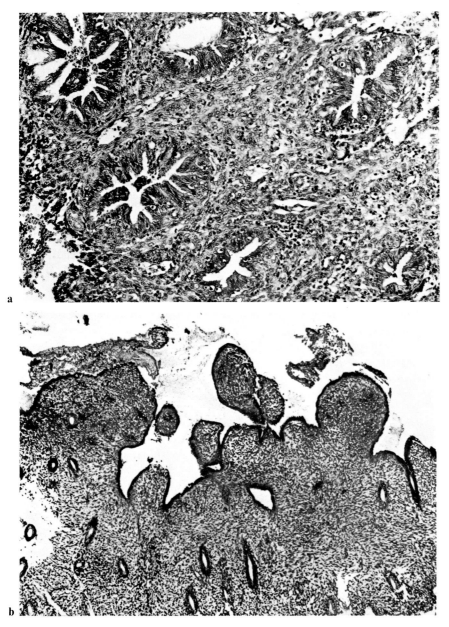

Fig. 78. a Irregular shedding, advanced stage. The typical star-like shape of the glands is conspicuous. The surrounding stroma is dense and rich in fibers. **b** End stage of irregular shedding that developed after use of oral contraceptive agents. The humped remnants of the old mucosa rest on newly proliferating parts

clarified in most cases, or at least inferred, if information about the duration of endometrial bleeding, about pregnancy tests and about urinary excretion of hormones is correlated with the results of the histological studies.

Irregular shedding may also follow a persistent, but previously insufficient corpus luteum, which may develop post partum or during the climacterium. If such an insufficient corpus luteum persists, the endometrial histology varies slightly from the classical picture of irregular shedding: some of the collapsed glands still reveal signs of abortive secretion while neighboring glands may show no such evidence although surrounded by focal hemorrhagic necrosis. This variety of irregular shedding is usually recognized only by the experienced pathologist; its identification, however, is important for correct treatment of the patient.

β) Dysmenorrhea Membranacea

Within the spectrum of irregular shedding dysmenorrhea membranacea represents a special entity. According to DEELMAN (1933) that term was first used by MORGAGNI in 1723. Pathologically, what is meant is a spontaneous slough of the endometrium in one cylindrical piece or in large membranous pieces that retain the shape of the uterine cavity (Fig. 79). Histologically, the tissue consists of corpus endometrium in either the predecidual or the decidual state. It is variably infiltrated with polymorphonuclear leukocytes and is in the process of dissolution. The decidual cells may disclose advanced retrogressive changes and often have spindly shapes. The endometrial granulocytes are generally very numerous and retain their granules. The glands are lined by low cuboidal cells whose small, rounded nuclei appear like a chain of beads. – The causes for this condition are the same as those for irregular shedding. GREENBLATT et al. (1954) and PANELLA (1960) observed the discharge of a decidual cast after administering progesterone (hormonal discharge). The associated dysmenorrhea is probably due to the failure of the tissue to undergo dissolution. Relaxin is not released since the level of progesterone fails to decrease. A decidual cast may be expelled under similar conditions after an abortion. It remains unclear, however, how despite the elevated level of progesterone the decidualized endometrium spontaneously detaches without first undergoing dissolution. One may postulate that the fall in progesterone takes place too late, at a refractory phase when dissolution of the tissue cannot occur. The only response possible is the complete discharge of the intact endometrium.

If the progesterone fails to fall, then with time it stimulates the stromal cells to transform into decidual cells, although no pregnancy exists. The decidua that forms cannot be distinguished from that of a pregnancy. Such cases are reported from time to time. SPECHTER (1953) found a typical decidua in two young women who had persistent corpora lutea, and once in a 71-year-old woman with carcinoma of the ovary. We have seen similar cases. On the other hand, decidual transformation of the stroma may develop concurrently with atrophy of the glands, resulting in "arrested secretion" (see p. 162). That condition is seen only after stimulation with exogenous gestagens. One of our patients, a 60-year-old woman who had received medroxyprogesterone acetate over a long time for endometriosis, developed a perfect decidua that contained great numbers of granulocytes but atrophic glands. Such a decidua may also be detached in large membranous pieces.

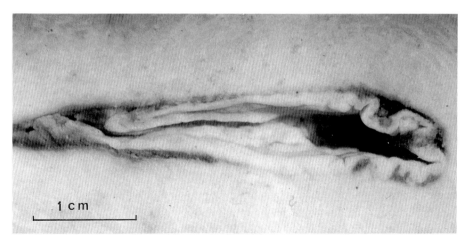

Fig. 79. Uterus containing sheets of dysmenorrhea membranacea in the process of shedding

γ) Secretory Hypertrophy

Occasionally one finds that patients in the preclimacteric or climacteric periods have a tall secretory endometrium, which may measure 1 cm or more in height, resembling the endometrium found about 10 days after successful implantation of a blastocyst. The glands are densely located, of irregular shapes, some cystically dilated, but most of them highly secretory even in the basal layer and directly underneath the surface epithelium. Their distribution is quite irregular. Some of their epithelial cells indicate excessive hormonal stimulation, thereby appearing unusually large and clear with prominent, irregular nuclei rich in chromatin. The stroma is predecidual, very loose and focally edematous (Fig. 80). The spiral arterioles are greatly hypertrophied and proliferated. We classify these changes under the term "secretory hypertrophy." Some patients show a predominance of glandular hypertrophy (glandular type of secretory hypertrophy, Figs. 80, 81b), others of stromal hypertrophy (decidual type, Fig. 81a), but intermediate forms do also occur. We surmise the condition results from a hormonal imbalance during the preclimacteric period, most likely from excess production of hypophyseal gonadotropin resulting in a hyperfunction of the corpus luteum (see p. 157).

f) The Endometrium Associated with Infertility

Normal implantation of the fertilized ovum depends on a precise physiological balance between numerous factors of structural and functional nature. Consequently, it is easy to understand how many different and unrelated disturbances can give rise to infertility. If we disregard disturbances causing infertility in the husband, then those arising in the patient may involve any part of her genital system or parts of her central nervous system that control the ovaries

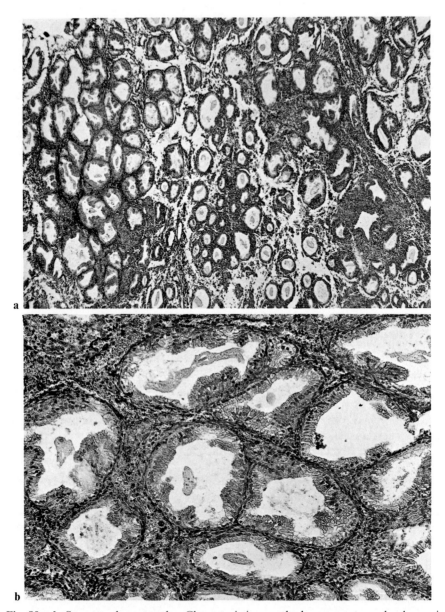

Fig. 80 a, b. Secretory hypertrophy. Characteristics are the hypersecretory glands varying in diameter and distribution; the surrounding stroma reveals either edema or predecidual change. **a** Low magnification; **b** high magnification

hormonally. Here I shall discuss only those causes of infertility that can be diagnosed from the characteristic changes they produce in the endometrium. We should emphasize, however, that if we exclude chromosomal abnormalities, then almost all disturbances of the genital organs can lead to structural changes in the endometrium.

To clarify causes of infertility, the clinician has available an impressive array of diagnostic tests to choose from. Because the newer methods for measuring

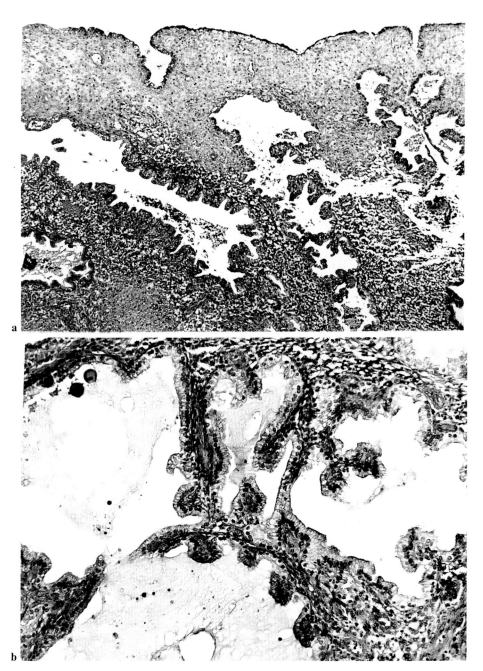

Fig. 81 a, b. Secretory hypertrophy; **a** decidual type; **b** glandular type

hormones in the blood are much more accurate than those used 15–20 years ago (GEIGER 1980), they have contributed much to our understanding of the secretion and interrelationships between hormones. Levels of hormones do fluctuate, sometimes only briefly, sometimes for longer circadian periods. Such fluctuations help to explain discrepancies occasionally noted between plasma hormone levels and histological dating of endometrial maturation. The most reliable method for diagnosing the cause of infertility, therefore, remains the histological study of an endometrial biopsy if performed by a pathologist experienced in this special field. Clinical investigators express the same opinion (ANNOS et al. 1980; ROSENFELD et al. 1980; LEDUC et al. 1981). The biopsy serves as a bioassay measuring the hormone at the tissue level (JONES et al. 1974). To be able to carry out his study accurately, however, the pathologist must know about the patient's menstrual cycle, on which day of her cycle the biopsy was made, and about any hormones she may have received. As a prerequisite for the clinician, he should obtain the endometrial biopsy at the end of the menstrual cycle; that is, premenstrually or at the onset of menstrual bleeding. If one finds a normal secretory endometrium, or a secretory endometrium undergoing normal involutional changes, corresponding to the day of the cycle, then the cause of the infertility is not in the endometrium but should be looked for elsewhere. We should not forget, however, that when the functional disturbances are slight, normal cycles may alternate with abnormal cycles. In such instances, it is advisable to repeat the endometrial biopsy in subsequent cycles. In addition to the functional diagnosis, the histological study may reveal unexpected inflammations of the endometrium, such as tuberculosis, or even polyps and tumors. – Moreover, the endometrial biopsy can supply tissue for determining progesterone receptors, which might help to explain a discrepancy between elevated serum levels of progesterone and a proliferative endometrium (DALLENBACH-HELLWEG 1984).

As indicated by the figures published by different investigators, the frequency of pathological changes of the endometrium in sterility varies greatly. No doubt the frequency depends to a large extent on the skill employed in preparing the histological sections of the endometrium, and on the experience and knowledge of the pathologist who studies them. According to VACZY and SCIPIADES (1949), HINZ (1953), and FOSS et al. (1958), 15%–20% of all infertile women have an anatomical or functional disturbance of the endometrium. STAFFELDT and LÜBKE (1967) specify 25%; KANTOR and HARREL (1953) 25.9%. According to SILLO-SEIDL (1971), the percentage is 46%. ROMAN and LABAEYE (1964) found endometrial disturbances in 54.8% of all infertile women. The disturbances manifest themselves in many different ways. In some instances, however, although the functional disturbances causing the infertility may subtly differ, the morphological changes they induce in the endometrium may be similar. Only by carrying out additional clinical, biochemical and endocrinological studies is it possible to clarify these subtle differences and precisely define the cause of the infertility (see Table 9).

The menstrual cycle may vary in length **(asynchronous cycles)** without the histological appearance of the endometrium deviating significantly from that of a normal cycle. Without a clinical history, therefore, it is impossible to diagnose variations in the cycle. Since both a short cycle and a prolonged cycle may be the only cause of the infertility, it is exactly for such abnormal cycles that the correlation of clinical data with the results of histological studies is

Table 9. Functional disturbances of the endometrium in infertility

Morphology	Possible causes

Atrophy	(a) Non-functioning ovaries
	    Gonadal dysgenesis
	    Deficient follicular development
	    Gonadotropin-resistant ovary syndrome
	(b) Hormone-refractive endometrium

Deficient proliferation	(a) Deficient follicular maturation or stimulation with deficient (and often prolonged) anovulatory cycle (b) Endometrium partially refractive to estrogen
Irregular proliferation or hyperplasia	(a) Central defect Polycystic ovary syndrome (repeated anovulatory cycles or persistent follicle) (b) Endometrium refractive to progesterone
Deficient secretory phase (a) With coordinated apparent delay (b) With coordinated true delay (c) With dissociated delay	Central defect (a) Persistent follicle and delayed ovulation (relative corpus luteum insufficiency) (b) Inadequate FSH stimulation (absolute corpus luteum insufficiency) (c) Inadequate LH stimulation with or without hyperprolactinemia
Abortive secretion	Non-ovulating, insufficient follicle with sporadic luteinization
Arrested secretion	Gestagen stimulation without ovulation, mostly exogenic
Asynchronous cycle	Disturbance of central regulation (direct or indirect by negative feedback mechanism)

of paramount importance. Only after the cause of the variation in the cycle has been clarified can a rational therapy be instituted.

Such a shift in a menstrual cycle, although the endometrium is otherwise normal, is enough to alter the attraction of the endometrial tissue for the blastocyst on the day of implantation (Foss et al. 1958; found by STAFFELDT and LÜBKE in 10% of their infertility cases). What conditions that attraction are the chemical and structural changes induced by the postovulatory rise in plasma progesterone. It must reach a precise level if the blastocyst is to be able to imbed at the proper time (BEIER 1981). Only with precise knowledge of the daily changes occurring during the menstrual cycle ("histological dating of the endometrium" – NOYES and HAMAN 1953) can such functional disturbances be detected. The asynchrony is usually due to a central dysfunction such as a juvenile hypofunction of the hypothalamus or a premature menopause, both of which may induce either deficient or excessive gonadotropic stimulation of the ovary (GEIGER 1980).

When the menstrual *cycle is shortened,* then ovulation may take place prematurely. The subsequent secretory phase, however, remains deficient since the endometrial tissues that normally differentiate under the effects of progesterone to prepare for nidation cannot develop completely because the preceding proliferation was inadequate. In other instances the proliferative phase may be of normal duration but the secretory phase shortened owing to premature regression of the corpus luteum. Under both circumstances we will find that the secretory phase is deficient shortly before menstruation (see p. 136). ROSENFELD and GARCIA (1976) reported that 36% of their 238 infertile patients had shortened menstrual cycles, whereas in only 3% were the cycles prolonged.

The *prolonged menstrual cycle* may also have various causes (PLOTZ 1950). On the one hand, the Graafian follicle may persist for about 3 weeks and be followed by a normal or abbreviated secretory phase. In that event, delayed ovulation may lead to intrafollicular overripeness of the ovum which results in infertility (see below). On the other hand, a persisting follicle tends to induce a protracted anovulatory cycle. Another possibility is irregular shedding of the endometrium associated with a persistent corpus luteum. As already mentioned, these various possibilities can be clearly differentiated if a curettage is performed premenstrually or just before the onset of bleeding, and the results correlated with those of vaginal cytology and with the clinical history (see Table 10).

If the menstrual cycles are of normal duration, then either a **deficient,** or **delayed** or **absent secretory phase** usually is responsible for the sterility. A major subdivision can be made into *anovulatory infertility,* usually caused by severe functional disturbance of the hypothalamus, pituitary, or ovary (see p. 103); and *ovulatory infertility* with failure in conception or implantation because of hypothalamic, pituitary, ovarian, or endometrial disturbances. The endometrium may fail to respond even to normally circulating progesterone (COOKE et al. 1972) because of the lack of progesterone receptors. Furthermore, habitual abortion may be caused by luteal insufficiency with decreased plasma progesterone levels, resulting in a deficient secretory endometrium incapable of holding (supporting) the implanted blastocyst. Since these abnormal cycles may occur regularly or may fluctuate with normal cycles (STEVENSON 1965), the histological proof of a normal secretory endometrium provides little information for prognosing the course of the next cycle. Only careful measurement of the basal temperature (RUST 1979) and repeated curettages or endometrial biopsies can clarify matters. Histochemically, the content of glycogen is usually diminished (HUGHES et al. 1964) and there is a discrepancy between the production of mucus and glycogen (STRAUSS 1963). DYKOVA et al. (1963) found in 93 of 270 infertile women that during the last 2 days of the menstrual cycle the predecidual change of the stroma was deficient or lacking, and was associated with poorly developed blood vessels. In addition, VACZY and SCIPIADES (1949) attributed importance to a decrease in the thickness and number of the collagen fibers as well as to their disordered arrangement, since these investigators found such changes in 72.4% of their sterile patients but in only 11.6% of their controls. One should also remember that occasionally a luteinized cystic follicle developing after a failed ovulation can cause infertility with a normal secretory endometrium (LUF syndrome). This syndrome cannot be diagnosed by endometrial biopsy or by plasma hormone assays. It can, however, be suspected in those women in whom the plasma FSH concentrations remain elevated for a few days after ovulation.

Table 10. Possible variations of endometrial function in infertility (for the numbers see Table 4)

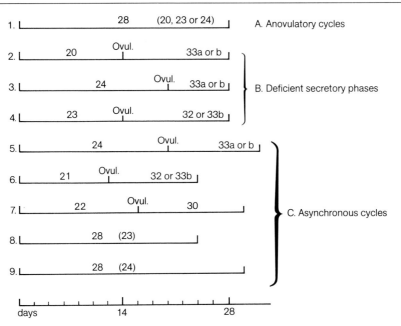

A1: Anovulatory cycle with cyclic (*20*), deficient (*23*) or irregular (*24*) proliferation.
B2: Apparently delayed, coordinated (*33a*) or dissociated (*33b*) deficient secretion following cyclic proliferation (*20*).
3: Truly delayed, coordinated (*33a*) or dissociated (*33b*) deficient secretion following irregular proliferation (*24*) with delayed ovulation and early breakdown.
4: Abortive (*32*) or deficient and dissociated (*33b*) secretion following deficient proliferation (*23*).
C5: Prolonged cycle, as in B3, but without early breakdown.
6: Shortened cycle with early ovulation following deficient proliferation (*21*), secretory phase as in B4, or shorter.
7: Prolonged, otherwise normal cycle (*22* and *30*) with delayed ovulation.
8: Shortened anovulatory cycle with deficient proliferation (*23*).
9: Prolonged anovulatory cycle with irregular proliferation (*24*)

If amenorrhea exists then the endometrium is usually *hypoplastic* or *atrophic*. In such cases a primary ovarian failure with a gonadotropin-resistant ovary syndrome must be suspected (RUSSELL et al. 1982). On the other hand, hypermenorrhea with *glandular-cystic hyperplasia* and a shift in the menstrual cycle can also prevent pregnancy. SILLO-SEIDL (1967) reported such a hyperplasia in 3.5% of 467 curettages and endometrial biopsies from infertile patients. Even commoner is the *irregular proliferation* elicited by a persistent follicle of short duration. MASSHOFF (1941) referred to that proliferation as "glandular hyperplasia" and alleged it caused infertility in 24.5% of his patients. In our series (SILLO-SEIDL and DALLENBACH-HELLWEG 1974) 28% of 1915 infertile patients had *polyps*; 2% were from the endocervix and 26% from the corpus endometrium.

After the polyps had been removed by complete curettage, 21% of the patients became pregnant.

In some countries, such as Spain and India (GAURIBAZAZ-MALIK et al. 1983) *tuberculous endometritis* is a major cause of infertility. In 3000 curettings of infertile women BOTELLA-LLUSIA (1967) found histologically that 10.6% had tuberculous endometritis. Signs of secretory changes were either deficient or lacking. In SILLO-SEIDL's series (Frankfurt, FRG) only 1.3% among 467 of his infertile patients (1967) and only 0.7% among 1000 (1971) revealed tuberculous endometritis. SHARMAN in Glasgow (1955) reported the disease in 5.6% of his patients, VACZY and SCIPIADES (1949, Budapest) in 7.1%. In addition to the endometrial changes, the tuberculous salpingitis that exists concomitantly in most of these patients also causes infertility.

According to STEVENSON (1965), the patients with endometrial atrophy or hypoplasia have the least chance (20%) of becoming pregnant after therapy, whereas women either with simple deviations in the length of the menstrual cycle or with deficient secretory phases have almost twice the chance (35%).

g) Functional Disturbances During the Climacteric

At the end of the childbearing period ovarian function does not cease abruptly. Rather, the secretion of ovarian hormones wanes gradually over several years in a way unique in every woman. All variations in the balance of the hormones may develop from the gradual and concomitant waxing and waning of both ovarian hormones to an irregular overproduction or deficiency of one or both hormones, to a persistent secretion of only estrogen beyond the menopause (see Table 5). Accordingly, the histological picture of the climacteric endometrium varies greatly. Consequently, the spectrum of changes regarded as still physiological is much broader than that for the reproductive years (see p. 86ff.). In addition, every investigator draws quite differently the boundaries separating the functional disturbances thought to be physiological from those clearly pathological. In our opinion a slight or even moderate functional variation in one or more menstrual cycles during the climacterium should not be judged as pathological. Hence, irregular proliferative changes may be the result of an occasional anovulatory cycle, or irregular, usually inadequate secretory changes the result of an insufficient corpus luteum. Preferably, only those persistent changes that can be classified with a well-recognized clinical entity should be regarded as abnormal.

Of these entities the most common is *glandular-cystic hyperplasia*. It usually develops during the climacterium when the production of progesterone gradually ceases but that of estrogen continues. The condition is prognostically important and must be followed clinically. Depending upon the hormonal balance of the patient, glandular-cystic hyperplasia may either revert to a regressive hyperplasia or progress to an adenomatous hyperplasia. Similar considerations are valid for all other functional changes occurring during the climacterium, since it is impossible to predict at that time just how the changes will end; their development depends entirely upon what happens to ovarian function.

Much less common than the glandular-cystic hyperplasia is the *secretory hypertrophy* of the climacterium. It probably is produced by overstimulation from excessive hypophyseal gonadotropin, which causes hyperactivity of a corpus luteum and extreme secretory changes in the endometrium (see p. 149f.). The basalis, which normally is functionless, participates in the secretion. The changes that develop almost always disappear with the cessation of ovulation at menopause.

Polyps of the corpus endometrium (LAU and STOLL 1962) are most frequent during the climacteric period. Their growth at that time is thought to be induced by the irregular stimulus of estrogen.

Most curettages performed during the climacteric period, however, reveal variations belonging within the broad spectrum of physiological changes expected at that time. The prognosis of these changes is therefore usually good, since they vanish as spontaneously as they appeared when the menopause sets in. Because the bleeding of these harmless cases cannot at times be distinguished from that of a more serious disturbance with dubious prognosis, a curettage during this critical period is indicated in every patient with bleeding. Carcinomas rarely develop at this time. In general they appear only after prolonged and total lack of progesterone.

h) The Effect of Hormone-Producing Ovarian Tumors on the Endometrium

The most common of these tumors are the estrogen-producing granulosa cell tumors and the thecomas. A group of other tumors, especially the cystomas but metastatic tumors to the ovary as well, may, by their growth and pressure, stimulate the surrounding ovarian stroma to produce increased amounts of estrogen. In most instances, the effect on the endometrium is the same: depending upon the amount of estrogen secreted, a glandular-cystic hyperplasia of variable intensity develops. If the production of estrogen is prolonged and unopposed the glandular-cystic hyperplasia becomes an adenomatous hyperplasia, which in turn may eventually develop into an adenocarcinoma. The changes produced are like those seen with a persistent follicle of long standing.

In comparison, only a couple of types of tumors produce progesterone; they are also less common. The major examples are the luteoma and the partly luteinized granulosa cell tumors. They generally induce a high degree of secretory hypertrophy of the endometrium, with glands that secrete excessively and a stroma that often shows decidual change. Occasionally an estrogen effect is also evident. Recently, a few sex cord stromal tumors with annular tubules have been observed in association with an arrested secretion of the endometrium, suggesting a production of synthetic gestagens by the tumor (CZERNOBILSKY et al. 1985; TRACY et al. 1985). If such changes are seen in an endometrium of a postmenopausal patient then one should think first of an ovarian tumor. But in the differential diagnosis the possibility of previous therapy with gestagens must be considered, as for example that used in the conservative treatment of endometriosis.

In contrast, all other ovarian tumors that produce hormones, particularly the androgen-secreting androblastoma and the gynandroblastoma are so rare that one seldom has the chance to study their effect on the endometrium. Clinically amenorrhea usually develops; the endometrium is hypoplastic or atrophic.

i) The Functional Disturbances of the Endocervical Mucosa

If a fractionated curettage has not been performed, then curettings of the endometrial cavity will often contain portions of the endocervix and transitional mucosa. Since the endocervix does not shed with menstruation, the functional disturbances induced in it by endogenous hormones are much less apparent than those seen in the endometrium. More important, however, is the fact that progesterone stimulates changes that are quite different from those produced by estrogen. The endocervical mucosa shows very little, if any, reaction to estrogen stimulation, but to elevated levels of progesterone reacts with *glandular and cystic hyperplasia,* as for example, with a persistent corpus luteum, or with pregnancy. The height of the endocervical mucosa increases, and its surface often becomes papillary. Its glands either grow, branching excessively, or dilate cystically, filling with mucus. Reserve cells of both the surface epithelium and the glands may proliferate intensely ("reserve cell hyperplasia"). – The transitional mucosa may show cystically dilated glands from the stimulation by both hormones; it represents a continuation of the hyperplasia of the endometrium and endocervix. Glandular-cystic hyperplasia of the cervical or transitional mucosa is of little clinical importance, since it is not desquamated and rarely causes bleeding. The excessive mucus secreted by the cystically dilated glands may occlude the endocervical canal or result in an annoying vaginal discharge.

3. Exogenous (Iatrogenic) Changes of the Endometrium

a) After Hormonal Therapy

As soon as an understanding of the menstrual cycle was achieved and it became obvious histologically that the ovarian hormones induced cyclic changes in the endometrium, attempts were made to treat patients who suffered hypophyseal dysfunction or deficient ovarian function by giving them ovarian hormones to compensate for their endocrine deficiencies. It soon became apparent, however, that every patient reacted uniquely, that the correct time, duration, dosage, and combination of hormonal therapy depended mainly on the state of the patient's endocrine system. When the doses of ovarian hormones exceeded physiological amounts, they caused characteristic histological changes in the endometrium different from those seen under endogenous stimulation. In addition, the effects of many of the synthetic estrogens and gestagens differ from their natural counterparts, depending on their chemical structure and biological potency.

α) Estrogens

The hormones grouped together and referred to as estrogens, although in their action similar, are chemically heterogeneous. The group includes various naturally occurring hormones, some of which are unique to certain species of animals, as well as synthetic steroids and non-steroidal agents. Of the estrogens secreted in the human, estradiol possesses the greatest affinity for the estrogen receptors. Because of their therapeutic advantages, orally active derivatives of estradiol (17α-ethinylestradiol, or its methyl ether, mestranol) are especially useful, for example as oral contraceptive agents. Other important prototypes of estrogens are quinestrol (Estrovis) and the conjugated estrogens (Premarin, Presomen, and Oestrofeminal), all of which have been used to treat estrogen deficiency. Because stilbestrol has been found to have carcinogenic side effects, it is not used anymore.

The estrogen potencies of these substances also vary even when they are administered by optimal routes (Table 11). The potencies, however, may be inversely proportional to the affinities the hormones have for estrogen receptors, since the substances are often slowly converted into estradiol, whereby their blood levels are maintained for long periods. Consequently, the estrogen potency of mestranol exceeds that of natural estradiol; and ethinylestradiol is one and a half times more active than mestranol when tested for its stimulation of stromal growth, and twice as active when tested for its stimulation of glandular growth (DELFORGE and FERIN 1970). These differences cannot be detected histometrically (BROSENS and PIJNENBORG 1976). Individual fluctuations in the responsiveness to hormones should be taken into account (HEMPEL et al. 1977). In contrast, estriol (for example, Ovestin), which is seldom used clinically, has only one-tenth the potency of either ethinyl-estradiol or stilbestrol (HASKINS et al. 1968).

Although the estrogens do show fine distinctions in their effects that are of clinical importance, most of these hormones are extremely potent, even in

Table 11. The potency of various estrogens ranked by the uterine weight test (after BRIGGS and BROTHERTON 1970)

Diethylstilbestrol dipropionate	14.37
Estradiol 17-cypionate	11.09
Estradiol benzoate	10.75
Estradiol dipropionate	10.00
Ethinylestradiol	9.72
Benzestrol	9.28
Diethylstilbestrol	8.76
Estrone	8.59
Estradiol	8.02
Dienestrol	7.73
Promestrol dipropionate	6.83
Diethylstilbestrol dipalmitate	6.60
Sodium estrone sulphate	4.00
Monomestrol	3.26
Hexestrol	2.48
Estriol	2.26
Control	1.00

tiny doses, since the target cells they stimulate are exquisitely responsive to low concentrations and promptly react by characteristic changes. On the other hand, prolonged high doses seem to overwhelm the receptors of the target cells and apparently exhaust the cytoplasmic structures that produce them (NORDQVIST 1970) so that specific enzyme systems become blocked (VILLEE 1961), and the cells become unable to respond to further estrogen. Atrophy ensues. An estrogenic effect also fails to develop when the receptors have been blocked by clomiphene or norethisterone. For example, in monkeys very high doses of estrogen lead to endometrial atrophy (HARTMANN et al. 1941), whereas in other animals (rabbits, mice) prolonged treatment with small doses promotes the induction of carcinoma (ALLEN 1942; DUNN and GREEN 1963; GRAHAM et al. 1980).

The oral or parenteral administration of estradiol alone from the 1st day of a menstrual cycle prolongs the proliferative phase and suppresses the secretion of gonadotropins by the pituitary, especially FSH. Development of a corpus luteum is inhibited until the estrogen is discontinued. Menstruation is consequently delayed (ZONDEK 1940). Treatment with estradiol during the secretory phase results in severe stromal edema (EGGER and KINDERMANN 1974), delay in secretory transformation of glands and stroma, and a disruption of the nucleolar channel system, an organelle normally found in the glandular cell nuclei of the secretory endometrium (see p. 26; GORDON et al. 1973). If the estrogen is discontinued after prolonged therapy, an estrogen "withdrawal bleeding" ensues; if the estrogen is given over a long period in consistently small doses, a spontaneous "breakthrough bleeding" occurs. Short-term treatment with progesterone prevents these two types of bleeding. The hemorrhage that follows after the progesterone is discontinued ("progesterone withdrawal bleeding") is never as profuse as with the estrogen withdrawal bleeding, which is due to tissue necrosis without dissociation of fibers. With only one injection of a depot estrogen the proliferation reaches its maximum after 3 weeks; thereafter the glands and stromal cells begin to degenerate (HEMPEL and BÖHM 1976). With prolonged administration of small doses of estradiol (20–100 µg daily) the endometrium responds with glandular-cystic hyperplasia (SCHRÖDER 1954; BLOOMFIELD 1957; GREENBLATT and ZARATE 1967; OBER and BRONSTEIN 1967; ROSENWAKS et al. 1979; and many others; see Fig. 57). Only estriol is less harmful to the endometrium (SJÖSTEDT and STRANDA 1971). From time to time portions of these hyperplastic endometria may undergo hemorrhagic necrosis and be discharged, but when the estrogen stimulus continues, unopposed by progesterone, they may progress to *precancerous adenomatous hyperplasias* (see p. 120). With the scanning electron microscope the superficial epithelium becomes furry with numerous, long microvilli. Their length is proportional to the potency of the estrogen administered (NATHAN et al. 1978). Droplets of fat appear in stromal cells of the upper layers of the endometrium (BLACK et al. 1941) and foam cells, which store estrogen metabolites or related substances (see p. 123) eventually develop. In contrast to the hyperplasias arising in the pre- and postclimacteric periods because of endogenous causes, those developing after many years of estrogen therapy are characterized by special morphological features: they develop multicentrically and even in the adenomatous stage may be circumscribed or polypoid. In the adenomatous regions the appearance of the nuclei and cytoplasm of the epithelial cells varies from gland to gland. Both flattened and nodular formations of metaplastic squamous epithelium as well as other types of metaplasia are especially common (HENDRICKSON and KEMPSON 1980). Consequently, treatment of patients in the climacterium or after the menopause for long periods merely because of annoying symptoms is not without danger. That danger can be minimized or eliminated when small doses of estrogen are combined with small doses of gestagen. If bleeding develops during therapy, it behooves one to find out why by histological studies.

β) Gestagens

The synthetic gestagens used clinically differ both chemically and metabolically from natural progesterone (JUNKMANN 1963; SUCHOWSKI and BALDRATTI 1964). Most are derivatives of 17α-hydroxyprogesterone or 19-nortestosterone (see Table 12). Although their gestagenic potencies vary considerably, most are more potent than natural progesterone. Norgestrel, which in its d-form is the most active gestagen known at present, is 80 times more active than progesterone. Its high potency may be due in part to its selective uptake by the endometrium, for as radioautographic studies have shown (ZALDIVAR and GALLEGOS 1971), more norgestrel localizes in the endometrium than does progesterone or chlormadinone. Accordingly, in contrast to the effects of natural progesterone, those produced by the synthetic gestagens depend closely on dosage, but what is really important is not so much the amount administered but the potency of the gestagen used. On the other hand, the potency varies depending on the chemical structure of the gestagen. To determine that potency, the demonstration of basal vacuoles of glycogen in the glandular cells ("the transformation dose") yields more accurate results than the "delay of menstruation test" (DICKEY and STONE 1976).

The administration of progesterone alone during the proliferative phase depresses the maturation of Graafian follicles, arrests endometrial proliferation, and postpones or prevents ovulation. If given during the secretory phase, progesterone prolongs the menstrual cycle. When progesterone is discontinued a with-

Table 12. Synthetic gestagens used in oral contraceptives

		Gestagen potency	Transformation dose (mg/cycle)
Derivatives of 17α-hydroxypro-gesterone	Megestrol acetate	2.0	35–50
	Chlormadinone acetate	20.0	20–30
	Medroxyprogesterone acetate	1.0	40–70
Derivatives of 19-nortestosterone	Norgestrel	80.0	12
	Norethynodrel	0.4	150–200
	Lynestrenol	2.7	35–70
	Ethynodiol diacetate	20.0	10–15
	Norethindrone (norethisterone)	1.3	100–150
	Norethindrone acetate	2.7	50–60
	Quingestanol acetate	5.4	

drawal bleeding occurs within a few days; when continued at low doses a breakthrough bleeding develops during therapy. If 5–6 mg chlormadinone acetate are given daily for 4 weeks or longer, then the secretory change is abolished and the endometrium remains in a state of *"arrested proliferation"* (BAYER 1965). With treatment beyond 6 weeks the arrested proliferation gives way to progressive atrophy of the glands and decidualization of the stroma. After 3 months of continuous therapy, amounting to a total dose of about 500 mg progesterone, a typical decidualized stroma develops with extreme or complete atrophy of the glands: *"arrested secretion"* (*starre Sekretion,* WINTER and POTS 1956; Fig. 82). The same picture can be produced experimentally in castrated monkeys after priming with estrogen (HISAW and HISAW 1961). Most likely, such exogenous progesterone, in the manner of a feedback mechanism, inhibits the secretion of FSH by the pituitary. If treatment is continued it may eventually lead to an irreversible *atrophy* with hyalinization of the stroma (CHARLES 1964; BAYER 1965; Fig. 83). Large daily doses induce similar results, but even then the duration of treatment is decisive. The various synthetic gestagens differ both quantitatively and qualitatively in their action. The dosage required to produce a transformation of the endometrium varies from preparation to preparation; with progesterone about 200 mg are needed, with the synthetic gestagens considerably less (see Table 12). Moreover, some gestagens may affect mostly the stroma, others primarily the glands. Following therapy with derivatives of 19-nortesterone, decidualization is more pronounced and the subsequent atrophy more extreme than with derivatives of progesterone (FRIEDRICH 1967). Since the glandular epithelial cells are more sensitive to progesterone and react to it earlier than the stromal cells do, the epithelium usually becomes refractory sooner to abnormal stimulation by gestagens, whereas the stroma begins to atrophy only after a prolonged decidualization (DALLENBACH-HELLWEG 1972).

In using gestagens in the treatment of endometriosis one not only takes advantage of their antiproliferative action (see GUNNING and MOYER 1967) but also of their effectiveness in producing a protracted delay in menstruation (CARTER et al. 1964). Even after the menopause, treatment with gestagens over a long period may lead to the development of a typical decidua, which differs from a decidua of pregnancy only by the atrophy of its glands (Fig. 84; see Table 23; p. 330f.). Occasionally, gestagen therapy is used to inhibit the progression of inoperable endometrial carcinomas and their metastases (see p. 272ff.). Natural progesterone is of value as substitution therapy, for example, for patients with deficient secretory phases during the last week of the menstrual cycle (GILLIAM 1955; GLASS et al. 1955; MOSZKOWSKI et al. 1962), and in supporting HMG-induced pregnancies (CHECK et al. 1985). Since estrogen is also deficient in some of these patients, they may require treatment with both hormones (ROLAND 1967). By administering gestagens to a patient with primary amenorrhea (the *progesterone withdrawal test*), it is possible to determine whether the patient produces estrogen or not. The test depends on the fact that the endometrium is unable to respond to progesterone without prior stimulation by estrogen ("estrogen priming"). If the patient does produce estrogen, then a progesterone withdrawal bleeding sets in 2–8 days after giving the gestagen. To evaluate the functional state of the endometrium, the *estrogen withdrawal*

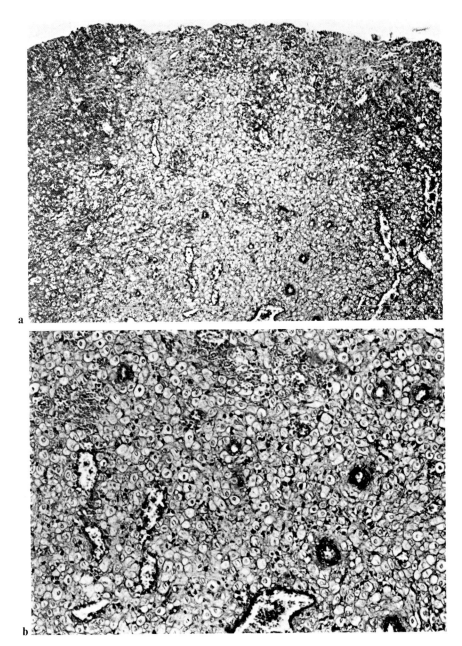

Fig. 82a, b. Stromal cells are transformed into decidual cells ("arrested secretion"). Advanced atrophy of glands and decidual change of stromal cells after many weeks of progestational therapy. a Low magnification; b higher magnification

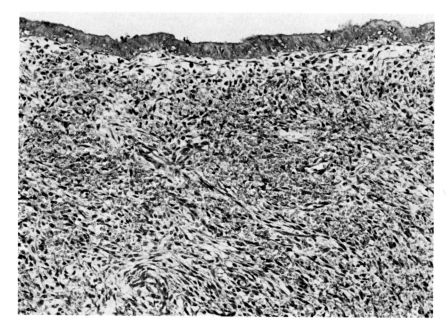

Fig. 83. Atrophy and fibrosis of the endometrium with complete loss of glands after several months of gestagen therapy

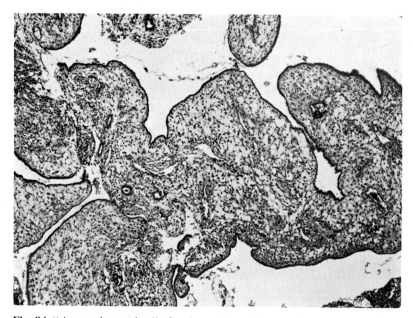

Fig. 84. "Arrested secretion" after 9 months of Orgametril

test may be performed. If the patient fails to bleed after discontinuing estrogen therapy, her amenorrhea is caused by anatomical (for example, aplasia, tuberculosis) or functional (for example, refractory target cells) abnormalities of the endometrium ("uterine amenorrhea").

γ) Both Hormones

By administering both hormones as they appear in a normal cycle, it proved possible to reproduce a regular menstrual cycle in castrated monkeys (HISAW 1935) and in castrated women (KAUFMANN 1933, 1939). What turned out to be important, however, was the relative amounts of the hormones (FERIN 1954; 1955, 1963; NEVINNY-STICKEL 1964; GOOD and MOYER 1968; see Fig. 85). Depending on the level of endogenous estrogen, the amount of gestagen needed was found to fluctuate considerably (RUDEL et al. 1964). Whereas 30 mg progesterone may be sufficient to induce a secretory transformation of an artificially induced proliferation phase, about 400 mg are needed to treat a glandular-cystic hyperplasia (GRUNER 1942). If the dose of estrogen given a castrated woman is too high or the dose of progesterone too low, then the secretory change may either be delayed up to 10 days or remain deficient (FERIN 1963). Because of these fluctuations the normal buildup of the endometrium should be checked histologically and controlled by repeating endometrial biopsies. By using the long-acting gestagens (e.g., 17-ethinyl-19-nortestosterone-onanthate) and depot estrogens, one application during a cycle is enough to elicit a menstrual-like breakthrough bleeding (DAVIS and WIED 1957; BOSCHANN and KUR 1957). These and other synthetic preparations are ideal for treating functional bleeding and

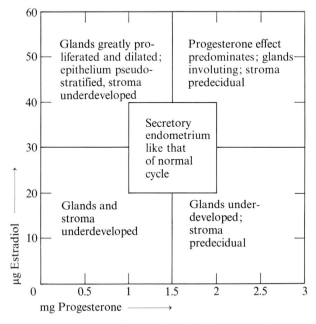

Fig. 85. Reaction of the endometrium to the administration of estrogen and progesterone. (Modified from GOOD and MOYER 1968)

secondary amenorrheas (BORGLIN 1962; DOMINGUEZ et al. 1962; CHARLES et al. 1964). Amenorrheas due primarily to ovarian insufficiency at times require a pretreatment only with estrogen (GOLD et al. 1965; OBER and BRONSTEIN 1967).

δ) Oral Contraceptive Agents

Hormonal therapy in gynecology, even today, is dominated by the oral contraceptive agents. Although these medications are occasionally used to correct abnormalities of hormonal regulatory mechanisms (functional bleeding, dysmenorrhea, endometriosis), their main use is for birth control. Based on experimental studies in animals (HABERLANDT 1921), BICKENBACH and PAULIKOVICS (1944) succeeded in suppressing ovulation in women by administering 20 mg progesterone daily, just as MISHELL et al. did later (1968). The same suppressive effect follows the administration of estrogen alone during the proliferative phase (BOARD and BORLAND 1964; and many others). Since studies soon showed that prolonged therapy with progesterone alone led to frequent breakthrough bleeding and eventual atrophy of the endometrium, and unopposed estrogen induced endometrial hyperplasia, combinations of both hormones in appropriate dosages were tried. As gestagen, derivatives of 19-nortestosterone or 17α-hydroprogesterone acetate were used, and are still in use. As estrogen, either 17α-ethinylestradiol or its methyl ether, mestranol, was selected because of its potent, prolonged effect. The doses of both hormones initially employed were reduced to the minimal concentrations still affording successful contraception, with the hopes of avoiding side effects that some patients treated with the first preparations had experienced. One should not forget that it is the potency of the hormones that determines how effective they act, not the dosage (HEINEN 1971). It is also important to remember that some women metabolize the gestagen components of some of the combination preparations into products having estrogenic and androgenic effects. It has been found that no direct relationships exist between the gestagen activity, that is, the dose of gestagen needed to produce secretory transformation, and the degree of ovulatory suppression (percentage of ovulations inhibited) (TAUSK 1969). Since 1953, PINCUS and coworkers have studied the use of many different preparations extensively (see PINCUS 1965). Since then, throughout the world, many investigators have introduced and tested countless new combination preparations of diverse chemical composition in varying dosages, and from the experience gained, have subsequently modified their preparations or developed newer ones. To list all of them now, as attempted in the first edition of this book, would far exceed the bounds set by its purpose, and the continual, rapid progress in developing new preparations would soon make such a list obsolete. What is important for diagnosing histological changes is not their names but their chemical composition (see Tables 11 and 12). Most hormonal contraceptives are administered as "combination" preparations, containing both estrogen and progestin, or as "sequential" preparations. The combination agents are taken either as pills for 20 consecutive days each menstrual cycle, usually from the 5th to the 24th day, or are given as a single injection or pill that lasts for the same period. Treatment with the sequential agents mimics the natural secretion of hormones by the ovaries, and involves taking a pill of estrogen alone from the 5th to 19th days (or 5th–14th days) to suppress ovulation. Thereafter, a pill containing both estrogen and progestin is taken until the 24th day to produce a secretory change and a menstrual-like breakthrough bleeding (KAISER 1963; GOLDZIEHER et al. 1964).

Another method is the use of progesterone alone, either orally as a "minipill", to be taken each day, or parenterally as a depot injection. New developments are the three sequence preparations, which provide minimal doses of both estrogen and progestin not possible with previous agents. Not only do these preparations reduce the overall burden with exogenous hormones, they also interfere less with the secretion of FSH and LH. They have not been used long enough, however, to allow adequate long-time evaluation of the histological changes they might induce.

As the use of all these preparations by healthy women has become more widespread, so have reports about their side effects bourgeoned to a voluminous literature, covering not only a wide spectrum of changes in many organs and tissues but also disturbances of hematological, endocrinological and neurological function. Since extensive reviews of these innumerable reports are available (for example, KIRCHHOFF and HALLER 1964; BORELL 1966; BARBER et al. 1969, HILLIARD and NORRIS 1979) there is no need to concern ourselves with them further. What primarily interests the gynecologist and pathologist, however, are the morphological effects of the oral contraceptives on the female reproductive system, and as regards this monograph, their effects on the endometrium.

As we have already noted (see p. 50), the endometrium is our most sensitive indicator for gauging the levels and proportions of the sex hormones in the blood. In healthy women the endometrium responds to exogenous hormonal therapy by very definite histological changes. The mass experiment now being carried out by the users of the antifertility agents has shown beyond all doubt that these endometrial changes take place with a precision that is astounding for a biological system. Consequently, by studying the endometrium and knowing about the hormonal state prior to therapy, it is possible with practice to determine how much and what type of antifertility agent the patient has received. Because most of the oral contraceptives used at present are similar in composition, the endometrium reacts to most in much the same way. Nevertheless, one can detect differences in the effects of some preparations (particularly differences between combination agents and sequential agents) when their dosages and chemical compositions vary (see JACKSON 1963; ROLAND et al. 1964, 1966; MEARS 1965; YANEVA et al. 1965; MORF and MÜLLER 1966; OBER 1966; RUDEL et al. 1966). One may also perceive distinctive variations that depend upon the patient's state of hormonal equilibrium, and these may vary within physiological limits between "predominately estrogen" to "predominately gestagen" (TENHAEFF 1971). Further variations in response among patients may occasionally be seen even when the same preparation is used to treat functional disturbances, since the response depends on the differences in endocrine dysfunction from patient to patient existing prior to treatment.

With almost all **combination preparations** the proliferative phase of the first few cycles is characteristically shortened, consequently the glands and stroma fail to develop completely. Equally characteristic is the premature appearance of persistently deficient secretory changes in the glands and stroma, with the glands remaining uncoiled. These abnormal changes can be readily explained: to reach its peak of proliferation and full development a normal endometrium needs 14 days of continuous stimulation by estrogen. By using a combination antifertility pill from the 5th day of the cycle on, that estrogen stimulation is prematurely interrupted by the gestagen component, inducing an early arrest of both growth and differentiation of the glandular epithelium at its incompletely developed stage. Continued therapy prevents further development and the epithelium remains immature. Another distinctive feature of the artificially arrested cycle is the remarkable intermingling of glands and stroma in very different stages of maturity, none of which corresponds to the true day of the cycle. As a result, the surface of the endometrium becomes uneven, eventually growing rough through knobby outgrowths and polypoid excrescences (Fig. 86). This colorful picture resembles in part that of the deficient secretory phase, which in its hormone levels also shows certain similarities to the artificially inhibited levels (Fig. 87).

In general, the following changes are observed to occur *during the first cycles of therapy*. The *endometrial glands* are unevenly distributed and vary greatly in their development, the degree of variation depending on how long treatment has lasted. Some glands are distinctly atrophic and narrow; others are enlarged and at times even cystically dilated, lined usually by small, low cuboidal epithelial cells, rarely by proliferated, tall columnar cells (Fig. 87b, 88). Near these glands one will often encounter other glands that are moderately dilated, composed of low epithelial cells with scanty cytoplasm and small, rounded nuclei. Occasionally small or larger vacuoles of glycogen may be found

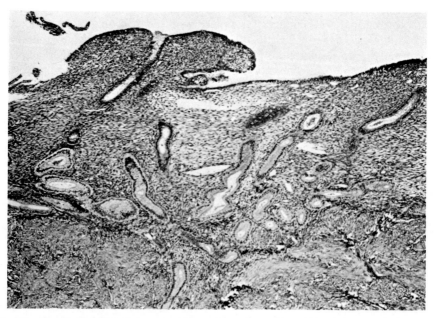

Fig. 86. After 6 months of Anovlar the endometrial surface is nodular, stromal edema is spotty, and the glands are variously developed: abortive secretion

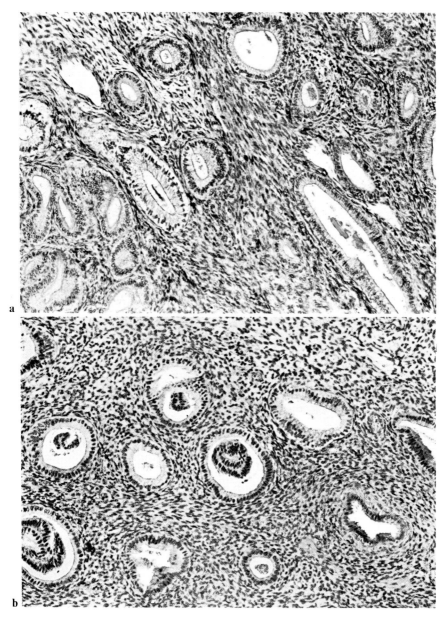

Fig. 87a, b. A prematurely deficient secretory phase. The glands are in various stages of abortive secretion. The stromal cells are spindly. **a** After 6 months of Anovlar; **b** after 6 months of Ovulen

near the nuclei, which are then located at random. The quantity of glycogen formed will vary, depending on the dosage and composition of the gestagen component of the agent used. After derivatives of progesterone there is more glycogen than after nortestosterone (SIEGEL and HEINEN 1965). In contrast, gly-

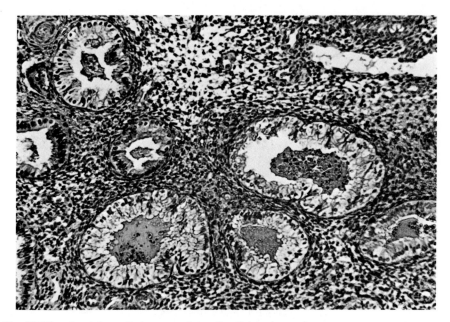

Fig. 88. The glandular cells become clear after Primosiston therapy

cogen in the lumen is virtually always lacking because its secretion from the cells is inhibited; the apical margin of the cell is always smooth and sharply defined. Acid mucopolysaccharides appear only after derivatives of progesterone, and then merely in small amounts. In the first half of the cycle mitoses are rare. The glandular nuclei contain small nucleoli which electron-microscopically appear rarefied and reveal no nucleolar channel system in the second half of the cycle (CLYMAN 1963). The cytoplasmic structures remain poorly developed throughout the cycle (ANCLA et al. 1965; FRIEDRICH 1967). The mitochondria are reduced in number and size, have only a few cristae (CLYMAN 1963), and are electron-optically dense owing to changes in their membranes which contain lipids. The granular endoplasmic reticulum is extremely sparse and protein synthesis is reduced accordingly (VERHAGEN and THEMANN 1965, 1970; TOTH et al. 1972). In contrast, the cells contain abundant lipid granules.

The spotty edema of the *stroma* is striking, accentuated by the non-edematous parts composed of dense small or spindly cells (Fig. 89). The ratio of glands to stroma is shifted in favor of the stroma. Depending on the dosage of gestagen in the preparation used (see TAYMOR 1961), a distinct predecidual or decidual change may take place prematurely (15th–20th day of the cycle) and abundant granulocytes appear (Fig. 90). After therapy with 17α-hydroxyprogesterone the synthesis of DNA by the stromal cells is measurably increased (FETTIG 1965). Ultrastructurally, the rough and smooth endoplasmic reticulum as well as the Golgi apparatus are hyperplastic; glycogen begins to accumulate (WIENKE et al. 1969). Occasionally, with the breakthrough bleeding that follows, decidual casts of the endometrial cavity are shed, resembling those discharged in dysmenorrhea membranacea. The differentiation of the stromal cells into

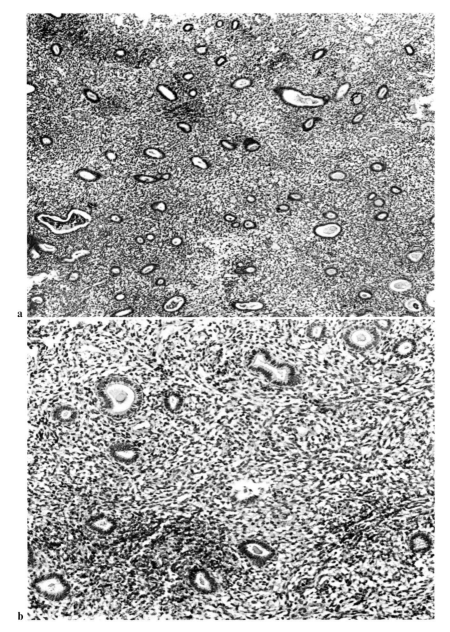

Fig. 89a, b. Beginning atrophy of the endometrium after 6 months of Anovlar. **a** Low magnification; **b** higher magnification

predecidual cells and granulocytes is not always coordinated, and even regions composed of small stromal cells may contain abundant granulocytes. In other parts of the stroma the cells may exhibit no evidence of differentiation. The development of the *reticulum network* varies greatly from region to region.

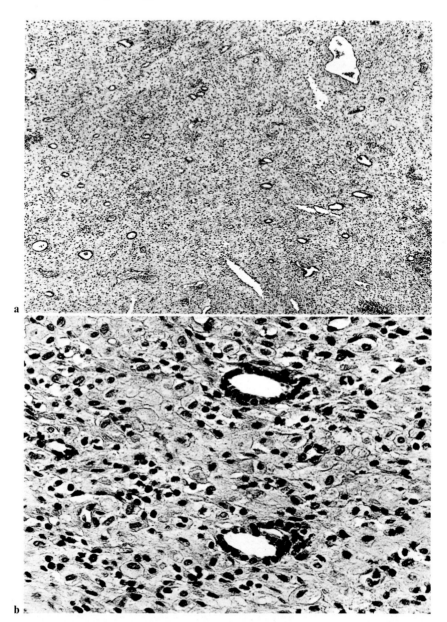

Fig. 90 a, b. Arrested secretion after combined hormonal therapy, the gestagen component however predominating. The glands are strikingly small and atrophic, the stroma has undergone decidual change. **a** Low magnification; **b** high magnification

Stroma containing well-formed, dense fibers may merge with stroma in which the fibers are either sparse or not demonstrable. WAIDL et al. (1968) drew attention to the absence of a normal reticulum network, particularly in the second half of the cycle.

The *blood vessels* undergo extraordinary changes. Generally the spiral arteries fail to develop. In their stead we find small or dilated capillaries. In rare instances a spiral artery may proliferate but does so prematurely and incompletely. The development of the vascular branchings in the superficial endometrium, especially of the subepithelial sinusoids, parallels the predecidual change of the stromal cells, and is therefore often focally intensified. ANCLA et al. (1965) were impressed by the proliferation of the endothelial cells in these vessels; it resembles that seen during pregnancy or that produced experimentally in the endometria of monkeys by relaxin (DALLENBACH-HELLWEG et al. 1966). BLAUSTEIN et al. (1968) found such vascular proliferations in 48% of endometria of patients taking the combination agents and in 73% of them receiving sequential agents. Perhaps fluctuations in hormones stimulate the abundant granulocytes, which are found focally in the predecidually changed stroma, to release their relaxin prematurely, thus causing the endothelial cells to proliferate. Some authors (OBER et al. 1964; CROWSON et al. 1965; OBER 1966, 1977; IREY et al. 1970) have even reported finding intense dilatation of stromal vessels and thromboses. Characteristic are small, or even large, focal hemorrhagic necroses of the stroma that probably account for the *protracted breakthrough bleeding* which often necessitates curettage. The breakthrough bleeding is a manifestation of the disturbed hormonal balance and is caused by a temporary, dose-dependent, relative or absolute deficiency of either of the two hormones administered. Accordingly, it may represent an estrogen-withdrawal bleeding like that of an anovulatory cycle, or it may represent a progesterone withdrawal bleeding with release of relaxin like that of menstruation, except it is protracted and develops focally. Because it develops so irregularly and imperfectly, the endometrium most likely does not shed normally, in some cases it may not shed at all, the retained portions merely shrinking. As a result the roughness of the endometrium is intensified. The lack of shedding may be recognized by finding slightly dilated glands filled with old inspissated blood, telltale evidence of a previous cyclic bleeding. Although most of the blood from such hemorrhages is probably discharged from the uterine cavity, some apparently seeps into patent glandular lumina of the adjacent, nondesquamated mucosa, to coagulate and remain there for long periods (cf. p. 98, Fig. 41), rarely even forming psammoma bodies (VALICENTI and PRIESTER 1977).

The *variations* in the histological picture, which depend, as already implied, on the dosages and types of preparations, are readily seen electron-microscopically (FRIEDRICH 1967). After using the combination agents the principle alterations found are the predecidual reaction and the concomitant sinusoidal dilatation of the vessels, the thromboses and the breakthrough hemorrhages. After higher doses of gestagens (5–10 mg) and after 19-nortestosterone these alterations are more intense than after using lower doses of gestagens (0.5–2 mg) and after 17α-hydroxyprogesterone acetate. As mentioned before, some synthetic gestagens are up to 80 times more active than natural progesterone (SUCHOWSKY and BALDRATTI 1964; VOKAER 1964; see Table 12). The frequent breakthrough bleeding after higher doses of gestagen can probably be explained by the development of many granulocytes in the predecidual stroma. With the fall of the gestagen these granulocytes liberate their relaxin, causing dissolution of the stromal fibers. Equivalent breakthrough hemorrhages can be produced in the endometria of monkeys by hormonal means (DALLENBACH-HELLWEG et al. 1966).

Therapy with *monthly injections of 17α-dehydroprogesterone and estradiol* results in proliferative changes with glandular mitoses during the first 9 days of the cycle, followed by irregular and insufficient glandular secretion and predecidual stromal transformation during the remaining part of the cycle (CZERNO- BILSKY et al. 1969). The secretory suppression is less pronounced than with the oral combination contraceptives, although great individual variances may be observed. These may be explained by individual differences in absorption rates of both hormones from cycle to cycle.

Since such a wide spectrum of histological pictures may develop, it is obvious why an accurate *dating of the endometrium* is impossible and why the daily changes advance imperfectly. For instance, during a cycle inhibited by oral contraceptive agents we may find only minimal variations, limited principally to differences in glandular development and in extent of focal breakthrough bleeding. Basal secretory vacuoles usually appear on the 7th or 8th day of the cycle, and the secretion may reach its "maximum" by the 13th–15th day. Thereafter the glands generally regress to a resting afunctional state. The focal predecidual reaction oridinarily either begins on the 20th day (RYAN et al. 1964; STARUP 1967) or fails to develop (KRAUSE et al. 1968). Invariably there is striking discrepancy in the development among the glands as well as between the glands and stroma.

In contrast, the *prolonged use* of contraceptive agents results in further histological changes. The abortive secretory changes gradually subside from cycle to cycle, and finally disappear (see GOLDZIEHER et al. 1964; RYAN et al. 1964; CROWSON et al. 1965; AZZOPARDI and ZAYID 1967; ROBEY et al. 1968). In some women the *endometrium atrophies,* and with its sparse and tiny glands it is indistinguishable from that of a non-treated, castrated woman (see CHARLES 1964; SHEFFIELD et al. 1969; Figs. 91 and 92). Somewhat later the glands may disappear, or their indistinct remnants, lined by flattened endothelial-like cells, may readily be confused with capillaries. The stroma becomes poor in cells, consisting primarily of collagenous fibers. A protracted breakthrough bleeding may supervene in these atrophic endometria. Such bleeding is probably due in part to the associated atrophic changes in the walls of blood vessels, in part to the focal refractoriness of endometrial tissue for one of the hormones (receptor function lost), causing a relative and real decrease in hormonal action locally. Immunohistochemically, no estrogen receptor-positive staining is detectable with the ER-ICA assay in the glandular or stromal nuclei of these atrophic endometria. The secondary amenorrhea that occasionally develops in these women can easily be explained by a complete refractoriness of the endometrium to hormones (Fig. 93). We have observed several patients in whom massive doses of hormones, given to induce ovulation, failed to produce any change in the refractory endometria (see also SHERMAN 1971, 1975), results similar to those obtained experimentally in monkeys (see HISAW and HISAW 1961). Thus this iatrogenic atrophy differs not only histologically from the physiological atrophy of ageing but also functionally by failing to respond to treatment. Physiological atrophy always responds to hormonal therapy and still possesses estrogen receptors detectable immunohistochemically. In contrast, iatrogenic atrophy does not always react, perhaps because the few surviving endometrial

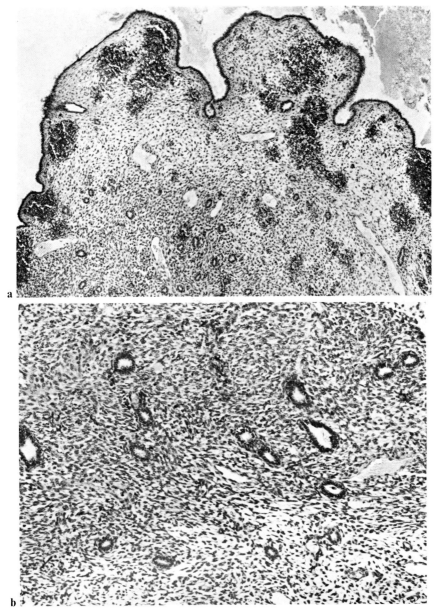

Fig. 91a, b. Advanced atrophy of the endometrium after Anovlar therapy for 9 months. **a** Survey view to show irregular surface and focal withdrawal hemorrhages. **b** Higher magnification

cells are unable to produce receptors for estrogen, a result of genetic injury or mutation caused by the protracted therapy with the synthetic hormones (contraceptive agents). DODEK and KOTZ (1967) have described an anovulatory syndrome developing in women after use of antifertility agents. Such extreme

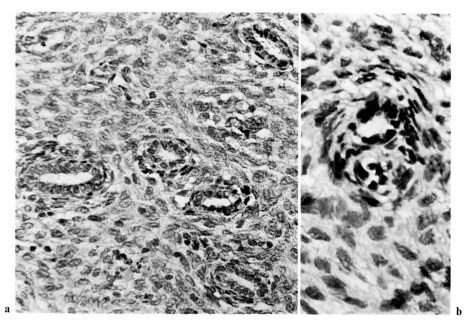

Fig. 92a, b. Same case as in Fig. 91. Some glands atrophic (a), others wasting away (b)

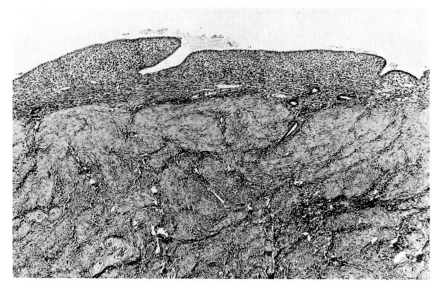

Fig. 93. Advanced atrophy of endometrium of a 41-year-old patient after continuous use of oral contraceptives, combination type, for 3 years

consequences, however, are rare, limited to single cases. Generally in atrophic endometria, between the regions without glands there are regions of reactive basal hyperplasia, from which regeneration still seems possible. – Other patients react to the long-term hormonal therapy with hyperplastic changes of the endo-

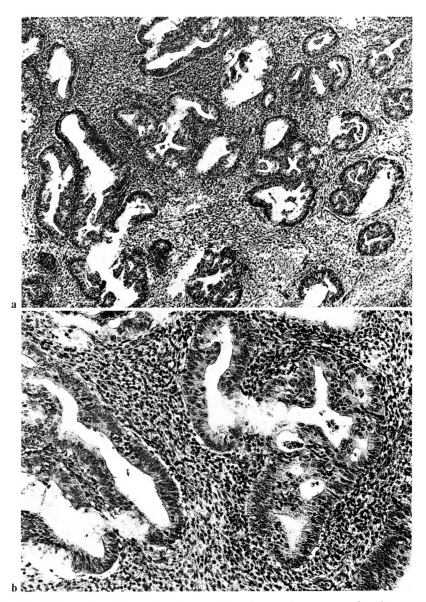

Fig. 94a, b. Beginning adenomatous hyperplasia after continuous use of oral contraceptives for 4 years. **a** Low magnification; **b** high magnification

metrial glands. That reaction may in rare instances lead to glandular-cystic (LAUFER 1968) or *adenomatous hyperplasia,* indicating that only the endometrial sensitivity to estrogen has persisted (or that the gestagen component of the therapy, for one reason or another, failed to exert its effect on the endometrium) (Fig. 94). Such glandular proliferation primarily develops after prolonged treatment with agents that contain high doses of estrogen, e.g., after sequential agents, or after metabolic conversion of gestagens into compounds with estrogenic action (CHARLES 1964; GOLDFARB 1964; HENZL et al. 1964). Squamous metaplasia of the hyperplastic endometrial glands is occasionally observed after prolonged use of certain agents (for example, after norethisterone) and may persist as long as 4 months after therapy has been stopped. SCHMID (1968) described atypical and precancerous hyperplasia of the endometrial glands with papillary proliferation and evidence of cellular secretion after long-term therapy with Lyndiol.

On the other hand, DOCKERTY et al. (1959) pointed out that when the gestagenic component predominates, the predecidual reaction it induces may assume a pseudosarcomatous appearance after prolonged use. Even the development of true endometrial sarcoma with pronounced nuclear pleomorphism, abundant abnormal mitoses and "positive cytology" has been observed after use of both Norlestin and Provest for 3–5 years (SONG et al. 1970). More frequently a nodular *stromal hyperplasia* with hyperchromatic, enlarged nuclei, with excessive formation of reticulum fibers, and with capillary or arteriolar proliferation may be found in patients taking oral contraceptives (Fig. 95). These changes should not be confused with the rare presarcomatous stromal hyperplasia (cf. p. 134). What the long-term prognosis of these nodular stromal hyperplasias might be we cannot state or predict at the present. We will only learn by experience whether these hormone-induced changes will eventually evolve into the presarcomatous variety of stromal hyperplasia. If they do, then we should expect a great increase in the frequency of endometrial sarcoma in the next 10–20 years.

Therapy with the **sequential agents** (for example, Estirona) produces still other histological pictures, because the first progestational stimulus acts on the endometrium at a later phase of the cycle. The most prominent changes are the prolongation of the proliferative phase induced by the estrogen and the delay in the appearance of secretion. Although the secretory changes may develop uniformly, they persist as deficient. Often there is pronounced stromal edema but in spite of it the endometrium remains low, that is, its height reduced. In their rather large series of women who received sequential contraceptive agents, GOLDZIEHER et al. (1964) and MAQUEO et al. (1964) found no evidence of secretory changes by the 22nd day of the inhibited cycle (2 days after beginning the progestational agent). On the 26th day, that is, shortly before onset of withdrawal bleeding, the endometrial glands resembled those of the 2nd day after a normal ovulation; they revealed no signs of involution. From our experience, a predecidual change usually fails to occur and endometrial granulocytes are rare. The spiral arteries remain poorly developed (BOARD and BORLAND 1964). OBER et al. (1966) were able to confirm these results with the sequential type of contraceptive agents when their patients took the progestational component for only 5 days. In contrast, after 10 days of progestational therapy (2 mg chlormadinone daily) these investigators found a decidual reaction at the end of the sequential cycle in 10% of their patients. After 20 days of such therapy the endometria of most of the women displayed a decidual reaction but the spiral arteries remained poorly developed.

Prolonged therapy with the sequential type agents leads to similar histological changes. An endometrial atrophy, as seen with the combination agents, rarely

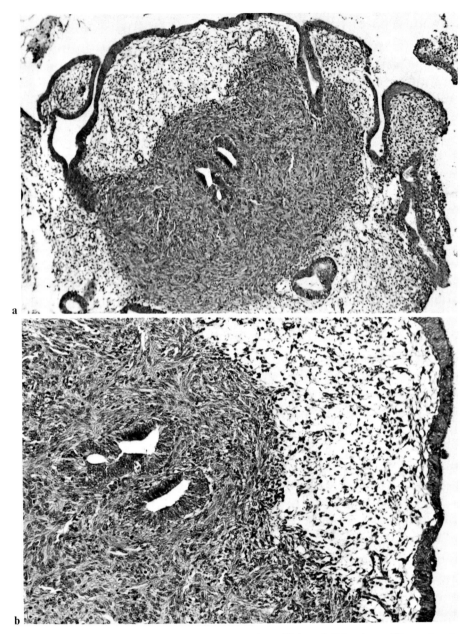

Fig. 95a, b. Focal stromal hyperplasia ("stromaloma") in a deficiently proliferated endometrium after oral contraceptives. **a** Low magnification; **b** higher magnification

occurs. Nevertheless, as successive biopsies will prove, the sensitivity of the endometrium (especially the glands) to the hormones gradually diminishes from cycle to cycle. The histological pictures may show an irregular proliferation or resemble a deficient secretory phase of a moderately severe ovarian insufficiency (FETTIG and KOPECKY 1968). Because the estrogen effect predominates, many investigators report finding that glandular-cystic hyperplasia (up to 50%), adenomatous hyperplasia (up to 13%) and more recently endometrial carcinoma develop more frequently than with combination therapy (LYON 1975; SILVERBERG and MAROWSKI 1975; VANDERICK et al. 1975; KELLEY et al. 1976; KREUTNER et al. 1976; LYON and FRISCH 1976; COHEN and DEPPE 1977; REEVES and KAUFMAN 1977; SILVERBERG et al. 1977). The sequential agents are less reliable contraceptives than are the combination agents; breakthrough ovulations occur in about 8% of the women who use sequential pills (MEARS 1965).

The effect on the endometrium of **daily small doses of a progestational agent** alone or of an injectable long-acting gestagen is more intense than that of combined preparations, and parallels that seen with gestagen treatment for endometriosis (cf. p. 162). Even during the first cycles after onset of therapy, the progestational agent severely retards the growth of the endometrium. A discordance in the development of the glands and stroma appears that varies in extent and quality, depending on the type of gestagen given, and leads to various degrees of arrested secretion.

Abortive secretion of glands may be seen as early as the 7th day of the cycle. The secretion of glycoprotein is diminished. The spiral arterioles remain underdeveloped. The reticular network appears fragmented or may not be visualized at all (KÜHNE et al. 1972). Treatment with quingestanol acetate, a potent gestagen, leads to pronounced histochemical abnormalities during all phases of the menstrual cycle (FLOWERS et al. 1974): diastase-resistant mucopolysaccharides accumulate at the apical border of the glandular cells. At their bases, small foci of glycogen persist throughout the secretory phase. The activities of succinic dehydrogenase, alkaline and acid phosphatases remain unaltered, suggesting that the transport ability of the epithelial cells is little affected. The cyclic variations in the acid mucosubstances also remain normal: the sulfomucins predominate during the proliferative phase and the carboxylmucins during the secretory phase. The endometrial blood vessels are dilated and may contain thrombi or aggregates of platelets, which are PAS positive and diastase resistant.

Pronounced changes also become apparent in the ultrastructure of glandular cells, which reveal signs of disturbed and premature differentiation and degeneration with elongated mitochondria, of irregularly developed endoplasmic reticulum, and of partial loss of the intranucleolar channel system during the secretory phase (FERIA-VELASCO et al. 1972; FLOWERS et al. 1974; MARUFFO et al. 1974). Many cells reveal abundant tonofilaments and microtubules associated with increases in ribosomes and granular endoplasmic reticulum. These suggest that the organelles needed for glycogen synthesis and transport are present, yet the amounts of glycoprotein and the transport systems within the cells are abnormal. After a single injection of medroxyprogesterone acetate, these changes are still reversible within 90 days (ROBERTS et al. 1975). As shown by scanning electron microscopy the ciliogenesis of the endometrial surface epithelium is defective, the number of cilia is reduced, and the non-ciliated cells close to the gland openings may exhibit destruction of their apical membranes (LUDWIG 1982). – Endometrial atrophy usually ensues earlier during continuous treatment with these progestational agents than with the combination type of contraceptives

(LEE 1969; KHOO et al. 1971). That is why a curettage usually proves unsuccessful, providing little to no tissue for histological examination.

Hence, contrary to previous assumptions, these agents do have an effect on the endometrium and on pituitary or ovarian function (MOGHISSI et al. 1973). In some of the patients taking low doses of gestagens, ovulation and fertilization may take place. The alteration of the endometrial architecture, however, renders normal placentation impossible, resulting in spontaneous abortion, primarily because of the underdeveloped decidua. A defective development of the blastocyst may also be regarded as a direct effect of the gestagen on the fertilized ovum (cf. p. 302). In addition, since peristaltic movement and secretory activity of the fallopian tubes are decreased (MALL-HAEFELI et al. 1976), there is a two- to five-fold risk of ectopic pregnancy (LIUKKO et al. 1977). In other patients chlormadinone has been noted to inhibit ovulation. Norgestrel almost regularly inhibits ovulation, and in addition alters endometrial structure, cervical mucus and hypothalamic-pituitary function (MOGHISSI and MARKS 1971); norethindrone acetate has a similar effect (MOGHISSI and SYNER 1975). The depression of gonadotropin secretion may well explain the persistent endometrial atrophy and subsequent amenorrhea these patients experience during and after treatment (COUTINHO et al. 1966; HASPELS 1970).

The contraceptive steroid *R2323*, which competes for the progesterone receptor, has an effect on the endometrium like that of progestational agents (AZADIAN-BOULANGER et al. 1976). The nucleolar channel system of the glandular epithelial cells remains rudimentary, giant mitochondria do not develop, and degradation of the glycogen granules by ergastoplasmic enzymes is delayed, resulting in a deficiency in glycoprotein secretion; all these signs point to progresterone insufficiency.

In monkeys the administration of estrogens after sexual intercourse (**"postcoital pills"**) delays the appearance of secretory changes in the endometrium only slightly (MORRIS and VAN WAGENEN 1966). Apparently these pills act as contraceptives not only by effects they have on the endometrium but by their stimulation of muscular activity in the fallopian tubes and uterus, thereby preventing nidation. The effectiveness of postcoital estrogens in women apparently depends on strict adherence to proper dose, which must be about 100 times that of the usual contraceptive pill, and to proper time schedules (BLYE 1973; HASPELS and ANDRIESSE 1973; SHEARMAN 1973). As to be expected, the endometrial epithelium proliferates intensely (HASPELS et al. 1977) and the differentiation of glands and stroma is retarded by 5 days (VAN SANTEN and HASPELS 1980). This retardation most likely explains how postcoital estrogen acts, disturbing the synchrony between blastocyst and endometrium (BEIER 1981). – The gestagenic "postcoital pills" produce severe side effects and often prove ineffective (LARRANGA et al. 1975). In contrast, the progesterone antagonist RU486 is well tolerated and induced early abortion in 85% of the patients (COUZINET et al. 1986). Histologically, it leads to decidual necrosis, probably by blocking the progesterone action at the receptor site.

Enzyme-histochemical studies (CONNELL et al. 1967; HESTER et al. 1968) give results that in part vary considerably from those of a normal cycle. After therapy with the combination type of contraceptive agents the activity of alkaline phosphatase is only slightly reduced; after sequential therapy it develops late, analogous to the other morphological changes. It finally increases in the second half of the cycle and reaches its maximum shortly before breakthrough bleeding starts. The concentration of the acid phosphatase, however, is reduced in both of the inhibited halves of the cycle. The succinic acid and lactic acid dehydrogenases as well as carbonic anhydrase are decreased, showing only slight fluctuations during the cycle. After therapy with the combination agents the activity of β-glucuronidase is lacking; after sequential therapy it is extremely low.

When added to the culture medium, oral contraceptive agents induce changes in human endometrium cultured in vitro similar to those produced by the natural hormones (CSERMELY et al. 1971).

Diagnostically it is difficult to classify these endometria, especially those after combination therapy. Nonetheless, the histological pictures are so characteristically abnormal, that with experience it is easy to recognize at a glance an endometrium from an inhibited cycle without knowing that the patient had taken contraceptive agents. We know of no endogenous endocrine abnormalities that are able to induce the same histological pictures. On the other hand, a conscientious pathologist endeavors to define the histological changes as precisely as possible, since from the degree of proliferative or secretory changes he finds he can draw important conclusions about the extent of hormonally induced alterations that have developed. These conclusions, in turn, provide clues for the prognosis and subsequent treatment. Accordingly, we classify the endometrium of an inhibited cycle under a numerical code in our diagnostic decimal system (see Table 4). An "ov" behind the two-digit number points to previous antiovulation therapy, thus with special ov-registry cards we can easily cull these cases from the files at any time, although their numbers vary. The numbers used most often are those for the deficient, shortened or irregular proliferative and secretory phases, and those for the atrophic endometrium or the anovulatory breakthrough bleeding. At times one finds the histological picture of an irregular shedding, which by the absence of endometrial granulocytes can be distinguished from irregular shedding due to other causes (DALLENBACH-HELLWEG and BORNEBUSCH 1969). If the estrogenic component predominates or the progestin is converted into estrogenic substances, a glandular-cystic hyperplasia results, occasionally even an adenomatous hyperplasia.

Resumption of Fertility After Discontinuation of Contraceptives. If therapy with the contraceptive agents is discontinued in good time or at least interrupted periodically, a return to normal cycles and a normal histology is quite possible (MAQUEO et al. 1963; RICE-WRAY et al. 1963; MEARS 1965; BREINL and WARNECKE 1967). Such restoration usually occurs in 91% of the women after an amenorrhea that may have lasted up to 4 months. The remaining 9% either experience longer periods of amenorrhea (RICE-WRAY et al. 1967) even up to 42 months (PLATE 1971; INGERSLEV et al. 1976) or the histological picture of a deficient secretory phase persists unchanged. The chemical composition of the contraceptive agent used greatly influences the duration of postcontraceptive amenorrhea (FERIN 1964). The injectable contraceptive agents (SCOMMEGNA et al. 1970) and the depot gestagens (GARDNER and MISHELL 1970; MAQUEO et al. 1970) produce the longest suppression of menstruation. In addition, women experiencing menstrual irregularities prior to taking oral contraceptives are more likely to develop prolonged amenorrhea (GOLDITCH 1972; RIFKIN et al. 1972;

BUTTRAM et al. 1974). The cause of such amenorrhea may be either anovulation from hypothalamic, pituitary or ovarian injury or endometrial atrophy and refractoriness. The occasional occurrence of amenorrhea with galactorrhea after oral contraception is thought to point to a depression of hypothalamic function, resulting in a prolonged decrease in the formation or secretion of pituitary gonadotropins (FRIEDMAN and GOLDFIEN 1969; HALBERT and CHRISTIAN 1969; STARUP 1972).

Mode of Action. The question of how the antifertility agents function has led for many years to the formulation of countless theories. As yet no one has provided a definitive answer. Most probably many factors are important. These may vary from patient to patient and may depend in part on the type of therapy, on the composition of the agent, and on the dosage of hormones used; then too, all of these factors may act either together or independently. It has been possible to prove that the contraceptive agents inhibit ovulation in some women (RAUSCHER and LEEB 1965) but such inhibition does not seem to be essential for the contraceptive effect.

The *structural changes induced in the histology of the endometrium* of most patients would be enough to explain the contraceptive action. As we have already observed during the discussion of functional disturbances, an endometrium morphologically modified by disturbed hormonal regulation becomes functionally altered as well, and is quite unable to accept or support a fertilized ovum. Numerous investigators have studied changes in various structures of the endometrium and concluded, these alterations were responsible for preventing nidation. HALLER (1966) referred to regressive changes in glands at the time of implantation; GOLDZIEHER et al. (1962), GOLDZIEHER and RICE-WRAY (1966), HESTER et al. (1968) emphasized the extensive atrophy of the endometrium; OBER (1966) pointed to the faulty development of the spiral arteries; WAIDL et al. (1968) stressed the inhibited development of intercellular fibers needed for supporting the blastocyst; HACKL (1968) was able to demonstrate that the glucose metabolism of the endometrium was reduced in vitro, and suggested that a similar change in vivo might be important. MORRIS (1973) considered the reduced endometrial anhydrase activity to be the basic mechanism of action. Furthermore, the inhibited development and ultimate incomplete maturation of the endometrium induced by the sequential agents, a state equivalent to a deficient secretory phase, is undoubtedly enough to prevent nidation (FETTIG and KOPECKY 1968; KALTENBACH et al. 1973). – Clinical studies have repeatedly shown that *the excretion of urinary gonadotropins is decreased* (EPSTEIN et al. 1958; BUCHHOLZ et al. 1962; DEMOL and FERIN 1964; WALSER et al. 1964; KAISER et al. 1966). With the combination agents the midcycle peak of LH, which normally induces ovulation, usually is flattened (BUCHHOLZ and NOCKE 1965). With the sequential agents it is chiefly the FSH that is decreased; the peak of LH remains unaffected (SWERDLOFF and ODELL 1968). Apparently the estrogenic component of the contraceptives suppresses the secretion of FSH (VORYS et al. 1965), whereas the progestins inhibit the production of LH (DICZFALUSY 1968; DICZFALUSY et al. 1969). In response to the fall of gonadotropins the ovaries begin to atrophy, as is readily evident from the increase in their stroma (fibrosis) and the failure of the Graafian follicles to mature. From these facts it seems most likely the contraceptive agents suppress ovulation by way of a feedback mechanism on the pituitary and hypothalamus (see also ARTNER and KRATOCHWIL 1965). We know from experiments in animals that the hypophysis enlarges, the chromophobe cells increase in number, and the acidophils and basophils lose their granules (BORELL 1966). From the studies of LUNENFELD (1964), however, it seems the contraceptive agents also *act directly on the ovaries by inhibiting certain enzyme-systems.* – Additional investigators indicate that other preparations may still be effective contraceptive agents although they fail to suppress ovulation (GOLDZIEHER et al. 1962; ERB and LUDWIG 1965). In such instances, especially after continuous administration of minute doses of progestins, the contraceptive effect is attributed in part to the endometrial disturbance (KÜHNE et al. 1972), in part to the *altered composition and increased viscosity of the cervical mucus* that retards passage of the sperm up to the endocervical canal (HALLER 1966; GARCIA 1967). Then too, some investigators believe these altered cervical secretions prevent *the sperm* from acquiring the capacity to fertilize (TAUSK 1969). Apparently the sperm need to stay at least 6 hours in the female genital tract to allow enzymes from the uterine mucosa to digest a protective coating on them before they are able to fertilize. Contraceptive agents also act on the *fallopian tubes,* affecting the secretory cycle of their epithelium, the size of their lumen, and the contractions of their musculature (see Table 13).

Table 13. Probable mechanisms of action of the oral contraceptive agents

Composition of the pill	Combination type of pill		Sequential type of pill		Pure progestational pill	
	Progestin + medium dose of estrogen	Progestin + high dose of estrogen	High dose of estrogen	Estrogen + progestin	Small dose of progestins ("luteal supplementation")	
Used – on days of the cycle	5–24 5–25 5–26	5–24 5–25	5–19+20–24 5–20+21–25 5–14+15–25		5–24	Continuously
Inhibition of gonadotropin	LH	LH (+FSH?)	FSH(+LH?)		None or irregularly	None or irregularly
Effect on the ovarian enzyme systems	Possible	Possible	?	?	?	
Endometrial factor	++	++	+	+	++	++
Cervical factor	++	++	none	+	++	++
Contractions of fallopian tube	Depressed	Depressed	Increased	?	Depressed	Depressed

The histological changes found in the endometrium after use of contraceptive agents are informative for many reasons. On the one hand, the changes give us a unique insight into how normal and abnormal endometria react to hormones; on the other hand, the changes show us what the limits of these reactions are. Like every other organ or tissue of the body, the endometrium changes its mode of reaction, depending on the duration, intensity, and type of stimulus affecting it. As experiments in monkeys carried out continuously for many years showed, the endometrium has, as HISAW so cogently expressed it, "a memory like an elephant", that is, it never forgets previous hormone therapy and reacts later accordingly. Long-term studies of human endometrium have been made after protracted therapy with contraceptive agents. The results suggest that because of injury to specific genomes the endometrial cells gradually lose their sensitivity to hormones and eventually atrophy or they remain responsive only to estrogen. Even though all of these changes may be reversible in a majority of patients after therapy is stopped, the very fact some changes are irreversible in a small percentage of women should cause concern. A discussion of the numerous deleterious consequences of hormonal therapy observed clinically, although important, is not pertinent to our subject at hand.

From our present knowledge of the action of hormones on the endometrium, we can formulate the following hypothesis about the possible late consequences of a continuous, truly long-term therapy:

1. By binding to specific receptors in their target cells, *estrogens* activate genomes, thereby inducing mitosis and cellular proliferation. From these facts several possibilities may occur:
   a) During a normal cycle progesterone causes estrogen-primed target cells to differentiate, inhibiting further growth
   b) Continuous, unopposed estrogen in small or moderate doses may lead to *uninhibited growth* (glandular-cystic hyperplasia → adenomatous hyperplasia → eventual carcinoma, see HERTZ 1968)
   c) Prolonged large doses of estrogen may injure the target cells and destroy their ability to produce receptors, terminating in atrophy of the endometrium (as proven by animal experiments)
2. *Progesterone* acts on the target cells to stimulate their differentiation and to suppress their uptake of estrogen:
   a) In physiological doses it induces the target cells to differentiate, thereby inhibiting their proliferation
   b) When a synthetic gestagen effect with its greatly increased progestagenic potency predominates continuously the action of estrogen is persistently blocked, and the endometrium eventually undergoes irreversible *atrophy*

Fortunately the modern combination preparations with their greatly reduced concentrations of hormones rarely induce the adverse reactions described, and if reactions do occur they are less severe. It should be emphasized, that these adverse reactions appear only when the patient's hormonal balance is profoundly upset. If the pathologist knows about them, it is he who generally recognizes them first. A precise histological diagnosis of the changes and their causes (from estrogens or gestagens?) is of paramount importance. From the kind of endometrial abnormalities he sees, the pathologist can provide the gynecologist with important information on how to treat the patient with another hormonal preparation, whose composition is deemed right for bringing about hormonal balance.

The **endocervical mucosa,** portions of which are often included in curettings (see p. 18), reacts to hormone therapy quite differently from the endometrium. Estrogens alone have very little, if any, proliferative effect on the endocervical glands but enhance differentiation with mucus production and secretion, and they may induce squamous cell metaplasia of the surface epithelium. In contrast, gestagens alone call forth and excessive adenomatous or microglandular proliferation of the endocervical glands (Fig. 96a). Often the reserve cells proliferate luxuriantly as well (Fig. 96b). The adenomatous hyperplasia of the endocervical glands closely resembles the glandular hyperplasia evoked in the corpus endometrium by estrogen, but surpasses by far the hyperplasia induced by excessive endogenous stimulation with progesterone, as for instance, during pregnancy. When both hormones are given, the changes brought about by the gestagens usually predominate. Since intensive therapy with gestagens leads to endometrial atrophy, such curettings may consist almost exclusively of large portions of hyperplastic endocervical mucosa with only tiny fragments of atrophic endometrium.

ε) Gonadotropins

In the monkeys (HISAW 1944) and in humans chorionic gonadotropin (HCG) alters the menstrual cycle by prolonging the secretory phase. The corpus luteum persists. More relaxin is produced, as the proliferating endothelial cells of small stromal vessels and the deciduomata indicate. Treatment of hypogonadotropic ovarian insufficiency with hypophyseal gonadotropin (HHG) has proved worthwhile. By giving their patients 400 units a day for 10–14 days, BETTENDORF and BRECKWOLDT (1964) succeeded in inducing follicles to mature and to ovulate. For stimulating the maturation of follicles, other authors (VAN DE WIELE and TURKSOY 1965; SCHMIDT-ELMENDORFF and KAISER 1967) pretreated with menopausal gonadotropin (HMG), then administered HCG (4000–5000 IU) to bring about the ovulation. In one large series of patients, 91% of the women ovulated and 51% became pregnant (LUNENFELD 1965). Occasionally, several follicles may mature and ovulate at the same time, resulting in multiple pregnancies (GEMZELL 1966). The endometrium may undergo partial secretory changes (see BUXTON and HERRMANN 1961), whereby some of its overstimulated glandular cells may develop such large polygonal nuclei and swollen, clear cytoplasm that they resemble cells of the Arias-Stella phenomenon (see Fig. 154b). The longer HCG is continuously given, the more intense these abnormal changes become.

ζ) Clomiphene

Clomiphene is also useful for regulating the length of the cycle and for inducing ovulation (GREENBLATT et al. 1961) (50 mg daily until the basal temperature rises or 100–150 mg daily for 5 days; KISTNER 1965). In fact, it often proves effective, especially then, when previous treatment with gonadotropin failed

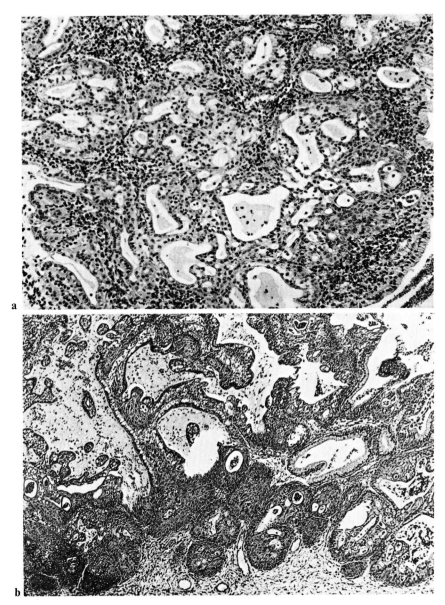

Fig. 96a, b. Adenomatous and microglandular hyperplasia of the endocervical mucosa. **a** Proliferation and branching of glands as small alveoli formed by poorly differentiated glandular epithelium. **b** Where glands confront stroma an excessive hyperplasia of reserve cells develops

(DÖRING 1965). In contrast, in primary hypogonadotropic ovarian insufficiency it may have no effect (BETTENDORF et al. 1965). To decide which drug should be used, either the "progesterone test" can be performed or a measurement made of the urinary estrogens before therapy is started. If the progesterone test is negative or the urinary excretion of estrogen for 24 h is below 10 μg, then gonadotropin should be administered. If the progesterone test is positive or the hourly value for urinary estrogens exceeds 10 µg, then clomiphene is the drug of choice. That would suggest that clomiphene affects the ovary directly and is able to induce ovulation only when the controlling hypophyseal centers are functioning, as for example, in a normo- or hypergonadotropic ovarian insufficiency caused by the Stein-Leventhal syndrome. About 70%–80% of the amenorrheic patients treated ovulate, particularly those with the Stein-Leventhal syndrome. Ovulation usually occurs within 2–41 days after onset of treatment; in more than 50% of the patients it occurs within 2 weeks.

Clomiphene stimulates the ovaries and adrenal glands to synthesize more estrogen (PILDES 1965) by acting directly on the enzymes (particularly 3β-ol-dehydrogenase) needed for converting the steroids (CARLSTRÖM and FURUHJELM 1969). Furthermore, because clomiphene is chemically similar to the synthetic estrogen chlorotrianisene (TACE), it binds to the estrogen receptors of the target cells, preventing the natural estrogens from binding. These then accumulate and by means of a feedback mechanism stimulate the anterior pituitary to secrete more gonadotropins (primarily FSH) (BUHL-JØRGENSEN et al. 1976). Thus, depending upon its dose and how long it is administered, clomiphene may act as estrogen or as an antiestrogen.

The percentage of patients that become pregnant, however, varies widely (WHITELAW et al. 1964; DÖRING 1965; CHARLES et al. 1967; TAUBERT 1969; refer to BIRKENFELD et al. 1986 for more recent statistics). The average is about 20%. If HCG and clomiphene are given together (COX et al. 1968), or if the dose of clomiphene is increased (GORLITSKY et al. 1978), then about 50% of the patients become pregnant. The discrepancy between the frequency of ovulation and that of pregnancy may be explained by postulating pseudoovulations due to luteinization of thecal cells of an unruptured follicle (VAN HALL and MASTBOOM 1969). A biphasic curve of the basal (body) temperature may result as well and be misconstrued as a sign of ovulation. Although the basal temperature rises, the endometrium may remain unresponsive and non-secreting because of its primary, inherent refractoriness to ovulatory stimulation (WHITELAW et al. 1970). Furthermore, and probably even more important, the discrepancy between the ovulation rates and the pregnancy rates cen be explained by the fact that clomiphene acts not only directly on the embryo and ovary, but on the endometrium as well. Clomiphene competes with estrogen for the estrogen receptor. In the absence of estrogen receptors, as for instance in atrophic endometrium, clomiphene cannot act without estrogen priming, which is needed to induce estrogen receptors. These, in turn, are necessary for the expression of the antiestrogenic effect of clomiphene. This antiestrogenic effect, when induced in the early proliferative phase, mimicks and enhances the preovulatory estrogen decrease (BIRKENFELD et al. 1986). Thereby clomiphene acts in a similar way to the synthetic gestagens of oral contraceptives by causing premature secretory transformation of endometrial glands. As a result, endometrial secretion remains deficient. These intricate facts help to explain why reports in the literature about the action of clomiphene are so conflicting, especially those regarding the question whether clomiphene can induce luteal phase defects or be useful in treating them. Like oral contraceptives, clomiphene will induce an abortive or deficient secretory phase in a normally ovulating woman (COOK et al. 1984). On the other hand, it may compensate for a deficient luteal phase by stimulating secretion (DOWNS and GIBSON 1983; FUKUMA et al. 1983). In about 50% of the patients, however, secretion remains deficient (VAN HALL and MASTBOOM 1969; GARCIA et al. 1977; WENTZ 1980; BALASCH et al. 1983; DALY et al. 1983). Furthermore, karyotypic studies of women after clomiphene therapy revealed an increase in heteroploidy and in chromosomal aberrations of endometrial tissue, results that may explain the persistant infertility of some of these patients (CHARLES et al. 1973).

The different effects of clomiphene in the deficient luteal phase are related to the various causes of inadequate secretion (cf. p. 136 ff.). The best clomiphene effect can be expected in a deficient luteal phase with coordinated delayed secretion due to follicular persistence with elevated estrogen levels and a resulting relative corpus luteum insufficiency (see Table 8), since clomiphene will counteract (compete with) the excessive estrogen to normalize the secretion. Similarly, an endometrium which is anovulatory before clomiphene treatment may show after treatment a secretory change like that of a normal cycle (CHARLES et al. 1963). In contrast, a deficient luteal phase preceded by a deficient follicular phase will not improve with clomiphene therapy, but instead worsen under the additional antiestrogenic action of clomiphene. These differences emphasize how important the correct histological evaluation of the endometrial biopsy is for selecting the proper therapy.

For in vitro fertilization such proper therapy for inducing ovulation is of decisive importance for the success of that procedure. Excessive failure rates are best explained by the fact that although clomiphene induces an ovulation the endometrium remains functionally retarded. In addition to determining the hormonal status biochemically prior to in vitro fertilization, it is essential that an endometrial biopsy be functionally evaluated histologically. Depending on the type of hormonal deficiency determined, treatment with HMG/HCG should be provided (when cycles are normal or estrogen deficiency is present) or with clomiphene (when estrogen overstimulation causes a relative corpus luteum insufficiency resulting in deficient secretion).

Clomiphene may be used not only to induce ovulation but also in large doses (200–400 mg daily for from 1 month to 2 years; WALL et al. 1964, 1965) to treat glandular-cystic hyperplasia and endometrial carcinoma after the menopause. Such intense therapy, like therapy with progesterone, serves to block the estrogen receptors, leading to a secretory change of the adenomatous or carcinomatous glands, and to their regression in some patients (KISTNER 1965). If the Graafian follicles still possess the potential to mature and ovulate, then continuous treatment with clomiphene (100–200 mg daily) will induce a secretory phase that may last 6–8 weeks. The stroma will show a definite, predecidual change. If therapy is continued without a pause, the endometrium gradually atrophies (KISTNER et al. 1966).

The **antigonadotropin** danazol, a derivative of 17α-ethinyltestosterone used for treating endometriosis, inhibits centrally the secretion of FSH and LH. Consequently, ovarian function dwindles and the endometrium becomes atrophic (DMOWSKI and COHEN 1975).

With **retrosteroid,** an agent capable of inducing ovulation and related to dydrogesterone, HERZER et al. (1969) were able to induce focal secretory changes only in the endometrial glands; the stroma remained unchanged. Even more remarkable, the drug produced that effect only during anovulatory cycles or after the menopause. In women with normal menstrual periods it stimulated focally the proliferative changes and inhibited the secretory changes.

The study of the effects and uses of **prostaglandins** has received much attention in recent years. These agents are best measured by biochemical techniques. It would go beyond the purpose of this monograph to review the vast literature on prostaglandins; we refer the reader to special articles dealing with them.

b) After Intrauterine Contraceptive Device

The intrauterine device as a contraceptive is not new. RICHTER (1909) and GRÄFENBERG (1931) first reported on the use of intrauterine rings or spirals for preventing pregnancy. Although these devices proved effective, they became unpopular because of the infections they induced. When it became apparent, however, that the oral contraceptive pills were not the ideal means for birth control among analphabetic peoples, the intrauterine device came under study again. In the early 1960s various designs of loops and coils made of plastics were devised and tested (Margulis Coil, Lippes Loop, Dalcon Shield). These were easy to insert compared with the ring device but proved unsatisfactory because of higher rates of pregnancy, expulsion and other complications. Consequently, in addition to these "inert" types, medicated progesterone and copper "T"-devices have been designed for adding local hormonal or chemical effects to the mechanical irritation of the devices. These have in general proved most effective in their protection against pregnancy. They also produce far fewer side effects than the rings, coils and loops (Fig. 97).

The histological reaction of the endometrium to the device varies with the type used. In the immediate vicinity of the **inert devices** the functional development of the endometrium is usually accelerated; electron-microscopic studies generally reveal premature secretory changes. During the proliferative phase giant mitochondria appear in the epithelial cells of the glands. Directly after ovulation the stromal cells undergo predecidual change (WYNN 1967, 1968). Mechanical injury of the endometrium often leads to decidualization of the surrounding stroma, not only in the experimental animal (for example, deciduoma of the rat) but also in women (SCHILLER 1925). Since one would expect a firm foreign body like an intrauterine device to injure the endometrium, it was not surprising when numerous histological studies revealed that these devices also induced focal decidualization (see illustrations of HALL et al. 1965, and WILSON et al. 1965; TAMADA et al. 1967). In about half of the women that change is already evident at the time of ovulation, and occasionally the dilated sinusoids of capillaries, so characteristic of the decidua, are also present (Fig. 98a). Even an Arias-Stella phenomenon may occur (HALL et al. 1965). In other instances, glandular development may be focally retarded but stromal differentiation advanced (NICOLAISEN et al. 1973). The endometrium directly beneath the device may show a pressure atrophy with focal fibrosis under the thinned surface epithelium (BONNEY et al. 1966). Large regions of surrounding endometrium may go unaffected and develop normally (KWAK 1965; ROZIN

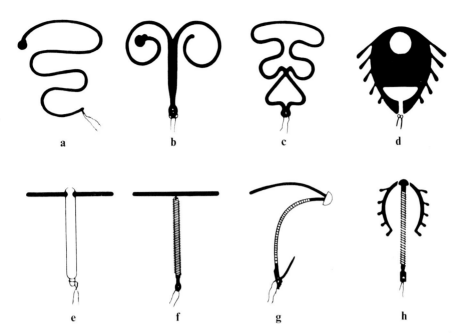

Fig. 97a–h. The various generations of intrauterine devices. *Upper row:* action purely mechanical, **a** Lippes Loop, **b** Saf-T-Coil, **c** Dana Super, **d** Dalcon Shield. *Lower row:* forms bearing medications, **e** Biograviplan containing gestagen, **f** Copper-T (Gyne-T), **g** Copper-7 (Gravigard), **h** Multiload

et al. 1967). – The endometrium adjacent to the device may contain sparse or, rarely, heavy infiltrates of leukocytes, lymphocytes and plasma cells, which may persist for many months even in the absence of bacterial infection (MOYER and MISHELL 1971). Leukocytes may also fill the glandular lumina beneath the surface. Some investigators have also found bacteria in the early stages (POTTS and PEARSON 1967). Occasionally there is a foreign body reaction with giant cells (BORELL 1966). We found the inflammation more pronounced following use of the Dalcon Shield than with the original loop and coil devices. In the regions involved by the inflammatory reaction the endometrial differentiation may be retarded, giving the false impression of a generally retarded secretory phase (LEE et al. 1967). In their studies ANCLA et al. (1967) described microthrombi of agglutinated platelets in small stromal capillaries. Histochemically, the endometria of women using the intrauterine device reveal no significant variations in enzyme reactions or in contents of nucleic acids and glycogen (KWAK 1965; SHAHANI et al. 1967), but acid mucins may increase throughout the menstrual cycle (HESTER et al. 1970). – A small percentage of the women using the intrauterine device develop a glandular-cystic or adenomatous hyperplasia, at times with extensive squamous metaplasia of the glandular and superficial epithelia. OBER et al. (1968) reported an adenocarcinoma occurring 57 months after insertion of an intrauterine device composed of polyethylene.

The premature secretory and decidual-like changes are reasons enough to explain the contraceptive action of the inert intrauterine devices. We know

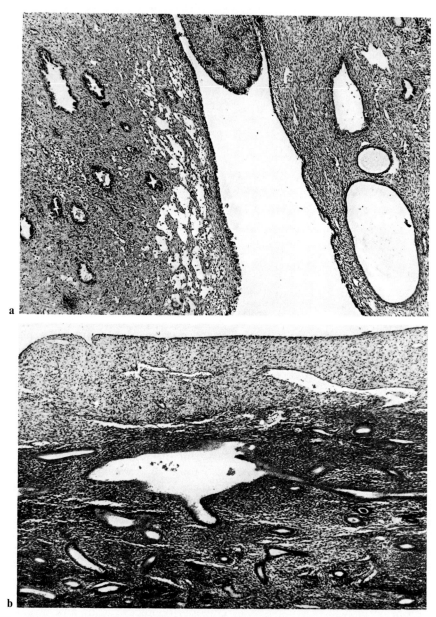

Fig. 98 a–c. Endometrium after intrauterine contraceptive device (IUD). **a** Inert device: mechanically induced focal decidual change of stroma (*at the left*) with secretory glands (cf. Table 23). *At the right,* the opposing endometrium consists of a fibrous stroma and cystically dilated glands. **b** Medicated device (containing gestagen): focal superficial arrested secretion with decidual change of stroma and atrophic glands. The underlying endometrium normally proliferative. Note the sharp line between the two layers. **c** Higher magnification of **b**

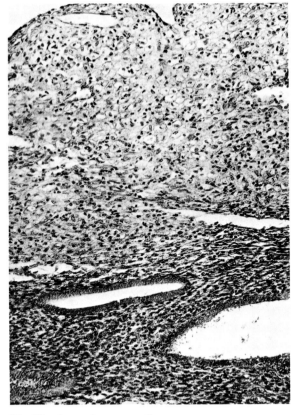

Fig. 98c. Legend see opposite page

from experience that a decidual change, as well as any alteration in the hormonal synchrony of the endometrium, alone suffices to prevent implantation of the blastocyst. Another reason for their contraceptive effect might be a local hormonal dysfunction secondary to the inflammation they induce. Alterations in tubal transport, mechanical interference with implantation, local chemotactic effects on the endometrium or a focal release of cytotoxic products formed by the surface interaction with the endometrium have also been suggested as the mechanisms preventing conception (DAVIS and LESINSKI 1970). In addition, macrophages induced by the inflammatory reaction may phagocytize spermatozoa or ova (DAVIS 1972; see also previous literature cited there).

Because the mechanically induced decidua develops only focally, it is easy to understand why pregnancy can occur when no inflammation is provoked. Pregnancy rates published for the Lippes Loop vary from 1.5% (LIPPES and ZIELEZNY 1975) to 10% (LAST 1974); for the Dalcon Shield from 1.3% (OSTERGARD 1974) to 5% (HASPELS 1973) and even 10% (PERLMUTTER 1974). The rates, however, fluctuate considerably between countries (Costa Rica: 8.4%, Guatemala: 2%, according to SANNUEZA 1975) and between investigative centers (SNOWDEN and WILLIAMS 1975). Further complications caused by the mechanical intrauterine devices are pelvic inflammatory disease (TAYLOR et al. 1975; DA-

WOOD and BIRNBAUM 1975; MEAN et al. 1976; BÖHM et al. 1977) with or without perforation of the uterus. Most perforations occurred when the device was inserted less than 8 weeks post partum (DAVIS 1972). Pelvic actinomycosis, observed particularly with the Dalcon Shield (LOMAX et al. 1976) produces irreparable disease in the pelvis and is therefore especially feared. Owing to its shape, the Dalcon Shield favors the growth of bacteria on its surface (WAGNER et al. 1976) and its pinnated tail promotes the ascent of bacteria into the uterine cavity. Because it was associated with an excessive rate of septic abortions, it was withdrawn from the market in 1974 (TATUM 1977).

The **mediated intrauterine contraceptive devices** (JOHANNISSON 1973; further literature see there) consist of a T- or 7-shaped strand of polyethylene, either impregnated with progesterone, which is slowly released, or wrapped with a fine copper wire. With this third generation of intrauterine devices, the harmful mechanical action is mitigated with a local hormonal (DOYLE and CLEWE 1968; SCOMMEGNA et al. 1970, 1974) or chemical action (ZIPPER et al. 1968).

The *progesterone-medicated T-shaped devices* carry in their main vertical stem a depot which gives off about 65 µg progesterone into the uterine cavity each day. That acts locally in a paracrine manner to induce perifocal decidualization and glandular atrophy of the superficial endometrium. The changes produced resemble an arrested secretion, and are sharply demarcated from the underlying functionalis, which proliferates or secretes normally, appropriate to the phase (Fig. 98b, c; DALLENBACH-HELLWEG 1975). If the patients had taken oral contraceptive agents before the intrauterine device was inserted, then the lower layers of the endometrium disclose a correspondent deficient maturation. Measurements of the DNA in the nuclei of glandular epithelial cells of the focally arrested secretion gave low values like those obtained after administering gestagens systemically (JOHANNISSON et al. 1977). Biochemical measurements, however, revealed no deviations in hormone levels as compared with normal control patients without intrauterine devices; they also revealed no influence on the hypothalamic-hypophyseal centers or ovarian function (TILLSON et al. 1975; WAN et al. 1977). Thus, when the gestagen is placed into the uterine cavity, it affects only the tissues in the immediate vicinity.

The perifocally arrested secretion induced by gestagen devices is characteristic in two chief respects. First, it is focal whereas the arrested secretion induced by administering gestagens either orally or parenterally involves the entire endometrium. Secondly, its glands are atrophied, whereas those of a decidualization brought about by the trauma of a purely mechanical device are normal. It is therefore possible in most cases to decide what type of device had been used (see Table 23). The contraception obtained is as good as that with systemically administered gestagens, giving a PEARL index below 1% (PHARISS et al. 1974; WAN et al. 1977), since the implantation of the blastocyst depends on the qualities of the upper functionalis. An important difference, especially for the endometrium, is that the basalis and basal functionalis remain uninvolved and are spared for the next regeneration. As compared with a simple mechanical device, the assurance for contraception is increased because of the glandular atrophy induced. At the same time, the hazards of a generalized gestagen effect are avoided.

In contrast with those after mechanical devices, the number of complications arising is very small. Inflammation of the endometrium rarely occurs since the decidua protects against it. The troublesome interval bleedings that at times develop (ZADOR et al. 1976) may be explained by the focal and variable release of relaxin from aggregates of granulocytes, analogous to the breakthrough bleeding associated with diffuse arrested secretion (see p. 173). The sinusoidal vessels concentrated in these regions facilitate and intensify those small breakthrough hemorrhages (see also SHAW et al. 1979, 1981). In addition ANCLA et al. (1967) described microthrombi in the vessels near the surface and HOHMANN et al. (1977) reported on defects of vascular walls associated with degenerating endothelial cells. After removal of the device, and independent of the duration of use, endometrial morphology returned to normal within 1 month (SILVERBERG et al. 1986).

The *devices entwined with a copper wire* 0.2–0.25 mm thick (T-, 7- and Multiload) give off copper ions from their surface of 200 mm^2 into the intrauterine milieu. These, like progesterone, are absorbed by the superficial layers of the endometrium and have been reported in the secretory vacuoles of the glandular epithelium (SALAVERRY et al. 1973). In contrast, electron-microscopic studies have failed to demonstrate the binding of copper ions to cell organelles, which might be related to their very rapid excretion (GONZALEZ-ANGULO and AZNAR-RAMOS 1976).

Biochemical measurements indicated that the concentrations of copper and protein in the endometrium increase and those of zinc and manganese decrease (HAGENFELDT 1972; HERNANDEZ et al. 1975). These results suggest that copper exerts a metabolic effect on the endometrial cells. LARSSON et al. (1974) found the fibrinolytic activity increased. The concentrations of DNA and RNA remain unchanged, but the activity of lactic dehydrogenase of the superficial endometrium is depressed (WILSON 1977). From the increase in the activity of acid phosphatase during the proliferative phase and the fall in the activities of alkaline phosphatase and β-glucuronidase during the secretory phase, one may conclude that glycogen metabolism is affected (ROSADO et al. 1976). Ultrastructural evidence of a disturbed catabolism of glycogen supported that conclusion (NILSSON et al. 1974). The values for the biochemical measurements, however, vary among the different authors (cf. e.g., MERCADO et al. 1972).

In contrast to the results of those biochemical analyses, light-microscopic studies with routine and special stains failed to provide morphological evidence that copper had an effect on the endometrium (DALLENBACH 1977; DALLENBACH-HELLWEG et al. 1979). If prior hormonal therapy or functional disturbances are excluded, the endometria are appropriately developed, the surface epithelium is almost always intact, even where the copper wires have pressed against and indented the surface (Fig. 99). The aggregates of polymorphonuclear leukocytes in the glandular lumina or under the superficial epithelium undoubtedly come from the uterine cavity. We should not regard them as harbingers of inflammation, since the glandular epithelium is uninjured and intact. True inflammatory infiltrates appear only when endometrial function is deficient; that is, when its development is delayed or abnormal, so that atrophy and functional insufficiency lead to reduced resistance (DALLENBACH-HELLWEG

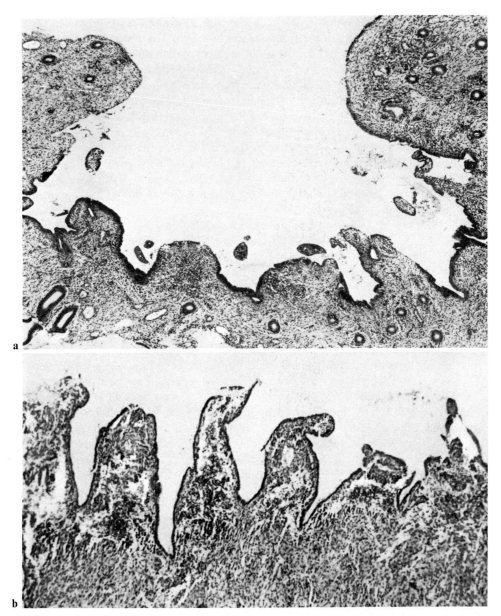

Fig. 99 a, b. Corrugated surface of the endometrium produced by copper coils of intrauterine device. **a** T-form with wire 0.25 mm thick. **b** 7-form with wire 0.20 mm thick

1980). Usually in such cases the use of oral contraceptives has preceded the insertion of the intrauterine device.

Granules of actinomyces may be found in endometrial specimens or on the surfaces of intrauterine devices. When endometrial function is normal, these colonies of microorganisms may represent an incidental finding. In rare instances, when endometrial function and resistance is decreased, the actinomyces may spread to induce ovarian or pelvic abscesses. They must be differentiated from lipofuscin granules of cellular origin described in mucus-rich tissues (O'BRIEN et al. 1985), including the endometrium.

The endometrial surface epithelium may be polymorphic with disturbed ciliogenesis (LUDWIG 1980), or may undergo metaplastic change, especially after long-time use of the intrauterine device. Foci of squamous or papillary metaplasia are most frequently observed. These metaplastic cells may be shed and may give rise to atypical cytological reports in Pap smears (RISSE et al. 1981).

The contraceptive action of the copper-bearing intrauterine device is, therefore, best explained by the biochemically detectable changes it produces in the intrauterine milieu (OSTER and SALGO 1975). We should also consider its possible effects on sperm (HICKS and ROSADO 1976).

The pregnancy rates published for large patient collectives vary between 1% and 2% (ORLANS 1974; AKINLA et al. 1975; JAIN 1975; PIZARRO et al. 1977), or even under 1% (TATUM 1973; LIEDHOLM and SJÖBERG 1974). The complication rate is comparably low. The rare perforations with the copper T- or 7-device occur typically through the endocervix (CEDERQVIST and FUCHS 1974; NYGREN and JOHANSSEN 1974).

The number of extrauterine pregnancies occurring with all types of intrauterine devices is clearly increased (LEHFELDT et al. 1970; TATUM 1976; ERKKOLA and LIUKKO 1977; TATUM 1977; ZIELSKE et al. 1977). The reasons given for that are: the intrauterine device acts only locally in the uterine cavity; it also promotes infections of the fallopian tube. Rare reports of ovarian pregnancies continue to appear (PANE et al. 1970; PUGH et al. 1973).

That fertility was not affected after removal of an intrauterine device was observed in two large series of patients (HATA et al. 1969; WAJNTRAUB 1970; PYÖRÄLÄ et al. 1982). Conception may be slightly retarded, but the length of use of the intrauterine contraceptive device made no difference. After 18 months, 93.1% of the patients had conceived.

c) After Intrauterine Instillation

Intrauterine instillation may be performed for two reasons; first, for hysterosalpingography: the procedure involves injecting a contrast medium of radiopaque oil (e.g., Lipiodol). Secondly, a liquid tissue adhesive may be instilled into the uterine cavity and into the lumina of the fallopian tubes to control persistent menorrhagia and to cause permanent sterilization. For that purpose, formaldehyde, hot waxes or cyanoacrylates have been used. STEVENSON and TAYLOR (1972) injected methyl-2-cyanoacrylate into 12 patients between day 1 and 16 weeks before hysterectomy. The liquid polymerized on the endometrium within about 20 s after the intracervical injection. It produced inflammation, necrosis and complete stripping of the superficial endometrial layers. With a high secretory endometrium the basal layers were preserved for later regeneration. With a low proliferative endometrium, the inflammation involved the basal layers as well, making regeneration impossible. A granulation tissue with multinucleated giant cells developed in some regions, whereas other portions usually showed stromal fibrosis with complete loss of glands.

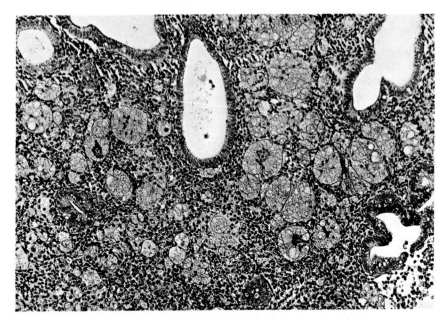

Fig. 100. Histiocytic storage disease. In the stroma of the functionalis between normal-appearing glands there are countless large and small clusters of histiocytic cells ladened with an unidentified foamy substance. The excessive accumulation of the foamy substance has displaced the nuclei of the histiocytes

Various histological changes may occur, depending upon the type of substance used for instillation, upon the individual reaction to it, upon the height of the endometrium, and upon the time that elapses between instillation and examination of the endometrium. Occasionally one may come across a peculiar histiocytic or granulomatous reaction with or without traces of foreign material in glandular lumina or in the endometrial stroma. The etiology of that reaction may be perplexing (see Fig. 100). In such instances, a previous intrauterine instillation (perhaps decades before) can only be suspected, since generally it is impossible to obtain a correct clinical history. We make our presumptive diagnosis only after excluding a systemic granulomatous disease (tuberculosis, sarcoidosis, etc.) and by comparing the changes we see with similar lesions known to be produced by instillation.

d) Regeneration after Curettage

If the endometrium is curetted during a phase of the cycle not followed by menstrual bleeding, then the mucosa that regenerates is without the hormonal stimulus normally acting during the postmenstrual proliferative phase. The question often asked – does a new cycle begin after a curettage or does the old continue according to plan – can be answered only in part. Studies of the effects of curettage in large groups of women with regular cycles disclosed that 82.6% menstruated at the expected time. In 7.2% the cycle was shortened, and in 10.2% it was prolonged (JÖRGENSEN and ENEVOLDSEN 1963). MCLENNAN (1969) found that regeneration after curettage was primarily delayed during the secretory phase, whereas during the proliferative phase or during a hyperplasia the endometrium promptly regenerated. In no instance did the cycle fluctuate more than a few days. From these results we may infer that the trauma of a curettage does not disturb the hormonal cycle of the ovary. If, however, a hormonal dysfunction existed beforehand, then a curettage may greatly prolong the cycle.

As histological studies indicate, the raw surface left after curettage regenerates very slowly, often remaining deficient since the processes of healing proceed independently, usually out-of-phase with the secretion of the ovarian hormones. A complete curettage may not be so complete as intended, as a hysterectomy specimen removed shortly after curettage may often show, with portions of endometrium remaining in the fundus or tubal recesses. These remnants will continue to undergo the regular changes of the cycle, which however may proceed faster than normal, being stimulated by the trauma. Thus, by the 20th day the stroma in these parts may show a predecidual or decidual change like that incited by an intrauterine device. Even a strip biopsy may cause the secretory phase to accelerate or, because of the mechanical stimulus, induce a spontaneous ovulation at the end of an anovulatory cycle. NOYES et al. (1950) reported that in two-thirds of their patients the first menstruation after curettage began a few days earlier than expected. The subsequent menstruations, however, occurred at the proper times.

A curettage performed with too much zeal, particularly when repeated several times or done after abortion or pregnancy, may result in so much basalis being removed that *intrauterine adhesions* (synechiae) develop *as a late complication*. According to several authors (ASHERMAN 1948; FOIX et al. 1966, see also for further literature; TURUNEN 1966) these adhesions, formed after total loss of the endometrium, not infrequently cause a secondary obstructive-type amenorrhea and sterility (Asherman's syndrome). Usually they are diagnosed by hysterography (SIEGLER 1962; TOPKINS 1962; HALBRECHT 1965; DMOWSKI and GREENBLATT 1969), seldom in the extirpated uterus, apparently because they are easily overlooked. As to be expected, if such a uterus is curettaged, few, if any, curettings may be obtained and these will chiefly consist of scar tissue and fragments of myometrium. The endometrial cavity may not be obliterated but instead crisscrossed by thread-like synechiae composed of endometrium, fibrous tissue or smooth muscle. The bands of endometrial tissue often undergo the same cyclic changes as the remaining endometrium or equivalent parts of the basalis. Usually by the time synechiae have formed the inflammatory changes have disappeared (FOIX et al. 1966). Adhesions that produce stenosis or occlusion only at the isthmus or in the endocervical canal may cause false amenorrhea with hematometra. If the patient remains fertile and becomes pregnant, then the likelihood the pregnancy will end with an abortion, miscarriage, placenta accreta or a pathological presentation of the fetus are great (JEWELEWICZ et al. 1976).

Besides an overly ambitious curettage, other causes for such endometrial adhesions are the less common necrotizing endometritis (after criminal abortion with soap solutions) or caseating tuberculous endometritis.

When the endometrium is totally destroyed, including the basalis, replacement by endometrial transplantation may prove beneficial. A few investigators have reported successful pregnancy following transplantations (REIFFENSTUHL and KROEMER 1965; TURUNEN 1966, see also for further literature).

Endometrial cryosurgery, a fairly new method and seldom used even today for the control of dysfunctional bleeding or for sterilization, produces extensive necrosis of the endometrium. Such necrosis may occasionally involve the myometrium, leading to the formation of an abscess (BURKE et al. 1973). The endometrium may regenerate focally if portions of the basal layer have been preserved. More experience with this method is needed before we can decide whether it is practicable.

e) With In Vitro Fertilization

Following follicular puncture in the procedure of in vitro fertilization, a normal secretory phase usually develops, provided the endometrial function was normal before the procedure (DALLENBACH et al. 1987). HAAKE et al. (1982) found only one endometrial specimen with a deficient luteal phase.

4. Endometritis

The histological concept of endometritis has changed considerably since the turn of the century. With the increase in our knowledge of the normal histology of the endometrium during the last decades, the concept has narrowed. Before HITSCHMANN and ADLER (1907, 1908) discovered the histological changes of the menstrual cycle, the physiological secretory phase was regarded as an "endometritis glandularis hypertrophica". In like manner, RUGE (1880, see RUCK 1952) distinguished glandular endometritis from interstitial endometritis. In the decades that followed, glandular-cystic hyperplasia was viewed as a hypertrophic, hyperplastic, or polypoid endometritis. There were two reasons for that: first, because in their searches for a lesion to explain the discharge in their patients, investigators often found a hyperplastic endometrium; secondly, because the hyperplastic endometria usually showed hemorrhagic necroses (see for example, R. MEYER 1923). It was only after glandular-cystic hyperplasia was associated with an elevated level of estrogen that the cause and effect of the entity became understood (SCHRÖDER 1928). RUCK's (1952) historical review offers detailed information on this subject. Until recently it was commonly believed that in the second half of the normal secretory phase polymorphonuclear leukocytes infiltrated the compacta of the endometrium, although an explanation for the unusual, presumed infiltration could never be stated. When accumulations of the leukocyte-like cells were encountered they were thought to indicate an endometritis. Such an endometritis, however, has disappeared from our catalogue of diagnoses, since we now know that these leukocyte-like cells are differentiated stromal cells (endometrial granulocytes), which have nothing to do with inflammation. The endometrial granulocyte is a normal component and product of the endometrial stroma (HAMPERL 1954; HELLWEG 1954). Similarly, the presence of lymphoid follicles in the endometrial stroma cannot be interpreted as evidence of an endometritis (for literature see RUCK 1952; RAHN 1968; see p. 34). Thus, the more we have learned about the histology of the endometrium the more we have had to reclassify conditions previously thought to be pathological as physiological or functional variations of the normal menstrual cycle.

In separating a true endometritis from apparent inflammatory changes, it is therefore necessary to apply strict criteria. These may be as clearly specified for the acute endometritis as for the chronic form; they correspond to the criteria ascribed to inflammatory reactions seen in other tissues and organs. Since the processes of inflammation chiefly involve the connective tissues and blood vessels, the inflammatory reaction in the endometrium takes place primarily in the stroma. An infiltrate of inflammatory cells is needed to make a diagnosis of endometritis. When strict standards are applied, endometritis is far less common than previously assumed. After excluding all postabortion and postpuerperal endometria, RUCK (1952) diagosed endometritis 70 times in 2759 curettings, that is, in 2.6% of the curettings. Women in the second half of the childbearing period had endometritis more often than did the younger women (see also WINTER 1956). In general, the normally functioning endometrium forms a barrier against acute infections if it is not severely injured, and since it is regularly shed every 4 weeks, there is little time for a chronic infection to develop.

a) Acute Endometritis

Most commonly acute endometritis is associated with an intrauterine abortion, which can be recognized by demonstrating the remnants of placenta and decidua. (Abortions are discussed more fully on p. 304 ff.) Further causes of acute endometritis are microorganisms, as well as physical, chemical and thermal agents. Examples of some of these are: foreign bodies inserted into the uterine cavity (intrauterine devices, talcum crystals, fragments of tampons) or necrotic remnants of tissue acting as foreign matter (twisted polyps, necrotic portions of leiomyomata, or cartilaginous and bony residua of a dead fetus). Besides the primary cause, which may either reach the uterine cavity from outside (for example, bacteria) or develop within the cavity (for example, sloughed remnants of necrotic tissue), a secondary cause, a wound of the endometrial lining, is necessary for the inflammation to become established. Such a wound occurs at every menstrual period, every abortion and every pregnancy, and is induced with every curettage. In all these conditions the cervical os is dilated, facilitating the ascent of bacteria into the uterine cavity (HOMMA 1955). Consequently, it is during these conditions that an acute endometritis usually develops.

Although the noxious agents causing acute endometritis vary greatly, the inflammatory reaction to them all is generally the same. *Histologically,* we find in the stroma heavy, focal infiltrates of polymorphonuclear leukocytes, which

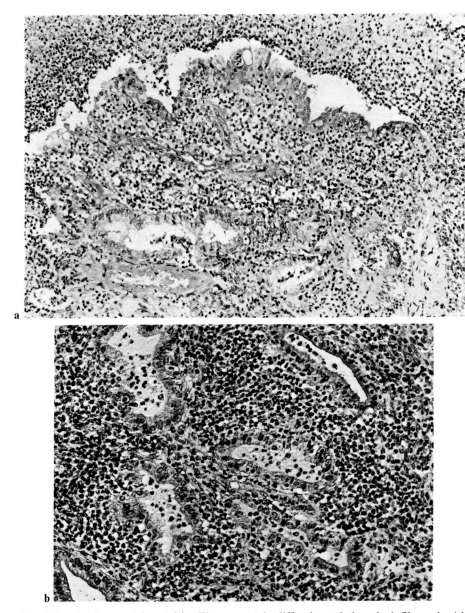

Fig. 101a, b. Acute endometritis. The stroma is diffusely and densely infiltrated with polymorphonuclear leukocytes. Glandular epithelium is destroyed (**a**) and glandular lumina contain leukocytes (**b**)

we can readily distinguish from the endometrial granulocytes since they penetrate and destroy the glandular epithelium and fill the glandular lumina (Fig. 101). The tissue at the leukocytic infiltrates undergoes dissolution and becomes necrotic, and the reticulum fibers disintegrate. The stroma about the infiltrates becomes variably hyperemic, edematous and hemorrhagic, in no way related, however, to the phase of the menstrual cycle. The reticulum fibers elsewhere remain intact (SEKIBA 1924). The hormonally induced changes that take place in the glands and stroma during the menstrual cycle need not be affected, and with the next menstruation the inflamed functionalis can be shed. In that way an acute, localized inflammation limited to the superficial endometrium may be discharged and the region heal. Often, however, the basal layers of the endometrium are involved, so that with the regeneration of the endometrium from below the inflammatory process again reaches the surface. In addition to the typical inflammatory changes of the endometrium described here, further changes may develop like those seen in other tissues. These changes (for example, edema, exudation, hemorrhage) cannot be regarded as characteristic of endometritis, since they may also be brought about by the physiological or pathological stimulation of hormones. A diagnosis of an endometritis can be made with assurance only if one limits oneself to those morphological criteria that are not induced by hormones.

b) Chronic Non-Specific Endometritis

Chronic non-specific endometritis develops in a woman who is still having menstrual periods only when the inflammation persists in the basalis or other parts that are not shed. The noxious agents causing chronic endometritis are the same as those that induce acute endometritis. CADENA et al. (1973) reported that in the 152 women they studied with endometritis, chronic inflammation was non-specific in 84%. Of these, it was caused by remnants of abortion in 41%, by postpartum factors in 12%, by intrauterine contraceptive devices in 14%, and by pelvic inflammatory disease in 25%. Primary chronic endometritis, however, develops only after the menopause, when the inflammatory process can persist and spread throughout the non-shedding endometrium. The incidence is low. In a recent report, chronic endometritis was diagnosed in 8% of all endometrial specimens (GREENWOOD and MORAN 1981).

Histologically, infiltrates of plasma cells and lymphocytes are characteristic, particularly the plasma cells, which can readily be detected with the methyl green-pyronine stain because it colors their abundant cytoplasmic RNA a bright red. Both types of cells are either scattered diffusely throughout the stroma or aggregated focally. Like the polymorphonuclear leukocytes, they can infiltrate and destroy the glandular epithelium (Fig. 102). They may also accumulate in the glandular lumina but do so less often than the polymorphonuclear leukocytes. In addition, a destruction of tissue is much less common. Often the endometrial architecture is so well preserved that under low magnification the infiltrates of chronic inflammatory cells may be barely evident. In contrast, the hormonally induced cyclic changes of the endometrium are usually profoundly affected, depending, however, on the severity of the inflammation. The postmenstrual epithelialization of the denuded endometrium is severely delayed at times and the regeneration of the endometrium greatly prolonged. If the secretory phase develops at all, it is deficient. Often the endometrium either remains in the proliferative phase or becomes afunctional. In light- and electron-micro-

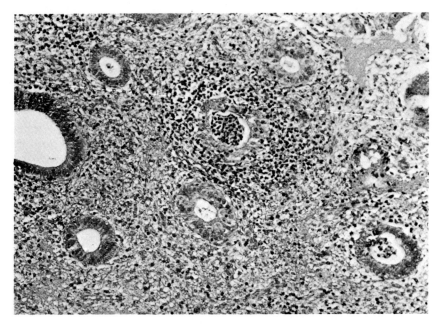

Fig. 102. Chronic endometritis. Lymphocytes and plasma cells have focally infiltrated the stroma and penetrated the glandular epithelium which is disintegrating

scopic studies, chronic productive changes in the connective tissue or in the blood vessels are seldom seen, since these structures in the endometrium are almost exclusively under hormonal control. It is exactly this responsiveness of the endometrium to hormones, however, that is affected by the chronic inflammation. On the other hand, the cause and effect may be reversed: nonfunctioning endometria act as a locus minoris resistentiae and are much more easily infected by microorganisms. Previously it was assumed that the chronic inflammation stimulated the glands to proliferate; the assumption has proved to be wrong. Instead, the epithelial cells undergo secondary degenerative changes; at first they swell, then they become necrotic and desquamate. After prolonged inflammation the endometrium fails to proliferate, reaching a histological state known as "endometritis atrophicans".

Senile endometritis is almost always associated with an atrophic endometrium, the relationship being like that between senile vaginitis and atrophic vaginal mucosa. Since senile endometritis may cause postmenopausal bleeding, it necessitates histological study to rule out a carcinoma. We usually find that the atrophic endometrium is diffusely infiltrated with lymphocytes and plasma cells; its surface may be ulcerated. Often the defect becomes covered with a metaplastic, squamous epithelium. In extreme cases when the entire uterine cavity becomes lined by such a squamous epithelium, the condition is referred to as "ichthyosis uteri". Although it most often persists as a benign metaplasia, it may become precancerous or even cancerous (see p. 244). Furthermore, it must be differentiated from the squamous epithelial components of an adenoacanthoma or a mucoepidermoid adenocarcinoma (see p. 240, Fig. 127).

If the endocervical canal or cervical os become stenosed (e.g., by a carcinoma or from scarring after insertion of radium or after cryosurgery or amputation of the cervix), then the inflammatory exudate cannot be discharged; it accumulates and a *pyometra* develops.

Before one finally decides to make the diagnosis of "non-specific endometritis" one should attempt to find the cause, which may be present as necrotic tissue or as a foreign body in an isolated fragment of the curettings. In any case, a search must be made for products of conception in suspected abortion, especially when the endometrium is undergoing a delayed involution.

In rare instances a dense infiltrate with large lymphoid cells may be misinterpreted as being a lymphoma; differentiation is possible by the heterogenous admixture of large lymphoid cells with plasma cells, mature lymphocytes, and neutrophils in severe chronic endometritis, in contrast to the rather uniform appearance of lymphoma cells (YOUNG et al. 1985).

c) Tuberculous Endometritis

In the Federal Republic of Germany, tuberculous endometritis has become uncommon, in the United States it is extremely rare (ISRAEL et al. 1963). In some European countries, however (Spain: BOTELLA-LLUSIA, 1967; Hungary: VACZY and SCIPIADES 1949; Britain: SUTHERLAND 1958, 1982), it is more common, and in India quite frequent (MANNDRUZZATO 1964; GAURIBAZAZ-MALIK et al. 1983). It is almost always associated with a tuberculous salpingitis, from which the bacteria descend to infect the endometrium. The denuded surface of the postmenstrual endometrium is especially susceptible to infection by the bacteria in the tubal secretions. The uterus is involved in about 49% of the cases of genital tuberculosis (THOM 1952). Endometrial involvement is most frequent during the third to fourth decade; it may also occur, although rarely, in the postmenopause (HASSELGREN and BOLIN 1977). During the past 30 years, the age incidence has changed: the proportion of postmenopausal patients is now much higher (SUTHERLAND 1982). A primary infection of the endometrium, which is produced by hematogenous spread from a pulmonary focus, is exceedingly rare. A latent, chronic tuberculous endometritis may acutely exacerbate after a pregnancy (MEINRENKEN 1949). Occasionally it is possible to demonstrate the bacteria in the endometrium with the fluorescent microscope (FINKE 1950) but rarely with bacteriological methods (ERIKSEN 1947). Generally, however, neither fluorescent microscopy nor the cultural techniques prove successful, thus the diagnosis must rest entirely on the histological diagnosis of the biopsy specimen.

The extent of the tuberculous inflammation in the endometrium may vary profoundly. As in non-specific, chronic endometritis, the most prominent features may be the diffuse or focal infiltrates of lymphocytes and plasma cells in the stroma with involvement and destruction of the glands. These may be the only changes seen in latent or treated tuberculosis. Often in such instances the tuberculous etiology of the chronic endometritis first becomes evident only after the fallopian tubes are removed and found to be involved by a typical

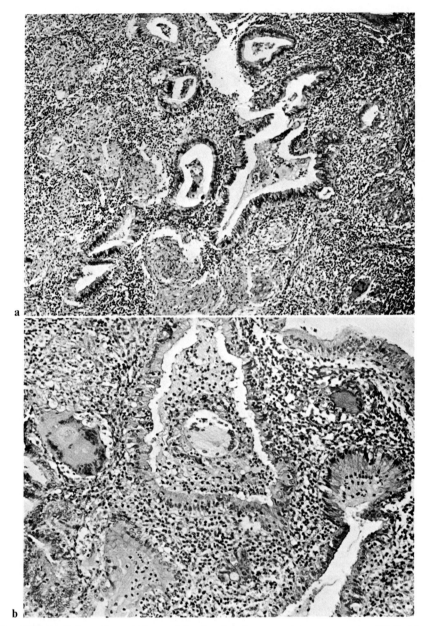

Fig. 103a, b. Tuberculous endometritis. A tubercle, comprising compact epithelioid cells and Langhans' giant cells, breaks through into the glandular lumen. a Low magnification; b higher magnification

caseating tuberculosis. Occasionally the endometrial infiltrates contain typical granulomata with variable numbers of epithelioid cells and a few Langhans' giant cells, all surrounded by a dense zone of lymphocytes. Under low magnification these granulomata can be detected in the densely cellular stroma as pale-

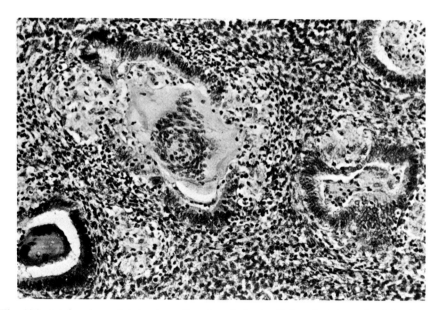

Fig. 104. A tubercle containing large Langhans' giant cells breaks into a glandular lumen

staining, indistinct, rounded lesions: the epithelioid tubercle. Frequently such lesions erode through the epithelium of a neighboring gland and fill its lumen (Figs. 103 and 104). The adjacent intact epithelial cells often respond by atypical proliferation, showing irregular stratification and metaplasia; some cells may contain prominent vacuoles of mucus (SCHRÖDER 1920). At times the stromal cells also become hyperplastic and decidual-like, a change perhaps representing a widespread transformation into epithelioid cells (ZANDER 1949). In severe infections the endometrial surface may ulcerate or undergo extensive caseation necrosis. If the endocervical canal becomes blocked, preventing discharge of the inflammatory exudate, a pyometra results. A curettage under such conditions may cause miliary dissemination of the infection (BÜNGELER 1935). In 20% of their cases of tuberculous endometritis NOGALES et al. (1966) found involvement of the basalis. Only in the severest cases does the infection spread to the myometrium (DE BRUX and DUPRÉ-FROMENT 1965). At the other extreme, if only a few tubercles exist and are localized to a small fragment of the curettings not included in the plane of section, then the tuberculous endometritis will go undiagnosed. When tuberculosis is suspected clinically or when a chronic endometritis exists without evident cause, then the paraffin block should be sectioned at deeper levels and a search made of all tissue fragments for a possible tuberculous granuloma. It is obvious why a simple strip biopsy is unsuitable for diagnostic purposes in these cases.

Often the tuberculous infection greatly suppresses the sensitivity of the endometrium to ovarian hormones. Infertility, which is primary in 94% and secondary in 6% of cases, almost always results (SILLO-SEIDL 1967; NOGALES-ORTIZ et al. 1979) from either the functionally altered endometrium or the associated tuberculous salpingitis. The endometrium is often functionally inert or monophasic, although it may exhibit a deficient secretory phase with a defective secretion of glycogen and an irregular distribution of glycogen and mucopolysaccharides. The stroma may, however, appear almost normal. As the literature indicates, the incidence of a coexisting glandular-cystic hyperplasia varies greatly (NOGALES et al. 1966: 1.1%; KIRCHHOFF 1955: 1.4%; BEHRENS 1956: 6%; NEVINNY-STICKEL 1952: 24%; STÜPER 1955: 30%; SCHAEFER et al. 1972: in all of their postmenopausal cases). The fibrosis about the tubercles, nevertheless, inhibits endometrial shedding during menstruation (NEVINNY-STICKEL 1952). Since a tubercle requires about 15 days to develop and tubercles are frequently found in the early proliferative phase, it is evident in such instances that at least those regions with tubercles could not have been discharged during menstruation. Most likely, the involved regions remain for several cycles (NOGALES et al. 1966). Supporting that opinion is the rare discovery that a polyp may contain tubercles but the remaining endometrium is free of tuberculosis. The proliferating endometrium becomes reinfected either from persisting foci or from recontamination of the surface by infectious discharges from the fallopian tubes.

Infertility may be the only clinical symptom of tuberculous endometritis. Not infrequently tuberculous endometritis is found incidentally at autopsy (THOM 1952); occasionally the diagnosis made from curettings comes as a surprise for the gynecologist.

If fertilization takes place, the blastocyst usually implants in the fallopian tube. According to DE BRUX and DUPRÉ-FROMENT (1965), 5% of all extrauterine pregnancies are caused by a chronic or healing tuberculous salpingitis. If, however, intrauterine implantation does occur, then the mother (WALTHARD 1933; MEINRENKEN 1949) or the child (KAPLAN et al. 1960) may die after delivery or after induced abortion from a miliary tuberculosis.

Tuberculous endometritis may be cured with specific therapy. The tubercles heal as hyalinized fibrous tissue and scars; the infiltrates of chronic inflammatory cells, however, persist in the endometrium for years.

d) Specific Endometritis Caused by Rare Microorganisms

Sarcoidosis of the endometrium, although rarely reported in the literature, may not be as rare as it seems (TAYLOR 1960). Spread by ascending reflux may occur, especially after an intrauterine abortion (BURKMAN et al. 1976). Because sarcoid granulomata so closely resemble those of tuberculosis, it seems likely sarcoidosis is not infrequently misdiagnosed as tuberculosis. All attempts should be made to distinguish it from tuberculosis, however, since therapy and prognosis for the two diseases are different (see Fig. 105). If the detection of acid-fast bacteria fails, then slight or absent necrosis in the granulomata of the fallopian tubes strongly suggests sarcoidosis (CHALVARDJIAN 1978).

Cryptococcus glabratus, an asporogenous budding yeast, may in rare instances produce a granulomatous endometritis that closely resembles tuberculosis (PLAUT 1950). Generally the organism, a normal inhabitant of soil, may be found as saprophyte in feces, urine and sputum. Equally as uncommon is the granulomatous endometritis caused by *Blastomyces dermatitidis* (FARBER

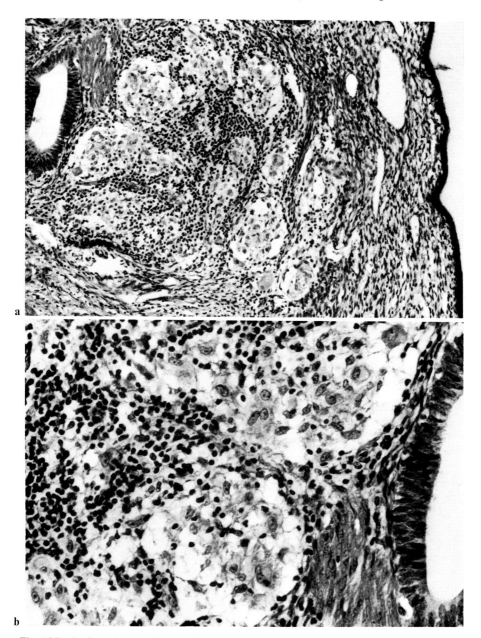

Fig. 105a, b. Sarcoidosis of the endometrium. Epithelioid cell granulomata without evidence of necrosis. **a** Low magnification; **b** higher magnification

et al. 1968). Blastomycosis often looks so much like tuberculosis histologically that in order to find and identify the fungal organisms special stains are needed; among these the Gridley stain (see HUMASON 1962), the PAS reaction, and the Gomori silvermethenamine stain are especially valuable. A granulomatous endometritis also closely resembling tuberculosis may be caused by infection with *T-Mycoplasma*. Although it usually produces few local signs or symptoms, this infection was reportedly associated with infertility or repeated spontaneous abortions (HORNE et al. 1973).

Actinomycosis of the endometrium is extremely rare. The actinomyces infect the endometrium by way of the vagina or by hematogenous dissemination from a focus elsewhere, e.g., an actinomycosis of the appendix (MACCARTHY 1955). The uterus may become a sac of granulation tissue filled with pus in which countless granules of actinomyces are found (HÜFFER 1922; for additional references see BLOCH 1931). LOMAX et al. (1976) reported actinomycotic endometritis developing after insertion of intrauterine devices. A mycotic endometritis consistent with *Candida* infection was observed in a 38-year-old female after prolonged therapy with progesterone (RODRIGUEZ et al. 1972). Endometrial coccidioidomycosis developed in a patient with a disseminated infection (SAW et al. 1975).

An infection of the endometrium with *herpesvirus* may occur. It has been described in patients with immune deficiencies following abortion (GOLDMAN 1970), with an intrauterine contraceptive device (ABRAHAM 1978), and with severe herpetic cervicitis ascending into the uterine cavity (SCHNEIDER et al. 1982). Enlarged ground-glass nuclei containing prominent rod-shaped viral inclusions were found in endometrial glandular and stromal cells, and verified by electron microscopy. There was focal necrosis, and chronic inflammatory cells infiltrated the endometrial stroma. Herpetic endometritis may be the cause of neonatal herpetic infection, and the initial step toward dissemination. MCCRACKEN et al. (1974) and DEHNER and ASKIN (1975) published similar cases of spontaneous abortion due to *cytomegalovirus endometritis* in which the endometrial glandular cells bore characteristic large inclusions. In rare instances, a papilloma virus infection may spread from the cervix to the endometrial cavity and cover the endometrial surface with a diffuse papillomatosis. This layer corresponds to an ichthyosis uteri containing coilocytes (see p. 216; VERKATASESHAN and WOO 1985).

Recently several cases of *chlamydial endometritis* have been detected. Chlamydial antigens could be localized with the immunoperoxidase technique in 4% of 90 cases of chronic endometritis (WINKLER et al. 1984). The antigens were localized in supranuclear intracytoplasmic inclusions of the surface epithelium and always associated with severe acute and chronic inflammation, stromal necrosis and epithelial atypia. Since the inclusions are difficult to localize in routine H&E stains, the immunoperoxidase technique should be used for all cases of severe endometritis to enhance early recognition and prompt application of correct antibiotic therapy in order to prevent further spread and its serious sequelae.

Toxoplasmosis of the endometrium is thought by some investigators to be more common than previously believed, yet one authority (PIEKARSKI 1970) doubts whether the entity really exists. WERNER et al. (1968), with the aid of the immunofluorescent method, reported detecting trophozoites in endometria and in smears of menstrual blood from patients with latent infection. Endometrial toxoplasmosis allegedly is the cause for congenital toxoplasmosis and for some habitual abortions (LANGER 1963, 1966), though proof of that contention is still lacking. Of 172 patients with abortions, toxoplasma were identified in only one by means of inoculation studies in animals (JANSSEN et al. 1970). Histologically, the organism was also seen only once among 87 patients with abortions (KRÄUBIG 1972). The infection supposedly develops as follows: the parasites reach the uterus by way of the blood stream (parasitemia), entering the basalis either directly or after invading from the myometrium. In the basalis the toxoplasma encyst. As the endometrium proliferates the pseudocysts are carried upwards into the functionalis. With menstruation the cyst wall may rupture, liberating the proliferating forms into the endometrial cavity, whence they may again invade the endometrium and form new pseudocysts in the basalis (WERNER et al. 1968). If toxoplasma do infect the endometrium as just outlined, it is strange that the histopathology of the infection has never been identified and reported.

Schistosomiasis of the endometrium is endemic in the Far East, Africa, and central America, but it may be found in the temperate zone in a patient who has once lived in any of these tropical regions (BERRY 1966). Diagnosis of the endometrial infestation is usually made by demonstrating the ova of the Schistosoma haematobium or mansoni in smears of vaginal or cervical secretions. The ova may also be found histologically in the endometrium or in the subepithelial stroma of the cervix. Here they induce either no reaction, or a decidual-like change in the surrounding stroma (WILLIAMS 1967), or a granulomatous inflammation resembling a tubercle, or a diffuse infiltration of eosinophils, histiocytes, lymphocytes, and plasma cells. The mucosal surface may ulcerate. Papillomatous growths may develop on the portio vaginalis (ectocervix). In rare instances the endometrium may be destroyed and replaced by a hemorrhagic granulation tissue. The patients are amenorrheic and infertile (MOUKTHAR 1966).

Gonorrheal endometritis is the result of an ascending infection from the cervix and represents a transitional stage in the development of gonorrheal salpingitis. Histologically it appears as a non-specific chronic endometritis with especially dense inflammatory infiltrates. The abundance of plasma cells is characteristic, but eosinophils may also often be unusually numerous. Reactive hyperplasia of the endometrial glands often ensues. The inflammation may spread to involve the myometrium.

A hematogenous infection of the endometrium by *pneumococci,* although extremely rare, may develop especially postpartum as a complication of lobar pneumonia (NUCKOLS and HERTIG 1938; MCCARTHY and CHO 1979).

Malakoplakia of the endometrium may be a rare cause of postmenopausal bleeding (THOMAS et al. 1978; CHALVARDJIAN et al. 1980; MOLNAR and POLIAK 1983; WILLÉN et al. 1983). The histological and electron-microscopic studies of the granulomatous endometritis reveal the typical Michaelis-Gutmann bodies and the rod-shaped bacteria in abnormal histiocytes. The histiocytic infiltrates may be misinterpreted as being neoplastic, since they may simulate clear cell carcinomas. A careful search for Michaelis-Gutmann bodies is advisable in doubtful cases and may also help to differentiate malakoplakia from non-specific chronic inflammation.

In 1960 PERKINS described a case of *"pneumopolycystic endometritis"* in which vesicles of gas, closely resembling those seen in colpitis emphysematosa, had formed in the endometrium. He believed the vesicles were the result of an infection with gas-forming bacteria.

e) The Foreign Body Granuloma

Various substances are capable of eliciting in the endometrium a foreign body reaction, which histologically resembles that seen in other tissues.

In those countries where *talcum powder* is still used, talcum granulomata may develop after intrauterine procedures. The particles of talc get carried into the endometrial cavity either by curettes or by probes (HAUDE 1956), which are contaminated with surgical dusting powder, or by the insertion of sulfonamide-containing suppositories in which talcum powder serves as a binding agent (BECKER 1950; MARTIN 1951; STRAKOSCH and WURM 1951; SCHUMACHER 1956; KNORR 1960). When the talc particles become embedded in the endometrial stroma, usually that of the basalis, they elicit a chronic inflammatory reaction of the granulomatous type. Histiocytes infiltrate to surround the particles of talc, and the multinucleated giant cells that subsequently form from them attempt to phagocytize the particles (Fig. 106). Vessels nearby proliferate; lymphocytes and plasma cells infiltrate the region. Depending upon the number and size of the talc particles and upon the extent of the inflammatory reaction induced, a chronic endometritis of variable intensity results. When it is severe, focal necroses may result and the granulomata may even erode into the myometrium. In hematoxylin-eosin stained sections the talc crystals are easily recognized as refractile, glass-like splinters or fragments. If torn away from the tissue during sectioning, the angular empty spaces they leave behind in the granulomata serve as important clues. Because the crystals are birefringent they can

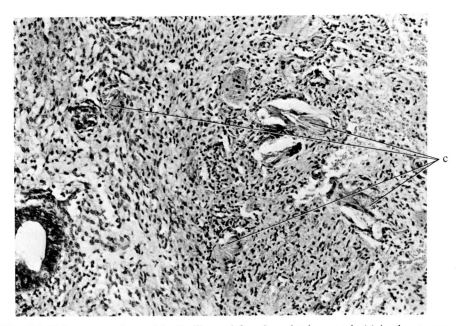

Fig. 106. Talcum granuloma. Needle-like and fan-shaped talc crystals (*c*) in the stroma are surrounded by foreign body giant cells and lymphocytic infiltrates

be readily distinguished from other foreign matter with the polarizing microscope. Talc crystals (hydrous magnesium tetrasilicate), however, resemble crystals of sulfonamide, which are also birefringent. The talc crystals, unlike the sulfonamides, are resistant to dilute hydrochloric acid and heat. Talc particles may remain in the uterine tissues for years, and if scanty, may produce no clinical symptoms. When the granulomata are large and numerous, however, the regeneration of the endometrium after menstruation may be disturbed either physically or chemically (through the liberation of silicic acid). Menorrhagia or a discharge may ensue (SCHUMACHER 1956). In the differential diagnosis all other types of endometritis should be considered, especially tuberculous endometritis and postabortal endometritis. The talc crystals must be identified before the diagnosis of talcum granuloma is made.

An *intrauterine contraceptive device,* a foreign body in the true sense of the word, induces in some patients (according to JESSEN et al. 1963, in 10.1% an acute or chronic endometritis of variable intensity. Where the device contacts the endometrium it may destroy the superficial epithelium. The surrounding stroma may become densely infiltrated with polymorphonuclear leukocytes, lymphocytes and plasma cells (see p. 191). The formation of foreign body giant cells about the devices occurs only rarely (BORELL 1966), probably because they are made of relatively innocuous material. The rather high incidence of endometritis induced by the older types of intrauterine devices was primarily related to their purely mechanical effect, which depended on shape, size, and chemical composition. In contrast, the modern copper T-devices or those containing gestagens injure a normal endometrium only rarely, leading at most to a light infiltration of polymorphonuclear leukocytes within the superficial spongiosa and the lumina of the glands. It is primarily when the endometrium is severely underdeveloped that a focal endometritis develops.

Intrauterine instillation (e.g., of a liquid tissue-adhesive to control profuse bleeding or to cause permanent sterility) may also be accompanied by acute or chronic endometritis (cf. p. 197).

f) Endocervicitis

Just as disease may be limited to the endometrium, so may an inflammation involve only the endocervix, often ending at the internal uterine os. The endocervicitis usually follows an infection that ascends from the portio vaginalis. Acute and chronic non-specific inflammation is common and develops after an inflammatory erosion of the portio or after an eversion of the endocervical epithelium. (Specific inflammations are much rarer.) Histologically the mucosa is papillary, edematous and densely crowded with polymorphonuclear leukocytes, lymphocytes and plasma cells (Fig. 107). Often the superficial columnar epithelium is replaced by metaplastic squamous epithelium. A gonorrheal infection more often causes a severe inflammation in the endocervix than in the endometrium. The frequency and histology of tuberculous endocervicitis correspond to those of tuberculous endometritis.

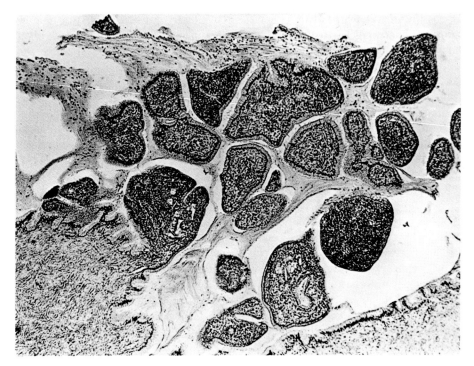

Fig. 107. Chronic endocervicitis. Lymphocytes densely infiltrate mucosal papillae

5. Metaplasias and Related Changes

The pluripotency of the Müllerian epithelium may give rise to various types of metaplasia along the line of Müllerian differentiation. Accordingly, the endometrial epithelium may be replaced focally, seldom diffusely, by any other epithelium of Müllerian type. The same holds true, although much less frequently, for the endometrial stromal cells. The metaplastic changes (growth) may be stimulated by endogenous or, more frequently, by exogenous estrogenic hormones [75% of all patients with metaplasia in the series of HENDRICKSON and KEMPSON (1980) had been previously treated with estrogens], by chronic inflammatory reactions or mechanical irritation. Consequently, metaplasias occur more frequently with increasing age of the patient, in non-menstruating endometria, mostly in the postmenopause.

a) Epithelial Metaplasia

The various types of epithelial metaplasia may occur separately, or combined in various regions of the same endometrium. The importance of their recognition lies in their distinction from early carcinomatous growth. This distinction may be difficult since the metaplastic changes are often associated with cystic or adenomatous hyperproliferation of the endometrial glands owing to the same hormonal stimulus. The accompanying endometria are hyperplastic in approximately 50% of the metaplasias, and atrophic or proliferating in the remaining 50%, whereas they are almost never seen in secretory-type endometria (HENDRICKSON and KEMPSON 1980). The distinction from malignant epithelium should always be based on the cytological structure, not on the metaplastic change per se: a bland metaplasia with eosinophilic cytoplasm within an adenomatous hyperplasia is no sign of an early carcinomatous change. If, on the other hand, a metaplasia shows clear cytological atypia, an early carcinoma developing within the adenomatous hyperplasia must be suspected.

α) **Squamous Metaplasia, Morules, and Ichthyosis**
Nodules of squamous epithelium arise from reserve cells of the glandular epithelium of irregularly proliferating or cystically dilated hyperplastic glands (BAGGISH and WOODRUFF 1967). Such nodules may develop focally or diffusely and may be found in all endometrial layers. All transitional stages are encountered, from a few small nodules to extensive metaplasia. The squamous epithelium may be mature and well differentiated, with distinct intercellular bridges and keratinized cytoplasm, or it may be immature and consist of small rounded cells with scant cytoplasm and poorly delineated cytoplasmic borders (Fig. 108 and cf. Fig. 56); such foci are called *"morules"* (DUTRA 1959). Since their cells may resemble large rounded stromal cells, their distinction from stromal elements may occasionally be difficult. The absence of reticulum fibers around individual cells helps to identify their epithelial nature. Larger morules may contain foci of central necrosis.

When the squamous metaplasia has involved the surface epithelium in a sheet-like fashion, an *ichthyosis* has developed. The ichthyosis may be combined with foci of squamous metaplasia or, in senile atrophy, the surface epithelium alone may undergo metaplasia. Such a sheet-like surface metaplasia may be

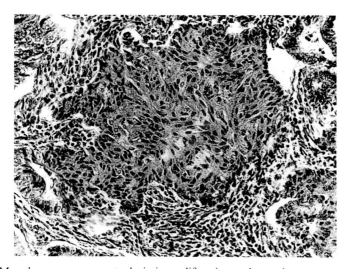

Fig. 108. Morular squamous metaplasia in proliferating endometrium

smooth or papillary, normally stratified and mature, occasionally covered with keratinized cells; or may show loss of stratification with cellular irregularity, depolarization, and enlargement of nuclei with occasional mitoses thus representing epithelial dysplasia. In rare instances, a koilocytic change within the squamous epithelium may be due to a papilloma virus infection ascending from a papillomatous koilocytic dysplasia of the ectocervix (VENKATASESHAN and WOO 1985; cf. p. 211). The stroma under the ichthyosis may contain chronic inflammatory infiltrates comprising mainly lymphocytes and plasma cells. Rarely, a dysplasia developing from an ichthyosis may give rise to a primary squamous cell carcinoma of the endometrium (HECKEROTH and ZIEGLER 1986). On the other hand, sheets of squamous epithelium found as components of curettings are always suspect of carcinoma, regardless of their stage of differentiation. Well-differentiated stratified squamous epithelium may occasionally line the uterine cavity and cover a mucoepidermoid adenocarcinoma in a postmenopausal women (compare Fig. 127). On the other hand, an ichthyosis over a senile atrophic endometritis may become dysplastic, probably as a reaction to injury or inflammation without underlying malignancy. Therefore, a thorough fractionated curettage is always required to determine the origin of ichthyosis.

β) Mucinous (Endocervical) Metaplasia

Within a proliferating endometrium small neighboring groups or larger areas of glands are found lined by high columnar mucinous epithelium of the mature endocervical type with small dense nuclei at the cellular base (Fig. 109). The abundant cytoplasm of the cells is pale in hematoxylin-eosin-stained sections and strongly mucin-positive with the PAS reaction. The mucin also stains me-

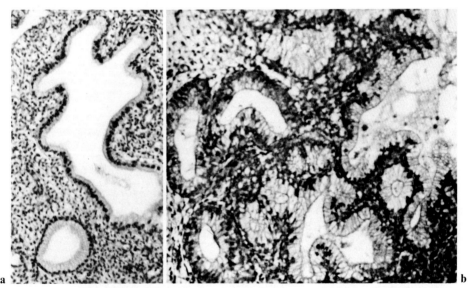

Fig. 109 a, b. Mucinous (endocervical) metaplasia of endometrial glands. **a** Low magnification; **b** high magnification

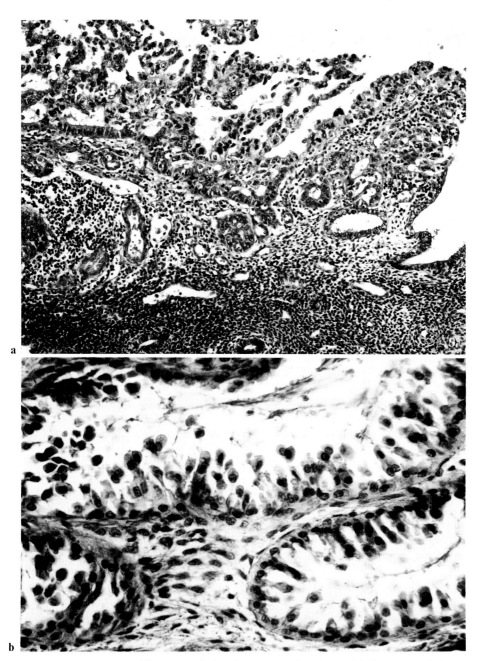

Fig. 110a, b. Serous papillary metaplasia of endometrial surface epithelium (a) and glands (b)

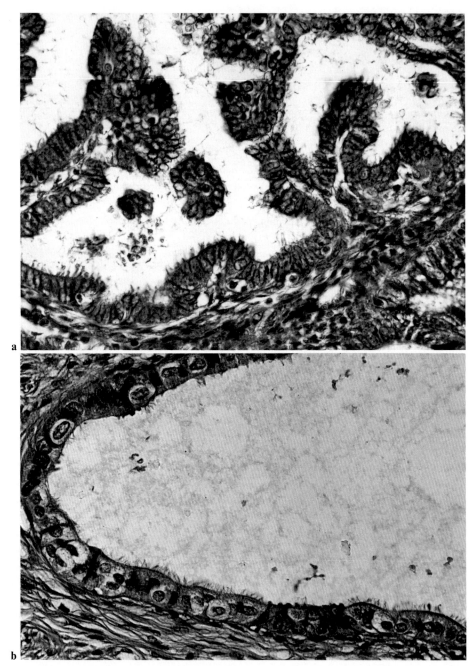

Fig. 111a, b. Ciliated cell change of endometrial glands; **a** pseudostratified type with papillary proliferation; **b** vacuolated type

tachromatically with toluidin blue at pH 2–5, whereas the endometrial cells surrounding the metaplastic foci are negative. The metaplastic glands have the architectural characteristics of the neighboring endometrial glands, but the histochemical and ultrastructural appearance of endocervical cells (DEMOPOULOS and GRECO 1983). The stroma around them is evenly spindle-celled and of the endometrial type. Occasionally, only parts of a gland are lined by metaplastic endocervical epithelium, whereas the remaining portions still represent endometrial-type epithelium. Mucinous metaplasia is usually associated with hyperestrogenism and frequently accompanied by irregular proliferation, endometrial hyperplasia or carcinoma (CZERNOBILSKY et al. 1980).

In rare instances, excessive mucinous metaplasia associated with endocervical stenosis in a postmenopausal woman may result in a myxometra (HONORE 1979). Excessive stimulation of the endocervical epithelium in these metaplastic foci must be differentiated from early mucinous adenocarcinoma of the endometrium.

γ) Serous Papillary Metaplasia

Syncytial aggregates of squamoid cells with papillary epithelial projections may replace foci of the surface or glandular epithelium (Fig. 110). Their nuclei are hyperchromatic, irregular, but mostly pyknotic and degenerated, and devoid of malignant criteria. Such metaplastic foci rarely occupy larger areas; if they do, however, they must be carefully differentiated from early serous papillary carcinoma. In carcinomas, the papillary structures possess fibrovascular cores, while those of serous papillary metaplasia are devoid of stromal support (HENDRICKSON and KEMPSON 1980). Serous papillary metaplasia occurs predominantly in postmenopausal women under exogenous estrogenic stimulation (RORAT and WALLACH 1984). This type of metaplasia must be differentiated from estro-

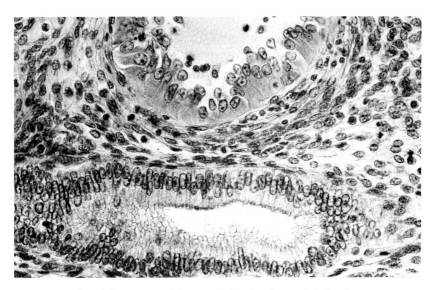

Fig. 112. Eosinophilic (oncocytic) metaplasia of endometrial gland

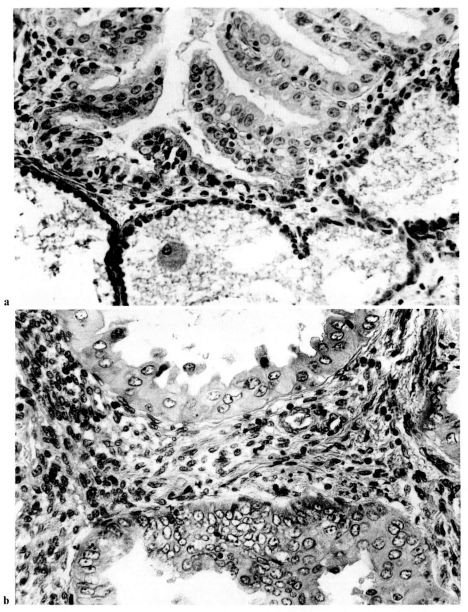

Fig. 113a, b. Eosinophilic (oncocytic) metaplasia with epithelial papillae (**a**) and hobnail nuclei (**b**)

gen-stimulated *papillary proliferation* of glandular epithelium (compare Fig. 111).

δ) Ciliated Cell Change

This type of metaplastic change resembles the mucosal lining of the fallopian tube (FRUIN and TIGHE 1967). These foci consist of single-layered or pseudostrat-

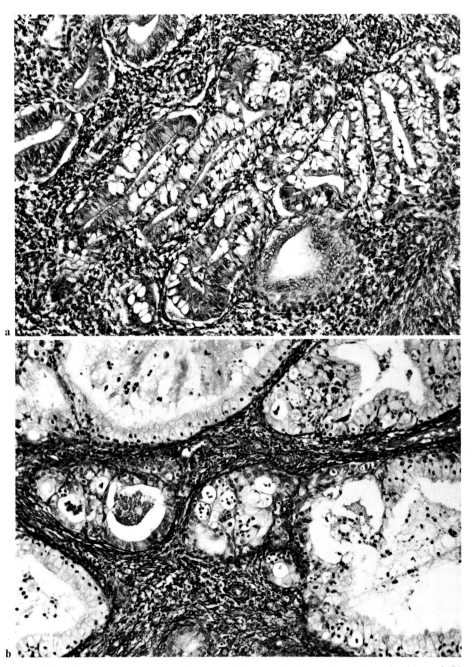

Fig. 114a, b. Clear cell change of endometrial glands; beginning (a), and advanced (b) cytological changes

ified tall columnar ciliated cells with eosinophilic, often vacuolated cytoplasm and may form intraglandular papillae (Fig. 111). They occur in proliferative or hyperplastic endometrium during estrogen stimulation (THORN et al. 1981). Since occasional ciliated cells are normal constituents of the endometrium, only larger accumulations of these cells should be called "metaplasia". Foci of ciliated metaplasia without cilia but with abundant cytoplasm may be called *"eosinophilic (onkocytic) metaplasia"* (Figs. 112 and 113).

ε) **Clear Cell Change**
These foci consist of cells with regular round nuclei and abundant clear cytoplasm which contains glycogen and scanty mucin (Fig. 114). They may be a prestage of eosinophilic or ciliated cell metaplasia. Such cells, however, may not always be truly metaplastic but instead functional variations of glandular cells or cells in disturbed mitosis (cf. p. 28 and 110).

b) **Stromal Metaplasia**

In rare instances the endometrial stromal cells undergo metaplastic changes. Small foci of *myogenic metaplasia* may occasionally be observed (Fig. 115), *cartilagenous, osseous,* or *fatty metaplasia* has rarely been found. All these foci may originate from endometrial stromal cells (ROTH and TAYLOR 1966; BHATIA and HOSHIKO 1982) and represent true metaplasia. On the other hand, in the morphological differential diagnosis fetal remnants following an abortion such

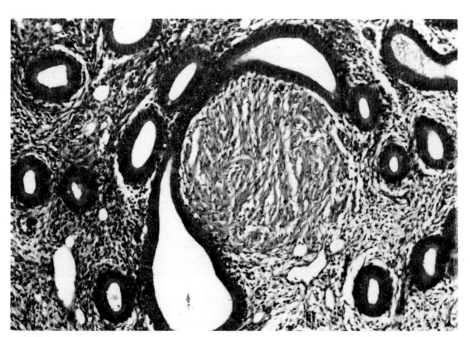

Fig. 115. Round focus of myogenic metaplasia in the endometrial stroma compressing the glandular lumen

as glial tissue (see p. 327) must be excluded. Areas of osseous metaplasia may also occur in the presence of retained necrotic tissue following calcification. Furthermore, all these foci must be carefully differentiated from mixed mesenchymal tumors by their minimal size and focally limited extension and by their benign histological and cytological appearance.

6. Neoplasms

a) Benign Tumors

In our experience benign neoplasms of the endometrium are very rare, primarily because we consider most **benign epithelial growths** of the endometrium (e.g., the polyps) as localized hyperplasias and not as true tumors (see p. 129ff.). The etiology and morphology of these epithelial growths requires that they be classified in the broad spectrum of polypoid glandular-cystic and adenomatous hyperplasias. The old expression "adenoma of the endometrium" has given way to the modern term "adenomatous polyp". The papillomas of the endometrium described in former times were actually exophytic, papillary carcinomas. There is no such tumor as an endometrial papilloma.

Since they originate from the endometrial stroma, the **benign growth of the mesenchymal tissues** also represent stromal hyperplasias in most instances. Sarcomas may arise directly from them without benign tumors developing as transitional stages.

Stromal nodules are a special form of focal stromal hyperplasia. They are well-circumscribed tumors that may arise in the endometrium or myometrium; about 5% are multiple (TAVASSOLI and NORRIS 1981). Histologically, they are composed of uniform cells closely resembling normal endometrial stromal cells. Mitotic activity is low, although not always reliable, since occasional nodules have up to 15 mitoses per 10 HPF but behave nonetheless in a benign fashion. Individual cells are enveloped by a dense reticulin network and occasionally by strands of hyalinized collagen. Most cells are diffusely arranged or form small cords which may have a gland-like appearance. True glands are, however, lacking. The nodules have rather sharp borders that compress the adjacent endometrium or myometrium. The nodules are generally regarded as benign, but may occasionally by presarcomatous. They can be distinguished from the low-grade stromal sarcoma only by their clearly demarcated margins and their expansile (non-invasive) mode of growth, they never invade the myometrium. An "endometrial stromaloma" described by ROSENBERG et al. (1964) may be reclassified as a "stromal nodule". Although this tumor grew so large and polypoid that it filled the uterine cavity, it remained nonetheless localized to the endometrium. Histologically, it consisted of uniform stromal cells enmeshed in reticulum fibers. There was no evidence of invasive growth or malignancy.

Hemangiomas of the endometrium and myometrium have been diagnosed from time to time (R. MEYER 1925; NEUMANN 1929; MARSH 1950; GRUND and SIEGEL 1954; HUNTER and COGGINS 1965). Grossly, these tumors resemble hemorrhagic polyps. Histologically, they usually arise from the inner myometrium and either grow into the endometrium or push it away. The endometrial stroma contains innumerable large and small, thin-walled blood vessels. One patient reported also had multiple cutaneous hemangiomata.

Hemangiopericytomas are rare stromovascular tumors deriving from the myoepithelial pericyte (GREENE and GERBIE 1954; SILVERBERG et al. 1971). They present a characteristic perivascular whorled pattern of proliferating spindle-shaped cells. These tumors are potentially malignant, despite low mitotic rates or lack of nuclear atypias (BUSCEMA et al. 1987). These tumors may arise in the myometrium or in endometrial polyps.

IRWIN (1956) described a primary *lymphoma* of the endometrium, which was polypoid and composed of many closely packed lymphoid follicles with prominent germinal centers. A few scattered endometrial glands could still be found within the tumor. SCHINKELE (1947) reported an *angiomyoma* of the functional layer of a secretory endometrium. Presumably the tumor had originated from smooth muscle cells of a blood vessel. Grossly the tumor appeared as a red nodule within the endometrium. HOLZNER and LASSMANN (1967) diagnosed as *"neurofibromatosis"* of the endometrium, circumscribed, fasciculated proliferations of Schwann cells that extended to just beneath the superficial epithelium. Similar proliferations were also evident in the myometrium. YOUNG et al. (1981) described a truly neoplastic *glioma* in a 15-year-old virgin girl. The tumor was a polyp 3 × 10 cm that filled the uterine cavity and invaded the myometrium. It was considered to be of either teratomatous or mesodermal (via heterologous neometaplasia) origin with aberrant cellular differentiation by transformation into other types of cell entirely foreign to the tissue from which they arise.

Benign Mixed Mesodermal Tumors. A rare benign variant of the malignant mixed Müllerian tumors is the papillary *adenofibroma (cystadenofibroma)* of the endometrium (VELLIOS and REAGAN 1973). This is usually found as an irregularly knobby or richly polypoid growth protruding into and filling the uterine cavity. Its elongated polyps are composed of closely crowded spindle-shaped fibroblasts or endometrial stromal cells, occasionally intermingled with smooth muscle cells (MILES et al. 1982), and are covered with an epithelium of cuboidal or columnar endometrial cells that may secrete mucus or show squamous metaplasia like that of the endocervix. Owing to the inherent growth potentialities of the epithelium and the profuse branchings of the polyps, buds of epithelium become caught up in the cellular stroma to form gland-like structures. The tumor resembles an ovarian adenofibroma. It must be distinguished from a well-differentiated homologous stromal sarcoma, which is not generally papillary, is better vascularized, and whose stromal cells often show mitoses (GRIMALT et al. 1975). The mitotic rate of the adenofibroma is below 4 per 10 HPF (ZALOUDEK and NORRIS 1981). The tumor never invades the myometrium, but it has a high rate of recurrence, and it may, after many years and frequent recurrences, undergo malignant change (see p. 288f.). The average age is in the late postmenopause.

A rare type of *stromal tumor with epithelial differentiation* was recently described in a 21-year-old woman (FEKETE et al. 1985). This benign polypoid growth arose from the endometrial stroma and penetrated superficially into the surrounding myometrium. It consisted of stromal cells closely intermingled with endometrial foam cells and epithelial nests. The tumor was interpreted as arising from multipotential mesenchyme which had differentiated toward endometrial stroma and epithelium, or from endometrial stroma which had retained the capacity to differentiate toward endometrial epithelium. Because they have different intermediate filaments, it is possible to differentiate these tumors from benign epithelioid tumors of myogenic origin using immunohistological methods.

Another variety of a benign mixed mesodermal tumor of the endometrium is the *atypical polypoid adenomyoma*. On gross examination this tumor resembles an ordinary endometrial polyp. It may be pedunculated or sessile and is then well demarcated from the underlying myometrium. Microscopically, it consists of irregularly arranged, highly proliferating endometrial glands with foci of squamous metaplasia surrounded by proliferating bundles of smooth muscle fibers, which present a well-differentiated ultrastructure (MAZUR 1981; DEL-PRADO et al. 1985; YOUNG et al. 1986). Despite the atypical adenomatous-like proliferation of the glands with architectural and occasional cytological atypias and loss of nuclear polarity, these small tumors do not invade the myometrium and do not recur after complete removal; consequently, they do not require a hysterectomy. In the curettings they have to be differentiated from fragments of an adenocarcinoma that invades the myometrium or is surrounded by a desmoplastic reaction, and from fragments of a carcinofibroma, which is usually

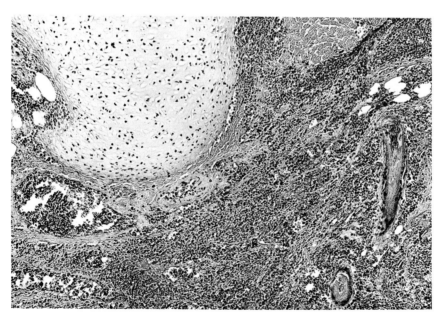

Fig. 116. Teratoma of the endometrium. Nodule of immature cartilage at *upper left* bounded by numerous blood-filled vessels and large infiltrates of lymphocytes. At *upper right* cross-sectioned skeletal muscle and a few vacuoles of fat; at *lower right*, abnormally developed hair follicles

devoid of smooth muscle cells (cf. p. 291). The relatively small size of the adenomyoma, its occurrence in younger women and its content of well-differentiated smooth muscle help to separate this entity from malignant tumors.

The polypoid adenomyoma originates in the endometrium, presumably by smooth muscle metaplasia of the endometrial stromal cells and by concomitant adenomatous proliferation of glands. Hence it is unrelated to the myometrium (MAZUR 1981).

We have seen a peanut-sized lesion of the endometrium that we diagnosed as a *benign solid teratoma* (DALLENBACH-HELLWEG and WITTLINGER 1976). It consisted of peculiar shaped portions of normal-appearing embryonal cartilage, thick-walled and tortuous vessels, twisted bundles of nerves, ducts of respiratory and intestinal epithelium, and sheets of skin, all of which were so scrambled together as to convince us the lesion was not the remnant of a malformed embryo (Fig. 116). In addition, we could find no traces of placental or decidual tissue in the surrounding endometrial tissues. MARTIN et al. (1979) reported on a benign cystic teratoma of the endometrium and suggested it may have arisen from an injured fertilized ovum or one that underwent parthogenesis.

b) Carcinoma of the Endometrium

The statistics in the literature on the **frequency** of endometrial carcinoma show that the tumor has increased considerably as compared with carcinoma of the cervix. Fifty years ago the ratio of endometrial carcinoma to cervical carcinoma was 1:14.8 (HINSELMANN 1930), and 30 years ago it was 1:3–4. More recently, however, in the larger gynecological hospitals endometrial carcinoma has been diagnosed as often as cervical carcinoma (GORE and HERTIG 1962; WYNDER et al. 1966; HELD 1969). The increase in the incidence of endometrial carcinoma is not just because women are living longer; there are other significant reasons but these will be discussed later. It should be mentioned now, however, that the relationship of endometrial carcinoma to cervical carcinoma is also racially dependent. For example, in Jewish women in New York City the ratio of these two carcinomas is 1:0.3 (they rarely develop cervical carcinomas); in all other white women the ratio is 1:1.29, and in negro women it is 1:5.2 (National Cancer Institute, Washington, 1952). In Japan the ratio is 1:24.4 (KAISER 1969), in Nigeria 1:40 (MORDI and NNATU 1986). Endometrial carcinoma predominately develops after the menopause (80%). As calculated from about 12000 cases, which were compiled from the literature (DALLENBACH-HELLWEG 1964) and supplemented by additional cases, the average age of the patients is 57.5 years. Only about 2% of all carcinomas of the corpus uteri are found in women under 40 years (SOMMERS et al. 1949; DOCKERTY et al. 1951; HUSSLEIN and SCHÜLLER 1952; KEMPSON and POKORNY 1968), and is very seldom associated with intrauterine pregnancy (SUZUKI et al. 1984). Endometrial carcinoma has been described in girls under 12 years but is extremely rare (MARTINS 1960).

A large percentage of the women who develop endometrial carcinoma have **endocrine disturbances;** it is particularly striking how many of them also have hypertension, diabetes mellitus, obesity, and are sterile (see Table 19). Even though the findings reported by the various investigators may not be quite comparable with one another, the large numbers of patients involved nevertheless allow us to obtain a fairly accurate survey of the subject. The menopause is often delayed (CROSSEN and HOBBS 1935; RANDALL 1945; GUSBERG 1947; TAYLOR and BECKER 1947; SPEERT 1948; PALMER et al. 1949; COSBIE et al. 1954; WAY 1954; PEEL 1956; KOTTMEIER 1959; DIEBELT et al. 1962, and others). The climacterium is free of disturbing signs and symptoms of hormonal insufficiency.

Usually when examined **grossly,** carcinoma of the corpus uteri is found in the fundus, arising from the mucosa of a tubal recess. Carcinomas originating in the region of the isthmus or just above it are uncommon; according to TAYLOR and BECKER (1947) they represent 24% of the corpus carcinomas. The reason for the low incidence here is probably the insensitivity of the isthmic mucosa to hormones. The tumors may project as spongy, polypoid or papillary masses into the uterine cavity. They may, however, be flat or ulcerated, or grow primarily into the uterine wall (R. MEYER 1930). With such invasion the uterus is not always enlarged (Fig. 117). Growth takes place relatively slowly, and metastases often appear late.

Various authors have suggested schemas for *classifying endometrial carcinoma by stages*. We use a modified version of the widely used JAVERT and HOFAMMANN (1952) classification (see HELD 1969) which is also identical with the International Federation of Gynecology and Obstetrics (FIGO) classification:

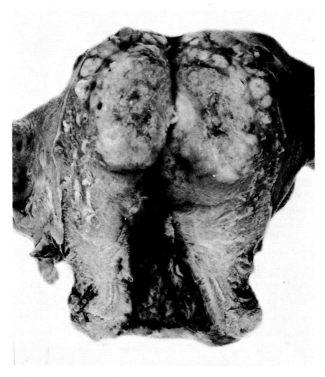

Fig. 117. A complete uterus opened to show an adenocarcinoma of the corpus endometrium that extends through the uterine wall to the serosa

Stage 0: limited to the endometrium
Stage 1: invasion of the myometrium
Stage 2: extension into any part of the cervix
Stage 3: extension into the fallopian tube, ovary or vagina; lymphogenous metastases, but limited to the small pelvis
Stage 4: spread to the urinary bladder or rectum, and/or hematogenous metastases

The extension into the endocervix may be either by direct downward growth from the uterine cavity, or more frequently, by spread along lymphatic channels (KADAR et al. 1982). A fractionated curettage should be made before treatment is started to determine whether the endocervix is involved or not, since the extent of the surgical procedure for stage 1 cancer differs considerably from that for stage 2. If cervical curettings contain tumor fragments showing no involvement of endocervical tissues, these may well represent tumor fragments shed from the uterine cavity. They should not be misinterpreted as involvement of the endocervix. For that diagnosis, direct invasion of endocervical tissues must be seen.

From the autopsies of 80 patients who had been treated for endometrial carcinoma, FISCHER (1957) found **metastases** in 80%. Structures and organs most frequently involved were: lymph nodes (47.5%), parametrium (30.5%), peritoneum (31.2%), liver (21.2%), pelvic connective tissue (18.7%), urinary bladder (16.2%), and rectum (13.7%). In 12.5% the vagina, bowel and pleura were invaded, the lungs in 10%. In only 2.5% of the cases were metastases disclosed in the ovaries, stomach and pancreas. Involvement of the kidney or brain was even less. Other investigators reported a higher incidence of ovarian metastases (JAVERT and HOFAMMANN 1952; 11.8%; RYDEN 1952: 8.4%; BERGSJÖ 1962: 9%; DAVIS 1964: 7%). According to HARNETT (1949), as well as to RANDALL and GODDARD (1956), distant metastases (stage 4) develop in only 9.4% of all patients with endometrial carcinoma. PIVER (1966) found, however, that 26.5% of patients with adenoacanthoma had metastases. The lungs (in 4% of DIETZ's cases, 1958) and liver were involved most often. Other authors emphasized the frequency of involvement of lymphatics and blood vessels (JAKOBOVITS 1956; BARBER et al. 1962) or the isolated metastases to the central nervous system (LIPIN and DAVISON 1947). Metastases to bones (VANECKO et al. 1967) and skin (DAMEWOOD et al. 1980) are rare. In HARNETT's (1949) series, the endometrial carcinoma remained localized to the body of the uterus in 65.6% of the patients. Compared with carcinomas of other regions, endometrial carcinomas metastazise infrequently but are more often associated with a second primary tumor, e.g., of the ovary, breast, or rectum. These may or may not resemble the endometrial tumor histologically. If they do, one should never forget that possibility to avoid misdiagnosing a second primary as a metastasis (JAHODA and TATRA 1972).

In the **histological characterization,** typing and grading are of importance as they influence prognosis and survival rates (POULSEN et al. 1975). For *typing,* endometrial carcinomas may be subdivided histogenetically, since these tumors, like those of other parts of the female genital tract, develop from descendants of the Müllerian epithelium (Table 14). Accordingly, a carcinomatous transformation may proceed from any stage of development of the endometrium or may follow a heterotopic differentiation, in which the transforming cell may be either fixed in its ability to differentiate further or be pluripotent. Each type of carcinoma may be preceded by structurally analogous precursors (Table 15). Variations in the histology of the precursor states are influences by age, constitutional factors of the patient, and exogenous factors, such as hormone therapy (GERSCHENSON and FENNELL 1982). All precancerous stages may be diffuse or focal, when only parts of the endometrium are still responsive to hormones while surrounding portions have lost their receptors. The carcinomas with endometrial differentiation develop from adenomatous hyperplasia

Table 14. Carcinomas of the endometrium

Histogenesis	Structure	Grading	Survival rate (%)	Relative frequency (%)
Endometrial	*Adenocarcioma*			59.6
	Glandular or	Grade 1	93	
	Glandular-papillary	Grade 2	76	
	Solid	Grade 3	61	
	Secretory	Grade 1	87	
	Ciliated cell	Grade 1		
	Adenocarcinoma with squamous metaplasia			
	Adenoacanthoma	Grade 1	87	21.7
	Adenosquamous carcinoma	Grades 2+3	47	6.9
Endocervical	*Mucinous adenocarcinoma*	Grades 1+2		
	Mucoepidermoid adenocarcinoma	Grades 2+3	47	
	Clear cell carcinoma			5.7
	Glandular or papillary	Grade 2	35	
	Solid	Grade 3		
Serous	*Serous papillary carcinoma*	Grades 1 / Grades 2+3	51	4.7
Ectocervical	*Squamous cell carcinoma*	Grades 1, 2, or 3		

Table 15. Possible origin of different types of endometrial carcinomas from respective metaplastic states

Adenomatous hyperplasia	→ Adenocarcinoma, endometrial type
With ciliated cells	→ Adenocarcinoma, ciliated cell type
With squamous metaplasia and morules	→ Adenoacanthoma
	→ Adenosquamous carcinoma
	→ Squamous cell carcinoma
With mucinous metaplasia	→ Mucinous adenocarcinoma
	→ Mucoepidermoid adenocarcinoma
With clear cell change	→ Clear cell carcinoma
With serous papillary metaplasia	→ Serous papillary carcinoma

and occur predominately during the early postmenopausal period. The carcinomas with ectopic differentiation develop from foci of corresponding types of metaplasia and occur predominately in the late postmenopausal period.

Histological *grading* should be based on the degree of structural differentiation and cytological atypia. According to the degree of structural differentiation, we distinguish, in accordance with FIGO, grade 1 (100%–70% well-differentiated carcinomatous glands), grade 2 (70%–30%), and grade 3 (30%–0%). The significance of cytological atypia within this grading system is still under study.

The **separation** of a well-differentiated (grade 1) carcinoma **from adenomatous hyperplasia** (grade 3) may be difficult because of the morphological similarities shared by both, such as back-to-back position of glands, epithelial stratification and nuclear atypia (WELCH and SCULLY 1977; TAVASSOLI and KRAUS 1978; HENDRICKSON and KEMPSON 1980). The most important and reliable criterion of the beginning of carcinomatous growth appears to be stromal invasion. This can be diagnosed by an altered fibroblastic (desmoplastic) stromal reaction around invading atypical glands, a confluent glandular pattern with microalveolar or cribriform proliferation and replacement of stroma (Fig. 119b), an extensive papillary pattern (Fig. 119a), or large areas of squamous metaplasia. One of these criteria, if it occupies an area 4.2 mm in diameter equaling one-half of a low-power field, would be sufficient for a diagnosis of stromal invasion (KURMAN and NORRIS 1982; NORRIS et al. 1983). A desmoplastic stromal reaction can be recognized by densely arranged spindle-shaped fibroblasts with elongated nuclei (Fig. 118). These fibroblasts are arranged in parallel about the

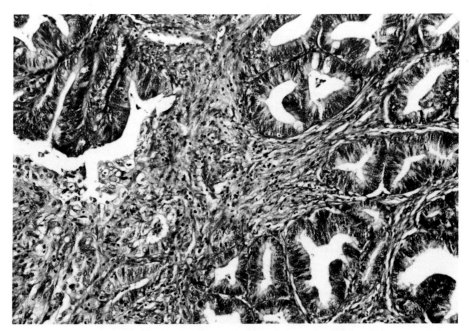

Fig. 118. Desmoplastic stromal reaction consisting of proliferating fibroblasts and sparse lymphatic infiltrates around invading carcinomatous glands

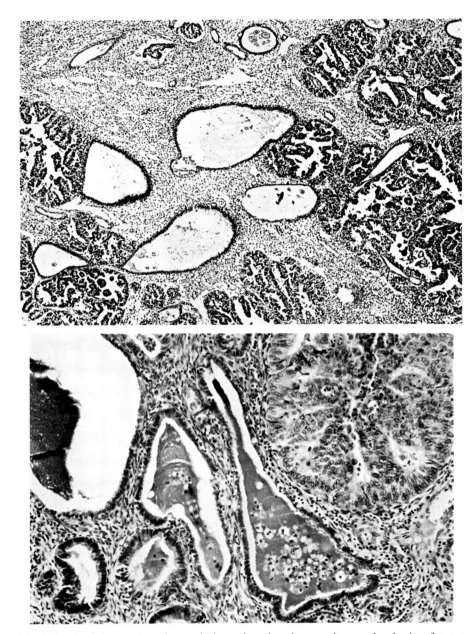

Fig. 119a, b. Adenomatous hyperplasia and early adenocarcinoma developing from a glandular-cystic hyperplasia

invading glands, thereby disrupting the glandular pattern. Such a stromal reaction must be distinguished from the stroma of atypical polypoid adenomyomas (cf. p. 225). The various glandular patterns diagnostic of stromal invasion need not include cytological atypias. Cells with a high grade of nuclear atypia may be, without regard to the area they occupy, highly suspicious of stromal invasion elsewhere in the endometrial specimen. Such atypical cytological changes are immediate precursors of early carcinoma (cf. p. 124f. and Fig. 66).

Early endometrial carcinoma exists for only a short time and consequently is rarely encountered. It develops either focally or multicentrically within an adenomatous hyperplasia by invading the stroma (Fig. 119). It is always limited to the endometrium. Within these foci, groups of glands are lined by multilayered, atypical epithelial cells which have depolarized, enlarged nuclei containing prominent nucleoli. They are frequently in mitosis. Their cytoplasm is pale or vacuolated. The stroma is rarefied and focally scant, particularly in regions with microalveolar change. The early carcinomatous foci have compressed borders and may be surrounded by lymphocytic infiltrates indicating stromal invasion. Most of these early carcinomas are glandular grade 1, but occasionally grade 2, or even grade 3 may be seen. Early adenocarcinoma has to be differentiated from grade 3 adenomatous hyperplasia (cf. p. 127, 230).

α) Carcinomas with Endometrial Differentiation

This most common type of endometrial carcinoma may be subdivided into the purely glandular or glandular-papillary adenocarcinoma of various degrees of differentiation, and into adenocarcinoma with squamous metaplasia or morules.

Adenocarcinoma. This type constitutes 86% of all endometrial carcinomas (HERTIG and GORE 1960). In deciding the type of therapy and in evaluating prognosis, not only is the staging of this tumor important, but also its histological grading (Table 14).

The *glandular or glandular-papillary adenocarcinoma* consists in its well-differentiated type (grade 1) of slender tubular glands. These are usually free of secretions and lined by a pseudostratified to stratified epithelium that may grow into the lumen or toward the tumor surface in a papillary fashion (Fig. 120). The nuclei are large, at times pleomorphic, and often contain several prominent nucleoli. Mitoses are numerous. The cytoplasm is sparse. In their fine structure, however, these cells do not differ strikingly from those of the normal or hyperplastic endometrium (THRASHER and RICHART 1972; AYCOCK et al. 1979). In cytological smears they are, therefore, usually recognized only with difficulty. A periglandular basal lamina is always developed. According to FERENCZY (1976), even poorly differentiated carcinoma cells may be suspected to be of endometrial origin from their abundant juxtanuclear microfilaments. Usually the stroma between the tubular glands is barely visible, being reduced to slips of scanty fibers of collagen and thin capillaries.

The poorly differentiated type (grade 2) may consist of well-differentiated (grade 1) regions sharply set off from poorly differentiated parts (grade 3) (Fig. 121), or may be a rather diffuse, moderately well-differentiated tumor composed of microglandular structures showing occasionally pronounced cribriform patterns. The glandular epithelium is lower, more cuboidal than that of the well-differentiated carcinomas. It is usually polymorphic, the cells have sparse cytoplasm and depolarized rounded nuclei. Mitoses are numerous. A basement membrane is rudimentary.

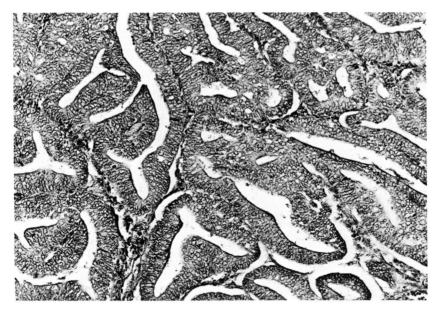

Fig. 120. A well-differentiated adenocarcinoma of the endometrium

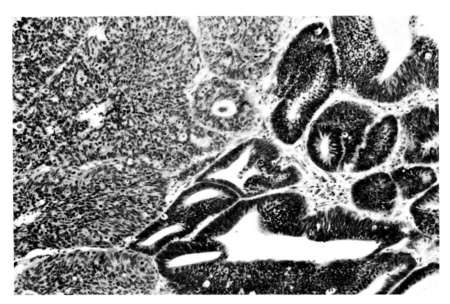

Fig. 121. Adenocarcinoma of the endometrium composed of mature and immature parts that are readily distinguished

The undifferentiated type (grade 3) is composed of solid sheets of cells in which one may often find primitive glands by using the PAS stain. These glands appear as pseudorosettes, containing in their centers small amounts of mucus about which the elongated tumor cells radiate (Fig. 122). Most nuclei are large,

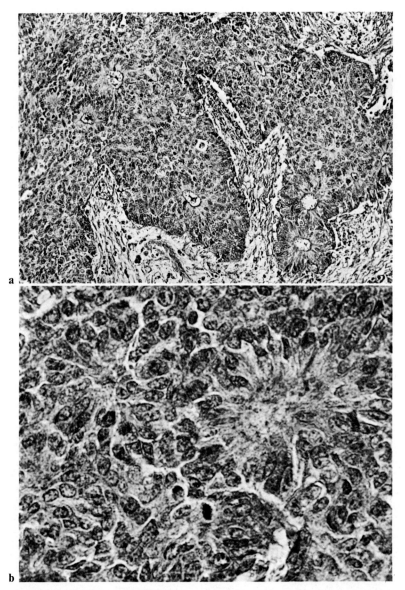

Fig. 122a, b. Immature adenocarcinoma of the endometrium, composed of solid cords of cells with some nuclei arranged in pseudorosettes and a suggestion of primitive gland formation. **a** Low magnification; **b** higher magnification

polymorphic, with clumped chromatin, and cytologically are clearly atypical. The cytoplasm is usually sparse.

The *secretory adenocarcinoma* consists of branching glands, whose cells secrete abundantly and contain irregularly depolarized nuclei arranged in a single row (Fig. 123). Except for its excessive secretory activity, this rare type of adeno-

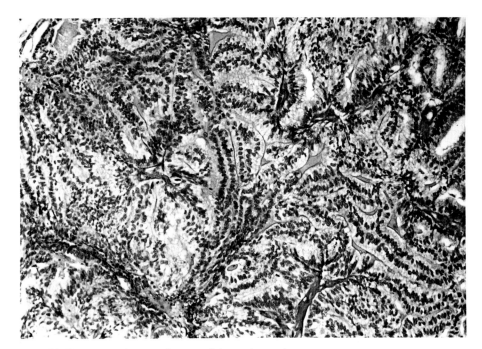

Fig. 123. Secretory adenocarcinoma of the endometrium

carcinoma differs in no other way from the well-differentiated type of adenocarcinoma. Some of the patients developing this tumor have received high doses of gestagens, suggesting the secretory activity is hormonally regulated. In the remaining patients, it may be difficult to detect the source of progesterone since most of them are in their late postmenopause (CHRISTOPHERSON et al. 1982). Secretory adenocarcinoma has to be distinguished from clear cell carcinoma because of its much more favorable prognosis (TOBON and WATKINS 1985).

The *ciliated adenocarcinoma* is a rare variant of the endometrial adenocarcinoma and is composed in large part of ciliated cells like those of proliferating endometrium (HENDRICKSON and KEMPSON 1983). The cilia have been shown to develop under estrogenic stimulation (SCHUELLER 1968; THOM et al. 1981).

Adenocarcinomas with Squamous Metaplasia. Depending on the thoroughness of the histological examination, the *adenoacanthoma* may constitute from 6.8% (MARCUS 1961) to 43.7% of endometrial adenocarcinomas (TWEEDDALE et al. 1964; DOBBIE et al. 1965: 5.5%; BOUTSELIS et al. 1963: 7%; HERTIG and GORE 1960: 14%; DAVIS 1964: 14%; JAVERT and RENNING 1963: 16%; CHARLES 1965: 37.1%; see the last for further references). NG et al. (1973) reported that over a 30-year period the adenoacanthomas had increased from 12.6% to 32.8%. ROBBOY and BRADLEY (1979) suggested that increase might be related to the growing use of estrogen therapy, since 51% of their patients with adenoacanthoma had previously taken estrogen.

The adenoacanthoma (adenocancroid: HERXHEIMER 1907) is a well-differentiated, often papillary adenocarcinoma of the endometrial type with nodular

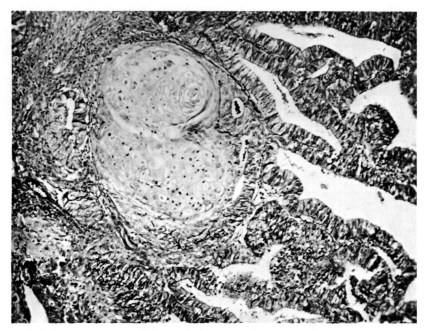

Fig. 124. Adenoacanthoma of the endometrium with nests of squamous cells among the glands

regions of squamous metaplasia or morules among the glandular structures (Fig. 124). The epithelium forming the glands, most of which are well differentiated, is pseudostratified or stratified and frequently grows as papillae. The glandular lumina are usually narrow and contain either scanty mucus or none at all. The nodules of squamous epithelium mingle with the cells of the glands from which they apparently arise; some nodules contain parakeratotic hornpearls, others often reveal intercellular bridges. Opinions vary greatly about the origin of these nodules of squamous epithelium (HENDRICKSON and KEMPSON 1980). Observations on their development and their morphological behavior suggest that they arise by metaplasia from the columnar epithelium (NOVAK 1929; TWEEDDALE et al. 1964; CHARLES 1965; WILLIAMS 1965). Because the histological structure of the nodules is so regular, most investigators assume they represent benign metaplasia within an adenocarcinoma. That they are potentially malignant is proved by the observation that some metastases of the adenoacanthoma not only consist of glands but often of squamous epithelium as well (CHARLES 1965). The scanty stroma present in the adenoacanthoma often contains abundant foam cells (DALLENBACH-HELLWEG 1964; TWEEDDALE et al. 1964; CHARLES 1965; see p. 251).

It is important to distinguish this well-differentiated form of carcinoma from the poorly differentiated adenosquamous carcinoma similarly composed of mixed types of epithelial cells, since the adenoacanthoma has a much more favorable prognosis with a 5-year survival rate of 87% (ALBERHASKY et al. 1982; CONNELLY et al. 1982); that for patients with adenosquamous carcinoma is 47%.

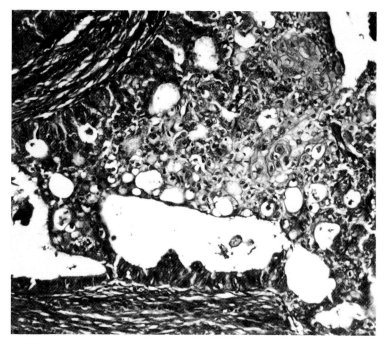

Fig. 125. Adenosquamous carcinoma of the endometrium. Moderately differentiated carcinomatous glands intermingled among poorly differentiated ill-defined foci of squamous metaplasia

The *adenosquamous carcinoma* is also increasing in frequency (SALAZAR et al. 1977) and is often associated with intraductal breast carcinoma (BLAUSTEIN et al. 1978). In this tumor, the glandular and solid-squamous portions are closely mixed (Fig. 125). Some glands are well-differentiated, others develop as compact small acini. The solid regions consist of immature squamous metaplasia with atypical nuclei, frequent mitoses, and variable abundant eosinophilic cytoplasm. Ultrastructurally, they show criteria of malignant cells, with chromatin-clumping of the nucleus and poorly formed tonofibrils in the cytoplasm (AIKAWA and NG 1973). Occasionally, these cells may have a glassy appearance (CHRISTOPHERSON et al. 1982). The most important criterion for distinguishing it from the adenoacanthoma is the disordered arrangement of the immature epidermoid components. Whereas the nuclei of the squamous cells of adenoacanthomas have diploid DNA values, those of adenosquamous carcinomas are aneuploid. In addition, the glandular component is often less well differentiated than that of the adenoacanthoma and usually contains no mucus. Immunohistological techniques for cell markers are of no help in differentiating the two types of carcinoma, since the mature and immature squamous metaplasias in these carcinomas show virtually identical cytoskeletons because of their common origin (WARHOL et al. 1984). Since adenosquamous carcinomas with a well-differentiated glandular component have an equally poor prognosis as those with poorly differentiated glands, it is the malignant squamous component that worsens prognosis and is responsible for early deep myometrial invasion (DEMOPOULOS et al. 1986).

β) Carcinomas Which Originate from Pluripotent Müllerian Epithelium

The **mucinous adenocarcinoma** of the endometrium is of the endocervical type and structurally and histochemically closely resembles the mucinous adenocarcinoma of the endocervical mucosa. The carcinomatous glands are generally cystic, filled with mucus, and lined by a tall, mucus-secreting epithelium with depolarized, polymorphic, and atypical nuclei (Fig. 126a). Elongated and branching intraluminal papillae develop. Microglandular and solid areas may occasionally be seen (Fig. 126b). Marked nuclear atypia is rarely encountered, mitotic activity is not prominent. The intra-cytoplasmic distribution of mucin is virtually identical to that of the endocervical adenocarcinoma. Two histological differentiation gradings may be distinguished, corresponding to grades 1 and 2. At the margins of the carcinoma, remnants of the endocervical metaplasia can often be found in the adenomatous hyperplasia that preceded the carcinoma. The distinction of the mucinous adenocarcinoma of the endometrium from that of the endocervix is difficult. It can only be made anatomically, since both produce almost identical acid mucopolysaccharides (CZERNOBILSKY et al. 1980; TILTMAN 1980; Ross et al. 1983).

The **mucoepidermoid adenocarcinoma** consists predominately of a mucoepidermoid component with mono- or multicellular mucus secretion and keratinization within solid cords of atypical epidermoid cells (Fig. 127). In addition to, and closely mixed in with, the solid components are well- or poorly differentiated carcinomatous glands of variable size formed by mucus-secreting cells of the endocervical type (Fig. 128). Depending on the degree of maturation, two grades of differentiation (grades 2 and 3) of this highly malignant type of carcinoma may be distinguished. It may be exceedingly difficult, if not impossible, to differentiate this endometrial tumor from a mucoepidermoid adenocarcioma arising in the endocervix, especially if the curettings consist only of carcinoma. A fractionated curettage may help in making the distinction but is not always reliable. The patient's age is important since mucoepidermoid adenocarcinomas of the endometrium occur chiefly in old women beyond the seventh decade, whereas mucoepidermoid adenocarcinoma of the endocervix has been found to arise in women of a mean age of 39 years (DALLENBACH-HELLWEG 1982). Careful study of the exstirpated uterus usually reveals the source of the carcinoma.

The **clear cell carcinoma**. This usually develops in the senile patient beyond the seventh decade of life. The tumor closely resembles the clear cell carcinoma of the ovary, cervix, and vagina both light- and electron-microscopically, and like these was incorrectly referred to as "mesonephroid adenocarcinoma" (JANOVSKI and WEIR 1962; VILLA SANTA 1964; DOBBIE et al. 1965; RUTLEDGE et al. 1965). Two possibilities exist for the origin of these clear cells: either they may originate from endometrial epithelial cells that secrete excessive amounts of glycogen (see cases of KAY 1957) owing to abnormal differentiation but unrelated to progesterone stimulation, or they may be tumor cells stemming from the Müllerian epithelium and still possessing multiple potentialities (see Table 21). In favor of a Müllerian origin is their ultrastructural similarity to

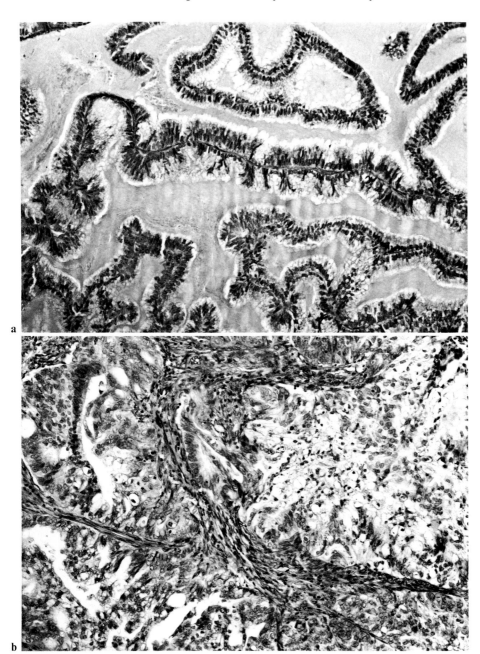

Fig. 126a, b. Mucinous adenocarcinoma of the endometrium; **a** well-differentiated type; **b** poorly differentiated type

the clear cell carcinomas of the ovary, cervix and vagina (SILVERBERG and DE-GIORGI 1973; RORAT et al. 1974; ROTH 1974; KURMAN and SCULLY 1976; HORIE et al. 1977). On the other hand, their structural identity is incomplete (EASTWOOD

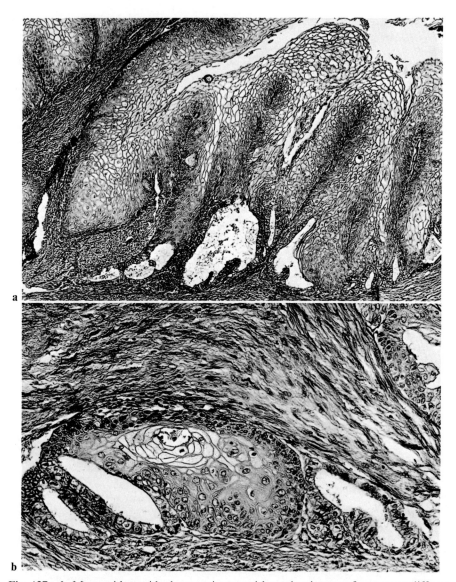

Fig. 127a, b. Mucoepidermoid adenocarcinoma with predominance of squamous differentiation. **a** Low magnification; at the surface it resembles an "ichthyosis uteri"; **b** high magnification: adenocarcinomatous cells differentiating into epidermoid carcinoma (so-called squamous metaplasia)

1978), perhaps owing to effects exerted by the respective tissue of origin. Occasionally some of their cells resemble those of an Arias-Stella reaction, presumably because of a hyperstimulation from postmenopausal secretion of gonadotropin. The clear cells are either arranged in solid nests or they form glands, cysts, or papillae. The enlarged nuclei are polymorphic and their chromatin is variably condensed (Fig. 129). Mitoses are common but fluctuate in number

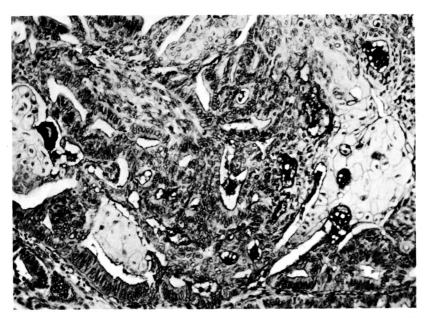

Fig. 128. Mucoepidermoid adenocarcinoma of the endometrium. Mono- and multicellular mucus secretion and keratinization within areas of squamous differentiation

from one region to another. The clear cytoplasm may contain glycogen or rounded PAS-positive, diastase-resistant hyaline inclusions. The cells of the papillary portions often contain nuclei in a hobnail position. To divide the tumor into different grades is of no value, since all grades have the same dismal prognosis, with a 5-year survival rate of only 35%. It may be impossible to distinguish the tumor microscopically from a clear cell carcinoma of the endocervix.

The **serous-papillary carcinoma** is of the serous type and develops almost exclusively in the senile patient. In LIU's (1970) series, the average age was 73, in the patient group of HENDRICKSON et al. (1982) it was 66. Grossly, this tumor often looks like placental tissue, but surrounded by a small atrophic uterus. Its histological appearance is almost identical to that of the serous-papillary carcinoma of the ovary: coarse fibrous or edematous stalks are layered with branching or complex epithelial papillae (Fig. 130). These consist of small, single or multilayered polygonal cells with elongated or rounded, often bizarre nuclei containing variable amounts of chromatin. Cellular and nuclear pleomorphism may be prominent, with occasional hobnail configuration of the nuclei. Mitoses are frequent and often abnormal. Psammoma bodies may be present. Ultrastructurally, the carcinomatous cells have fewer secretory granules and more prominent paranuclear microfilaments and tonofilaments than those of the endometrial-type adenocarcinomas (SATO et al. 1984). This tumor usually grows out profusely into the uterine cavity, may arise in polyps, and invades the myometrium early and extensively, without gross enlargement, mainly by lymphatic and vascular spread. The carcinoma cells invading the myometrium form irregular glands with infolding tufts. In addition, the tumor spreads frequently and early to the cervix, ovaries, and peritoneum. Its prognosis is less

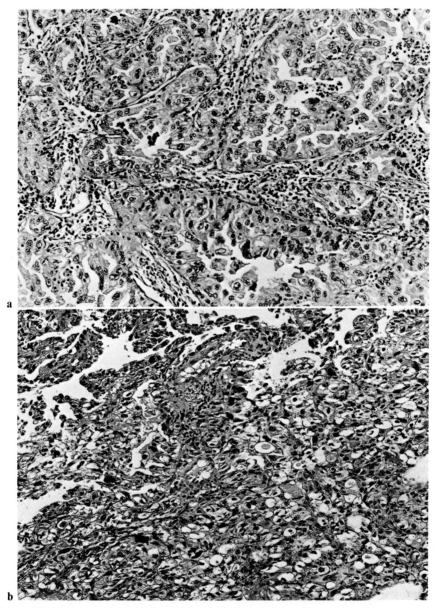

Fig. 129. a Clear cell carcinoma with nuclear changes like those of an Arias-Stella phenomenon. Patient 77 years old. **b** Poorly differentiated clear-cell carcinoma producing glandular structures

favorable than that of the endometrial type of adenocarcinoma, with a 5-year survival rate of only 51% (CHRISTOPHERSON et al. 1982; HENDRICKSON et al. 1982; JEFFREY et al. 1986) or even less: 45% for stages 1 and 2 and 11% for stages 3 and 4 (CHAMBER et al. 1987).

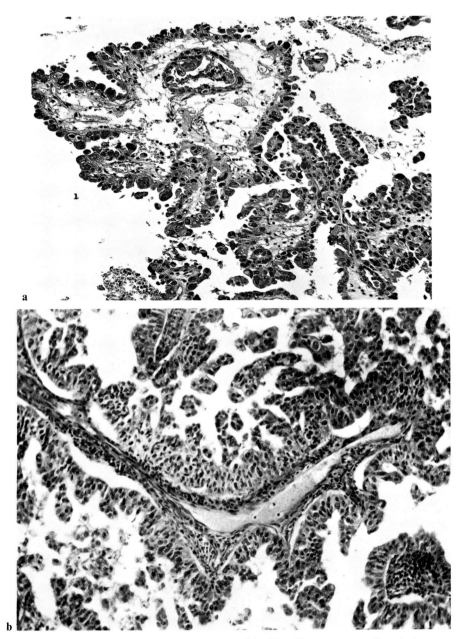

Fig. 130. a Serous-papillary adenocarcinoma with villus-like structures. Grossly it resembles placental tissue. Patient 72 years old. **b** A well-differentiated adenocarcinoma with intraluminal papillae. **c** Legend see p. 244

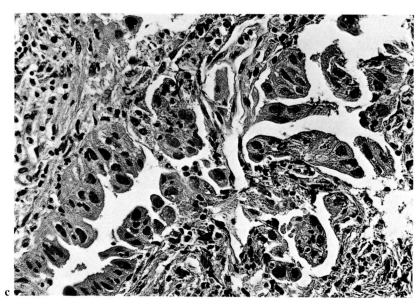

Fig. 130c. Oxyphilic ("oncocytic") appearance of glandular epithelial cells of a serous-papillary adenocarcinoma. Patient 74 years old

It is important to distinguish the serous papillary carcinoma from: (a) the papillary structures of a well-differentiated adenocarcinoma of the endometrial type (which are broader, have slender stalks, the carcinoma cells are columnar, more regular, and are usually pseudostratified to stratified) because of the much more favorable prognosis of the latter (CHEN et al. 1985); and (b) from the papillary type of clear cell carcinoma (in which most of the tumor cells are hobnail shaped and contain hyaline cytoplasmic inclusions) because of the even less favorable prognosis of the latter (CHRISTOPHERSON et al. 1982).

The primary **squamous carcinoma** of the endometrium represents the ectocervical type. It is extremely rare. KERGER (1949) suggested that such tumors arose from islets of squamous epithelium left behind as embryonic remnants of the Müllerian epithelium (for additional references refer to CORSCADEN 1956; CHU et al. 1958; PERIS et al. 1958; BARNETT 1965; WHITE et al. 1973; KAY 1974; MELIN et al. 1979). It is also possible these tumors develop from an ichthyosis uteri (RUGE 1918; HOPKIN et al. 1970; SELTZER et al. 1977; BERSCH et al. 1984; HECKEROTH and ZIEGLER 1986), the result of a generalized metaplasia of the glandular epithelium. RYDER (1982) observed a primary verrucous carcinoma of the endometrium. A primary squamous cell carcinoma of the endometrium has only twice been reported in a women before the menopause (YAMASHINA and KOBARA 1986). More often a squamous carcinoma or carcinoma in situ of the portio or endocervix grows upward into the uterine cavity where they may replace or infiltrate the entire endometrium (SCHMITT and SCHÄFER 1977). Consequently, a primary squamous cell carcinoma of the endometrium can be diagnosed only when the ecto- and endocervix are normal.

The **histological diagnosis** of a well-differentiated adenocarcinoma in **women under 40 years of age** must be made with great caution. Such rare endometrial carcinomas in patients of that age group may be diagnosed with certainty, with all therapeutic consequences implied, only if immature components predominate; that is, when poorly differentiated regions and nuclear atypia indicate without doubt that the tumor is malignant. Clinical experience has taught us that growths, which histologically would be classified after the menopause as unequivocal adenocarcinomas, in young women are able to regress and therefore should be regarded as adenomatous hyperplasias (ULM 1965; GRATTAROLA 1969, 1973; DALLENBACH-HELLWEG et al. 1971; FECHNER and KAUFMAN 1974; MOUKHTAR et al. 1977; NORRIS et al. 1983). It is in such cases that our ability to judge the biology of a tumor by its histology fails us; what is decisive is the patient's age. Typical for this young age group is the focal character of the adenomatous hyperplasia at multiple, segregated sites, which may be surrounded by almost normal endometrium (Fig. 131). Often foci of squamous metaplasia, morules (BLAUSTEIN 1982), or intraluminal papillary growth develop within the atypical glandular epithelium (Fig. 132), which shows structural, but no cytological atypias. Extensive metaplasia, referred to as "adenoacanthosis" (CRUM et al. 1981), may be seen. The limited and focal character of this adenomatous hyperplasia may explain why on occasion it can coexist with a normal pregnancy (KARLEN et al. 1972; SANDSTROM et al. 1979). Its misinterpretation as invasive carcinomas has led to surgical overtreatment in these young patients with no myometrial invasion in the excised uterus, and with 10 or more years' survival without recurrences.

γ) Histochemical Results

Most of the results described here were obtained before the histogenetic subclassification was introduced. Since, however, 86% of all endometrial carcinomas are of the ("usual") endometrial type, the results described here refer mainly to that type of tumor.

The *content of* **nuclear** *DNA* in the carcinoma cells is unrelated to the grade of their differentiation (ATKIN et al. 1959), but generally it is increased (FETTIG and OEHLERT 1964; FASSKE et al. 1965; FETTIG 1965). Studies of the *chromosomes* of the carcinoma cells have revealed that some of the cells are hyperdiploid, some hypodiploid to hypotetraploid (WAKONIG-VAARTAJA and HUGHES 1967); anomalous numbers are increased as compared with non-malignant endometria (BAKER 1968). In contrast, STANLEY and KIRKLAND (1968) reported endometrial carcinomas to be chiefly diploid or pseudodiploid, a result quite different from that for carcinomas of other organs. TSENG and JONES (1969) also found diploid or pseudodiploid sets of chromosomes in endometrial carcinomas that were like those sets found in glandular-cystic hyperplasia and adenomatous hyperplasia. From their results they concluded that endometrial carcinoma was biologically unique. Similarly, FEICHTER et al. (1982) found no cytophotometrically detectable differences between well-differentiated endometrial adenocarcinoma and adenomatous hyperplasia. TASE et al. (1985) found diploid and tetraploid DNA values in grades 1 and 2 and even in a part of the grade 3 adenocarcinomas, but aneuploid values only in some grade 3 tumors.

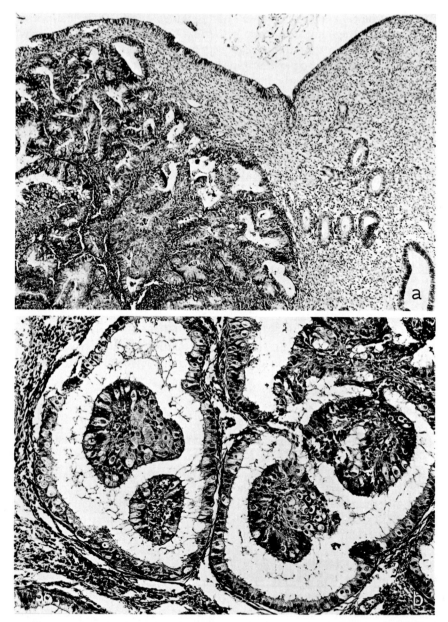

Fig. 131 a, b. Circumscribed carcinoma-like adenomatous hyperplasia in a 32-year-old patient, (**a**) replacing the stroma, (**b**) the hyperplastic epithelium forming distinct papillae in glandular lumina

The nuclear distribution of *estrogen receptors* can be visualized immunohistochemically with the ER-ICA assay using monoclonal anti-estrophilin antibodies (see p. 16). Whereas well-differentiated adenocarcinomatous glands show intense nuclear positivity, poorly differentiated carcinomas react heterogenously

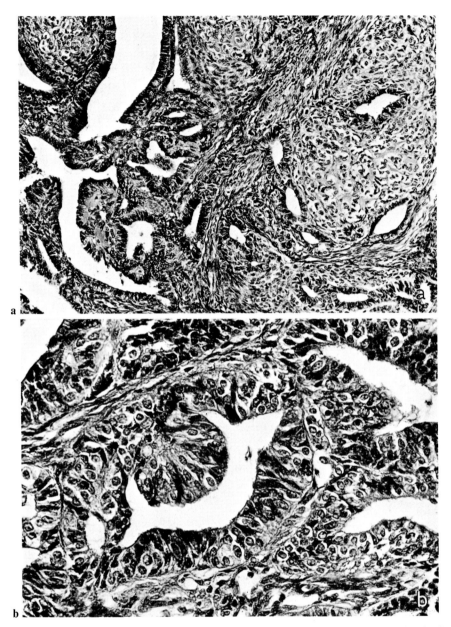

Fig. 132a, b. Carcinoma-like adenomatous hyperplasia, a borderline case, developing in a 37-year-old patient after 17 years of estrogen therapy. The glands are disarranged (**a**), some showing papillary overgrowth into their lumina (**b**)

(Fig. 133): solid or microglandular areas may be entirely receptor-negative, or contain only a few positive nuclei scattered widely among negative nuclei (CHARPIN et al. 1986; PERTSCHUK et al. 1986, personal observations). This incapability to produce receptor proteins indicates a loss of differentiation for the cancer

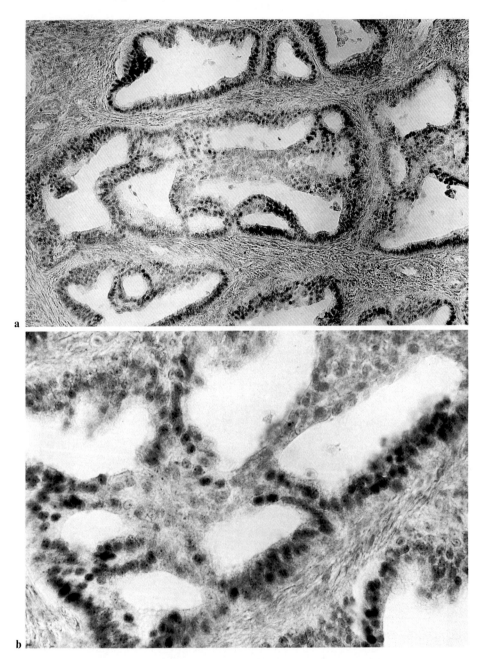

Fig. 133a, b. Immunocytochemical demonstration of estrogen receptor sites in the nuclei of carcinomatous glandular cells in a moderately differentiated adenocarcinoma of the endometrium: strong reaction in well-differentiated glandular portions as compared with weak reaction in poorly differentiated parts. ER-ICA assay. **a** Low magnification; **b** high magnification

cell. The cytoplasmic content of *progesterone receptor*, as measured in the cytosol fraction, changes almost in parallel with the concentration of nuclear estrogen receptor: it decreases with increasing tumor anaplasia (VIHKO et al. 1980; EHRLICH et al. 1981). Immunocytochemical measurements of the progesterone receptor with the PR-ICA assay will most likely yield more precise results in the near future.

Recently, an estrogen-related protein (24 K) was detected immunocytochemically with monoclonal antibodies in the cytoplasm of well-differentiated glandular and squamous cells of adenocarcinomas and adenoacanthomas, but was lacking in poorly differentiated cells (SLEDGE et al. 1985); the protein's value as a potential marker of tumor differentiation has yet to be proven.

The **cytoplasm of the carcinomatous glandular epithelium** may be either clear or dark, and may contain *glycogen* (ELTON 1942; ATKINSON et al. 1952; McKAY et al. 1956), glycoproteins, or mucus (DALLENBACH-HELLWEG and BRÄHLER 1960; SALM 1972) (see Table 16). Often the amount of mucus or glycogen parallels the degree of cellular differentiation (CRAMER and KLÖSS 1955; LEWIN 1961; STRAUSS 1963) and may vary greatly within a tumor or even within one carcinomatous gland.

In 80% of the well differentiated adenocarcinomas, as in the normal endometrium, the *acid mucopolysaccharides* are localized at the apical end of the glandular cells. Thus by staining for mucus it is possible to distinguish an endometrial carcinoma from an endocervical carcinoma, since the mucus in the cervical carcinoma is distributed in the majority of cases throughout the cytoplasm of the carcinomatous cells (SORVARI 1969). In addition, the acid mucopolysaccharides of the endometrial glands differ histochemically in quantity and quality (MOORE et al. 1959) and immunohistochemically in their composition of cytokeratin filaments (MOLL et al. 1983; CZERNOBILSKY et al. 1984) from those of the glands of the cervix. The most common type of mucins in endometrial carcinoma are sulphomucins. Difficulties arise in distinguishing the rare type of mucinous adenocarcinoma of the endometrium from the mucinous adenocarcinoma of the endocervix, since their sulfated and non-sulfated acid mucopolysaccharide contents are almost identical (CZERNOBILSKY et al. 1980; TILTMAN 1980).

Table 16. Histochemical results in benign and malignant conditions of the endometrium

	RNA	Phosphatase		Esterase	Glycogen	Glycoprotein	Lipid	Foam cells %
		Alkaline	Acid					
Proliferative phase	+	+ +	(+)	+	(+)	(+)	(+)	–
Secretory phase	(+)	(+)	+ +	+	+ +	+	(+)	–
Glandular-cystic hyperplasia	+ +	+ +	(+)	(+)	(+)	+ +	+ +	30.0
Adenomatous hyperplasia	+ +	+ +	(+)	(+)	(+)	+ +		53.0
Early carcinoma	(+)	(+)	+ +	+ +	(+)	(+)		40.9
Adenocarcinoma	+ +/(+)	+/(+)	+ +/(+)	+ +	+ +/(+)	+ +/(+)	+ +	38.2

Through loss of acidic groups the mucus in glandular lumina of the corpus carcinoma is often nonmetachromatic, thus contrasting with the extracellular mucus in the non-carcinomatous endometrium. – Endocervical and endometrial adenocarcinomas can also be distinguished with the immunoperoxidase reaction for *CEA*, since the intracellular distribution of CEA and mucus is quite similar (COHEN et al. 1982), and CEA has not been observed in most of the endometrial adenocarcinomas (UEDA et al. 1983). – The two carcinomas can be distinguished even more precisely with the reaction for *Vimentin* which is positive in 65% of the endometrial carcinomas but consistently negative in normal or neoplastic endocervical epithelium (DABBS et al. 1986). – The cytoplasmic *RNA* in the cells of the endometrial carcinoma is increased (ATKINSON et al. 1949; ATKINSON 1955; MOOKERJEA 1961; FRAMPTON 1963), but varies from one part of the tumor to another (GROSS 1964) as electron-microscopic studies have confirmed (NILSSON 1962). – The number and size of the *mitochondria* differ from cell to cell (FASSKE et al. 1965; WESSEL 1965), their cristae are few and irregular. Although the ends of the *Golgi complex* consist of ballooned, double lamellae, they show no secretory function. The *ergastoplasm* is poorly developed, containing an electron-dense substance. In the cytoplasm of well-differentiated carcinoma cells there are, in addition, numerous *osmiophilic granules*. The cells of poorly differentiated carcinomas have unusually well-developed, basal cytoplasmic processes.

Argyrophilic cells were detected in 26% (AGUIRRE et al. 1984) to 68% (BANNATYNE et al. 1983) of endometrial adenocarcinomas, some of which revealed neurosecretory granules ultrastructurally and reacted with HNK-1 antibodies against neuroectoderm immunohistochemically (UEDA et al. 1986). They were also positive for serotonin, dopamine, and ACTH. The authors consider argyrophilia mainly as an incidental finding which is not completely reliable in the detection of APUD cells. At least some of the argyrophilic cells appear to be without clinicopathological significance, since the patients had no corresponding hormonal manifestations (INOUE et al. 1982; SCULLY et al. 1984: review for further references). On the other hand, some carcinomas with argyrophilia could be related to APUDomas, or the argyrophilic cells might develop by derepression of the genetic code during carcinogenesis with aberrant cell differentiation toward hormonal function (UEDA et al. 1979; PRADE et al. 1982; SCULLY et al. 1984). Such transformation of malignant cells into cell types entirely foreign to the tissue from which they arise has been termed "neometaplasia" (YOUNG et al. 1981). OLSON et al. (1982) described a small cell carcinoma of the endometrium which, ultrastructurally, showed cytoplasmic neurosecretory-type granules and complex junctions consistent with a neuroendocrine tumor.

The activity of the *alkaline phosphatase* decreases as the carcinoma becomes less differentiated (ATKINSON and GUSBERG 1948; HALL 1950; MCKAY et al. 1956; MOOKERJEA 1961; LEVINE 1963; KUCERA 1964; PFLEIDERER 1968). The activity of *17β-hydroxysteroid dehydrogenase* also decreases as the carcinoma becomes less mature (POLLOW et al. 1975). The activity of the *acid phosphatase* is usually increased (MCKAY et al. 1956) but occasionally may also be decreased (GOLDBERG and JONES 1956). The *esterase* activity varies greatly (GROSS 1964), at times being increased (MCKAY et al. 1956). The same holds true for β-glucuronidase, phosphoamidase and most of the *dehydrogenases* (ISHIHARA et al.

1964; MOUKHTAR and HIGGINS 1965; TAKI et al. 1966; THIERY and WILLIGHAGEN 1967; FILIPE and DAWSON 1968; PFLEIDERER 1968). JIRASEK and DYKOVA (1964) reported an abnormal localization of esterase and acid phosphatase along the basement membrane of the glandular epithelium and concluded it indicated atypical metabolic processes. From the results of extensive studies, PFLEIDERER (1968) pointed out that there was no enzyme reaction characteristic of endometrial carcinomas. The results of the reactions vary greatly from one region of the tumor to another and depend as well on the age of the patient. Only in the actively growing parts of the tumor do enzymes become activated, participating either in oxidative catabolism or in the simultaneous proteolytic digestion of degenerating connective tissue.

Lipids and *cholesterol* are present in large amounts in the **stroma** of the endometrial carcinoma (ATKINSON 1955; LONG and DOKO 1959), a fact most likely correlating with the appearance of lipid-containing *foam cells* in the stroma of well-differentiated adenocarcinomas (STOERK 1906; DUBS 1923; SCHILLER 1927; NUNES 1945; CHIARI 1955). HARRIS (1958) found foam cells in 11% of endometrial carcinomas; KRONE and LITTIG (1959) in 13% and ISAACSON et al. (1964) in 43% of their cases. VON NUMERS and NIEMINEN (1961) also observed foam cells in some of their cases. SALM (1962) described lipophages (most probably foam cells) in the stroma of 7.5% of endometrial carcinomas but could detect none in normal endometrium. He proposed that when the cells were found they strongly suggested the presence of carcinoma. We detected typical foam cells in 25% of poorly differentiated adenocarcinomas, in 38% of well-differentiated adenocarcinomas and in 43% of adenoacanthomas (DALLENBACH-HELLWEG 1964; see Fig. 134, 135). Morphologically and histochemically they are identical with the foam cells of adenomatous hyperplasia (see p. 122ff.). One may encounter all transitions, from typical foam cells to hyalinized end-forms. With the progression from adenomatous hyperplasia to carcinoma not only do the number of foam cells decrease, but also the DNA content of the stromal cells (FETTIG 1965).

When *psammoma bodies* are found in an endometrial carcinoma, they may indicate that the tumor is a metastatic carcinoma, usually from the ovary (see p. 291). Primary *psammocarcinomas* of the endometrium (HAMEED and MORGAN 1972) or adenocarcinomas with psammoma bodies (FACTOR 1974; LIVOLSI 1977) likewise may occur, but are rare, and a small primary tumor in the ovary can never be excluded with certainty. According to HITSCHMANN (1903), psammomatous bodies can develop from degenerated and calcified cells of an epidermoid carcinoma or from shedding epithelial cells of a serous-papillary adenocarcinoma, which may resemble ovarian carcinoma (see Fig. 130a).

Prognosis. Apart from the extent of spread of an endometrial carcinoma at the time therapy is started, its prognosis is determined by the differentiation *(histological grading)* of its cells. According to earlier statistics, the 5-year survival rates of well-differentiated adenocarcinomas varied from 72%–86%, for poorly differentiated adenocarcinomas with uniform nuclei from 45%–79%, and for the immature carcinomas with pleomorphic nuclei they fell to 28%–58% (PÜSCHEL and MÖBIUS 1967; LIU 1972). Within the group of well-differentiated

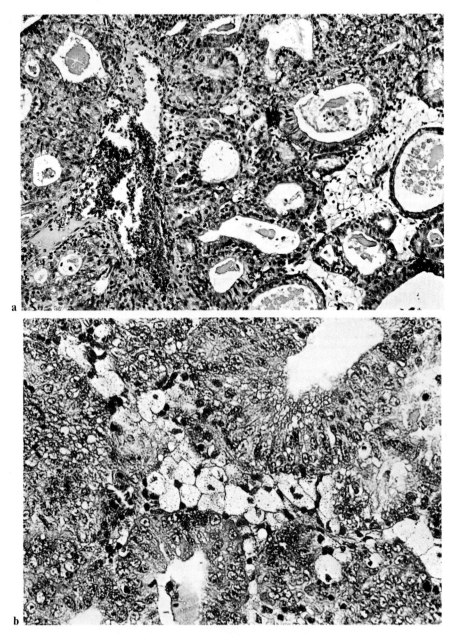

Fig. 134a–c. Well-differentiated adenocarcinoma with foam cells in the gusset-like stretches of stroma. **a** Low magnification; **b** higher magnification.

tumors, patients with mucus-secreting endometrial carcinomas proved to have a more favorable prognosis than those with non-mucinous tumors of like structure (LEVINE 1969); the clear cell carcinomas showed even a worse prognosis (PHOTOPULOS et al. 1979). In STOLL's series (1957) the cure rate for all cases was 61%; in the series of CLIMIE and RACHMANINOFF (1965) and NG and REAGAN

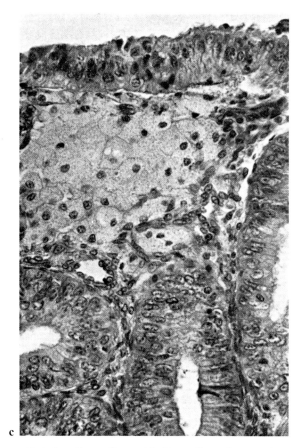

Fig. 134c. Foam cells below the surface epithelium of an adenocarcinoma

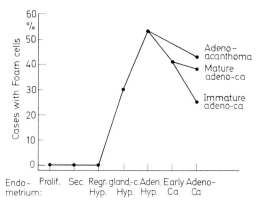

Fig. 135. Relative frequency of foam cells in hyperplasia and carcinomas of the endometrium

(1970) it was 63% and 69.7%, respectively. From earlier statistics the prognosis of adenoacanthoma varied greatly due to the failure to separate the unfavorable adenosquamous carcinoma from the adenoacanthoma (HAINES and TAYLOR 1962; TWEEDDALE et al. 1964; CHARLES 1965; WILLIAMS 1965; BADIB et al. 1970; NG et al. 1973). A more detailed judgement of the survival rates became possible with the use of the histogenetic tumor classification (CHRISTOPHERSON et al. 1982; see Table 14). – Independently of the histological type, a 5-year cure was observed in 80%–98% of the women with a tumor at *stage* 0. The cure rate for tumors at stage 1 was 66%–78%, at *stage* 2 6%–56%; at stages 3 and 4 no patients survived 5-years (BAILAR 1961; THIEDE and LUND 1962; JAVERT and RENNING 1963; DOBBIE et al. 1965; FRANZ 1965). Furthermore, the depth of myometrial invasion is of prognostic relevance. When correlated with the histological grade, there was a minimal risk for lymph node metastases in early carcinoma irrespective of grade, and with invasion limited to the inner one-third of the myometrium in grade 1. There was a substantial risk in grades 2 and 3, when invasion was limited to the inner one-third of the myometrium, and in all grades with deep myometrial invasion (BORONOW et al. 1984). – In addition to the histological differentiation and to the stage of the tumor, the *patient's age* and the *therapeutic management* influence the prognosis. As reported in a clinical study of 355 endometrial carcinomas, the 5-year survival rate following hysterectomy and bilateral salpingo-oophorectomy proved more favorale; 83% for tumors at stage 1, 79% at stage 2, 42% at stage 3 and 13% at stage 4 (MILTON and METTERS 1972). As compared with radical surgery, the prognosis after radiation therapy is much less favorable (SALL et al. 1970; and others). Adjuvant radiation therapy with hysterectomy provides no better prognosis than hysterectomy alone (FRICK et al. 1973; AALDERS et al. 1980). To review all reports of therapy studies for stages 1–4 published in recent years would far exceed the scope set for this monograph. The pathologist should realize, however, that besides a precise histological classification of the tumor, the clinician needs to know how far it has invaded the myometrium in order to select the best therapy for that patient (SÖDERLIN 1975; SALAZAR et al. 1978). The particularly favorable prognosis of endometrial carcinoma in women under 40 years of age may be related in part to the mistake in diagnosing adenomatous hyperplasia as cancer (see p. 245). Regardless of the stage of growth or the type of treatment, endometrial carcinoma recurs in about 14% of all cases (DEDE et al. 1968).

δ) Precursors of Endometrial Carcinoma
Like carcinomas in other parts of the body, most endometrial carcinomas are preceded by a precancerous state. To determine which lesions may occur as precursors, three approaches are available for investigation (HERTIG et al. 1949):
1. A retrospective approach by studying the development of the carcinoma from previous curettages
2. A prospective follow up of the patient after the first curettage revealed one of the types of hyperplasia
3. A coincidental (concurrent) study of changes in those regions of the endometrium not involved by the corpus carcinoma.

The compilation and review of such studies reported in the world literature revealed interesting results (DALLENBACH-HELLWEG 1964; SHERMAN and BROWN 1979). The *retrospective method of study* proved to be the most informative. Most authors found that in a large percentage of their patients the endometrial carcinoma had been preceded by adenomatous hyperplasia. The percentage in whom the tumor was preceded by glandular-cystic hyperplasia, "adenocarcinoma in situ", or polyps of the endometrium was somewhat smaller. In the *prospective studies* only a small number of women with glandular-cystic hyperplasia developed endometrial carcinomas; the number was significantly higher in those with adenomatous hyperplasia and highest for "adenocarcinoma in situ".

The values for the prospective method of study are generally low because once the diagnosis of hyperplasia is made the practice is to treat promptly, not to wait. *A study of the coincidental occurrence* of various forms of hyperplasia in regions of the endometrium uninvolved by the corpus carcinoma yield results comparable to those of the retrospective approach of study. Most of the changes found are those of adenomatous hyperplasia (see Fig. 136). In general the noncarcinomatous regions have a higher mitotic activity and a greater tendency to proliferate than an equivalent endometrium (KAISER and SCHNEIDER 1968).

How are we to explain why *glandular-cystic hyperplasia* in the prospective studies terminates as carcinoma in only a low percentage of cases but in the retrospective and coincidental studies is found in a higher percentage of carcinomas? The explanation is quite simple. Most of the glandular-cystic hyperplasias occurring before the menopause are harmless. That is, glandular-cystic hyperpla-

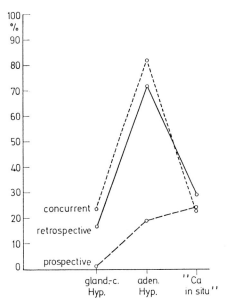

Fig. 136. The prospective, retrospective, and concurrent frequencies of hyperplasias associated with endometrial carcinoma

sia merely represents a transitory disturbance that develops during the short period of hormonal imbalance at the beginning and at the end of the reproductive years. Occasionally, however, glandular-cystic hyperplasia may persist, especially after the menopause, and under long-standing, unopposed hormonal stimulus may become an adenomatous hyperplasia, which may then undergo change to carcinoma. Consequently, we should not be surprised that in a fair percentage of corpus carcinomas (concurrent study) we would find a glandular-cystic hyperplasia in parts of the endometrium uninvolved by the tumor. Even when the adenomatous hyperplasia has already become a carcinoma, it is quite possible to detect remnants of a glandular-cystic hyperplasia of many years' standing in some regions of the endometrium. Applying the same assumptions, we may explain the higher percentage of glandular-cystic hyperplasia revealed by the retrospective study. From the studies of NOVAK and YUI (1936), NOVAK (1956) believed it was important for the prognosis to distinguish clearly between glandular-cystic hyperplasia *before* the menopause and that developing *after* the menopause, which he regarded as precancerous (36 of his 815 cases). In these 36 patients he observed endocrine disturbances like those seen in the patients with endometrial carcinoma. On the other hand, hyperplasia in young women, although a rare disease, should be considered a potential precancerous lesion, because of the frequent endocrine disturbances accompanying it. In a series of young patients (between 15 and 35 years old) with hyperplasia, 14% developed an adenocarcinoma 1–14 years after the initial diagnosis (CHAMLIAN and TAYLOR 1970). According to HERTIG and GORE (1963), women developing glandular-cystic hyperplasia before the menopause have a ten-fold greater chance of developing a carcinoma many years later than the average women. Although not common, the development of a carcinoma from a hyperplasia is certainly not merely accidental. The studies cited above indicate that when viewed from the aspect of the carcinoma, glandular-cystic hyperplasia is indeed a precursor although in itself in the great majority of occurrences (during adolescence, climacterium) a benign process. These two ways of looking at glandular-cystic hyperplasia often are not sharply defined in the literature, thus leading to misunderstandings about the prognostic importance of that type of hyperplasia (WINTER 1950; BEHRENS 1954; KOFLER 1954; RÜTTNER and LEU 1954; SCHRÖDER 1954; RITZMANN and HILLEMANNS 1977).

The situation is quite different for *adenomatous hyperplasia,* which was initially described under that term by GUSBERG (1947). With all three approaches of study (retrospective, prospective, and concurrent) the percentage of adenomatous hyperplasias is found to be very high. The possibility it is a precursor of carcinoma therefore is great. In support of that idea are the pronounced atypical proliferations of glands and glandular epithelium occasionally found in adenomatous hyperplasia that make it extremely difficult, if not impossible, to distinguish adenomatous hyperplasia from carcinomas (see Fig. 119). Patients with adenomatous hyperplasia present clinical manifestations, especially those of hormonal abnormalities, which are like those of early endometrial carcinoma (GUSBERG et al. 1954; GARNET 1958; GUSBERG and KAPLAN 1963; see Table 19). As the prospective studies suggest, in a small percentage of patients adenomatous hyperplasia does regress without therapy. That implies adenomatous hyperplasia is not an irreversible precancerous condition and probably depends on a hormonal stimulus for its progression. BEHRENS (1956) observed that the adenomatous hyperplasias with atypical epithelial cells but without atypical glands transformed later into a carcinoma much less often than those with both atypical cells and atypical glands. The glands of the adenomatous hyperplasia and those of the subsequent carcinoma are similar; that is, of the same variety. Numerous reports of large series of cases and single observations have been published on the progression of adenomatous hyperplasia into carcinoma (review of literature, see DALLENBACH-HELLWEG 1964).

"Adenocarcinoma in situ" (HERTIG et al. 1949) is most frequently found in the prospective method of studies, evidence strongly suggesting that it is an early but irreversible neoplastic lesion. From our follow-up studies of women with such lesions (DALLENBACH-HELLWEG 1979, cf. p. 127f.), and from analogies made with comparable early neoplastic changes in other organs (for example, the stomach), we recommend these endometrial lesions be regarded as *early carcinomas,* and the term "adenocarcinoma in situ" be abolished. That renaming seems all the more logical and valid, since its glandular cells are aneuploid and do push out into the surrounding stroma, explaining how metastases may occur even at this early stage.

From such considerations the majority of investigators (see review by SPEERT 1948; BEHRENS 1958; ANDREWS 1961; GRAY and BARNES 1964; FOSTER and MONTGOMERY 1965; SHERMAN and BROWN 1979; FENOGLIO et al. 1982) concluded, that adenomatous hyperplasia should be looked upon as a potential precursor of endometrial carcinoma. Even R. MEYER (1923) and SCHRÖDER (1928) referred to progressive transitions from hyperplasia to carcinoma. The transformation takes place gradually and may require years or even decades.

HERTIG and SOMMERS (1949) found that glandular-cystic hyperplasia was most common 6–13 years before the carcinoma became evident in curettings. Adenomatous hyperplasia was most common 1–5 years, and adenocarcinoma in situ 3–5 years before the carcinoma appeared. HALL (1957) observed similar intervals and concluded from them that the degree of atypia might serve to indicate how long the latent period would last before a carcinoma developed. BEUTLER et al. (1963) noted that with hyperplasia before the menopause there was an average interval of 12 years before the carcinoma manifested itself, but with hyperplasia after the menopause only 6 years were required before the carcinoma was diagnosed. MÜLLER and KELLER (1957) also found atypical hyperplasia 4–14 years before carcinoma became apparent; consequently they preferred to regard hyperplasia stage 0 of corpus carcinoma. Some authors (CAMPBELL and BARTER 1961; GUSBERG and KAPLAN 1963) ignored the terms "adenocarcinoma in situ", classifying instead their adenomatous hyperplasias into different groups of severity.

Only a few authors (JONES and BREWER 1941) have questioned the precancerous importance of the hyperplasias, since they have observed endometrial carcinomas in patients with a secretory or atrophic endometrium. Such cases do occur, but in most instances they indicate that the carcinoma has arisen either from a focus of *metaplasia* (see Table 15) or in a *corpus polyp*; that is, in a focal region of hyperplasia that has behaved like a diffuse hyperplasia (Fig. 137). At times the carcinoma is sharply demarcated from the normal basalis (Fig. 138 and cf. Fig. 140). It is not uncommon to find polyps prior to or with the carcinoma (SCHEFFEY et al. 1943; in 7.8%; KOTTMEIER 1947: in 20.7%, HERTIG and

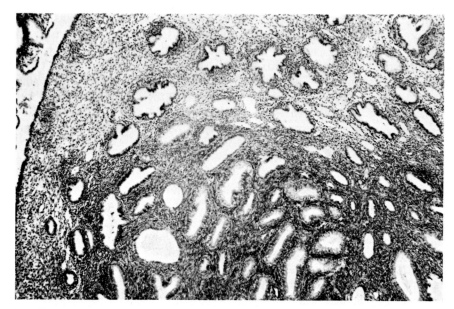

Fig. 137. Focal adenomatous hyperplasia with beginning carcinoma in the remaining secretory endometrium

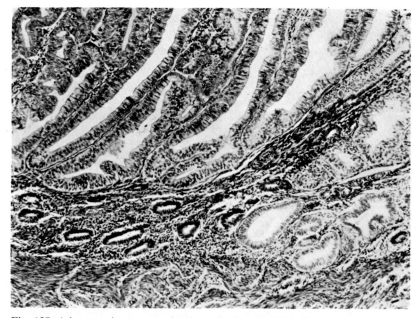

Fig. 138. Adenocarcinoma growing into the (stratum) basalis

SOMMERS 1949: in 12%; HENRIKSEN and MURRIETA 1950: in 26%; KINDLER 1956: in 19.3%; WEBER 1961: in 14.6%; BOUTSELIS et al. 1963: in 11.7% of all cases). An early carcinoma may still be limited to the polyp, but usually the polyp is only one of the multicentric foci of carcinogenesis (SALM 1972).

PETERSON and NOVAK (1956) reported that 15.5% of all corpus polyps after the menopause are involved by carcinoma. HUBER (1951) found the involvement in 58%, KREMER and NARIK (1953) in 16.3%, STOKES (1948), HUBER (1951), SCHRÖDER (1954), and PETERSON and NOVAK (1956) were able to show that some carcinomas had arisen in polyps. HERTIG et al. (1949) disclosed that 14 of their 64 adenocarcinomas in situ developed in a polyp. According to ARMENIA (1967), women with a corpus polyp have a nine-fold greater chance of developing a carcinoma within the next 12 years than the average women.

HERTIG and GORE (1963; GORE and HERTIG 1962, 1966) reported they had never seen a carcinoma develop in a normal endometrium.

If it is true that endometrial carcinoma does develop from adenomatous hyperplasia and the antecedent glandular-cystic hyperplasia, then one should expect a common etiology or at least common disposition for these diseases. Recent observations have suggested, however, that the carcinomas with differentiation anomalous for the endometrium should be separated from those showing an endometrial differentiation, not only because they differ histologically but also pathogenetically (BOKHMAN 1981; DELIGDISCH and COHEN 1985; DELIGDISCH and HOLINKA 1986; HACHISUGA 1986). The patients developing adenocarcinomas with endometrial differentiation are usually in their early postmenopause, about 50 years old, and show signs and symptoms of prolonged hyperestrogenism. Their carcinomas, which arise from the preceding glandular-cystic and adenomatous hyperplasias, are well differentiated, positive for estrogen and progesterone receptors, and are less invasive, showing thereby excellent survival rates. In contrast, the patients developing carcinomas of Müllerian (ectopic) differentiation (clear cell, papillary, anaplastic) are in their late postmenopause, of an average age above 60 years, and often show no signs or symptoms of hyperestrogenism. Their carcinomas develop from focal ectopic metaplasia which may be surrounded by resting or atrophic endometrium. Such tumors are poorly differentiated, negative for hormone receptors, grow aggressively with early myometrial and lymphatic invasion, and consequently show poor survival rates.

When the frequencies of these two main types of endometrial carcinomas are compared between countries, interesting *geographical differences* become apparent. In the United States, CHRISTOPHERSON et al. (1982) found that more than 88% of the carcinomas showed endometrial differentiation; only 10%–12% had developed from ectopic metaplasia and were poorly differentiated. In the USSR (BOKHMAN 1981) and in Japan (HACHISUGA 1986), the frequencies were about 65%–35%. The higher rates of the well-differentiated adenocarcinomas associated with hyperestrogenism observed in the western world may be related to the common use of estrogen therapy, which is seldom prescribed in the USSR or Japan. These geographical differences also influence survival rates in various populations.

ε) Etiological Concepts

The cause of the poorly differentiated carcinomas anomalous to the endometrium remains unknown. The carcinogenic mechanisms involved are probably similar to those causing cancers in other organ systems of old people, such as defective repair mechanisms for DNA or increased mutations. In contrast, the vast clinical and epidemiological experience of the past 50 years confirms the close relationship between hyperestrogenism and adenocarcinoma of endometrial differentiation (GUSBERG 1967; FOX 1984). A great many findings support such a conclusion:

Ovarian changes. The percentage of endometrial carcinomas associated with *granulosa cell tumors or theca cell tumors* is greater than that to be expected normally (SMITH et al. 1942; SPEERT 1948; WOLL et al. 1948; NOVAK and MOHLER 1953; KOFLER 1954; WAY 1954; PEEL 1956; RANDALL and GODDARD 1956; DAVIS 1964; GUSBERG and KARDON 1971). The percentage is even greater if one computes the opposite relationship – the percentage of ovarian tumors associated with endometrial carcinoma. Before the menopause that rate is 2.8% (as calculated from a compilation of many large series published in the literature; for review see DALLENBACH-HELLWEG 1964), when a corpus luteum (progesterone production) might be present to neutralize the estrogen effect. In contrast, after the menopause the rate is much higher – 23.3% – owing to an unopposed stimulation by estrogen. Although theca cell tumors (thecomas) are quite rare, they are more often associated with corpus carcinomas than are the more common granulosa cell tumors. The thecomas, moreover, may be so small they cause no palpable enlargement of the overy, being incidentally found after total hysterectomy for endometrial carcinoma (SCHRÖDER 1954; FATHALLA 1967). The thecomas produce larger amounts of estrogen than the granulosa cell tumors (BISKIND and BISKIND 1949; INGRAM and NOVAK 1951; JAKOBOVITS 1963). – The reason why the percentage of endometrial carcinomas associated with feminizing ovarian tumors is not higher is explained by the fact that other ovarian changes occur with endometrial carcinoma. In 1941 SMITH reported on a *stromal hyperplasia* of the ovary, which he found in 87% of his patients with endometrial carcinoma. Since then many subsequent investigators have confirmed his findings and checked them against control cases (see Table 17).

Table 17. Corpus carcinoma and stromal hyperplasia of the ovary

Author	Year	Number of patients with carcinoma	Stromal hyperplasia	
			Associated with carcinoma %	In control patients without carcinoma %
SMITH	1941	180	87.0	
WOLL et al.	1948	331	84.0	44.0
MCGARVEY, GIBSON	1952	85	55.0	
NOVAK, MOHLER	1953	64	54.0	21.0
BAMFORTH	1956	81	50.0	
SCHNEIDER, BECHTAL	1956	44	52.3	35.0
HERTIG	1957	389	90.0	
SOMMERS, MEISSNER	1957	38	73.0	36.0
MARCUS	1963	100	Twice as common as in the control patients	
Total number		1312	72.2	39.2

RODDICK and GREENE (1957) criticized the significance of these studies, contending that the control cases revealed less stromal hyperplasia merely because they were autopsy material. SOMMERS and MEISSNER (1957) were able to refute that criticism, however, by showing in autopsy studies that the ovaries of patients with endometrial carcinoma had greater stromal hyperplasia than did the ovaries of control patients. NOVAK and MOHLER (1953) noted that the more mature an endometrial carcinoma appeared, the more pronounced the stromal hyperplasia of the ovaries.

WOLL et al. (1948) described clusters of proliferating theca cells and small so-called granulomata (HERTIG 1944) in the hyperplastic cortical tissue. McKAY (1962) pointed out that the stromal cells of the ovary have the potentiality to produce estrogen and can be stimulated to do so with luteinizing hormone (LH). They are most likely the precursor cells of the thecoma (McKAY et al. 1953), and in animal experiments can be stimulated to proliferate by injecting LH after estrogen levels are reduced (BISKIND and BISKIND 1944, 1949; KULLANDER 1956). LEMON (1956) as well as LAJOS et al. (1963) proved by biochemical methods that stromal hyperplasia produced estrogen, and PROCOPÉ (1968) detected increased excretion of urinary estrogen in that condition. The ovaries removed from women with adenomatous hyperplasia or endometrial carcinoma revealed in vitro an excessive production of estrogen (PLOTZ et al. 1967). ZANDER et al. (1962) were able to demonstrate in polycystic ovaries with intense stromal hyperplasia that the formation of androgens was increased. Various investigators have been able histochemically to demonstrate steroids in the theca cells, but not in the inactive stromal cells of the ovary. MERKER and DIAZ-ENCINAS (1969) electron-microscopically found signs of steroid synthesis in the stromal cells of rats and rabbits after the animals had been stimulated with pregnant mare serum (PMS) and human chorionic gonadotropin (HCG). In his cases of diffuse thecoses, FIENBERG (1963) described transitions from stromal cells to theca cells and was able (1969) to demonstrate in all of his examples of endometrial carcinoma lipids and oxidative enzymes in the proliferating theca cells of the stroma. Likewise, MESTWERDT et al. (1972) reported groups of large polygonal stromal cells within the ovarian stromal hyperplasia of all endometrial carcinomas examined. The cells possessed abundant cytoplasm and showed typical ultrastructural characteristics of steroid producing cells: smooth endoplasmic reticulum, tubular-vesicular mitochondria and heterogenous lipofuscin granula, as well as enzymatic activities characteristic of steroid biosynthesis. NOVAK et al. (1965) found that 66% of postmenopausal women with enzymatically active stromal hyperplasia had either a hyperplastic endometrium or an endometrial carcinoma. It seems probable that stromal hyperplasia, clusters of theca cells, and thecomas are only various stages in the response to the same hormonal stimulus.

Several other investigators were impressed by the *hilar cell hyperplasia* in ovaries from patients with endometrial carcinoma (SHAW and DASTUR 1949; SHERMAN and WOOLF 1959; AMES and JANOVSKI 1963). Subsequent studies by others (GREENE and PECKHAM 1951; NOVAK and MOHLER 1953; ANTHONY and RODDICK 1962; MARCUS 1963), failed to confirm that association. In our own material, however, we have also found a close correlation between the extent of hilar cell hyperplasia and the degree of endometrial proliferation, up to including carcinomas. – Hilar-cell tumors (MOHAMED et al. 1978) and *Brenner tumors* (JOPP 1965) have also been related to the development of endometrial carcinoma.

Table 18. Corpus carcinoma and the Stein-Leventhal syndrome

Author	Year	Number of patients with carcinoma under 40 years of age	Associated with Stein-Leventhal syndrome	
			(n)	(%)
SPEERT	1949	14	3	21
SOMMERS et al.	1949	16	4	25
DOCKERTY	1951	36	7	19
Total		66	14	21.2
		Number of patients with Stein-Leventhal syndrome	Associated with carcinoma	
			(n)	(%)
JACKSON, DOCKERTY	1957	43	16	37.2

The rare patients in the childbearing period who develop endometrial carcinoma usually have abnormal ovaries; often there are signs and symptoms of the *Stein-Leventhal syndrome* (see Table 18; cf. also JAFARI et al. 1978). It is necessary to point out, however, that the discoverors of this syndrome found no endometrial carcinomas in the first patients they described, and they then doubted whether the syndrome is always correctly diagnosed (LEVENTHAL 1958). Certainly in all the combination cases reported in the literature the authors have specified polycystic ovaries without corpora lutea, a state functionally equivalent to an unopposed estrogen effect. Clinically, all these young patients with endometrial carcinoma exhibit pronounced endocrine disturbances with obesity, diabetes mellitus, sterility and hirsutism. A corpus luteum is found only rarely. DOCKERTY et al. (1951) noted that the ovaries in 50% of their cases were large and cystic. As to ovarian function, these young patients with endometrial carcinoma usually behave like women after the menopause. The simultaneous occurrence of pregnancy with endometrial carcinoma is extremely rare (SANDSTROM et al. 1979).

It is worth mentioning that endometrial carcinoma develops more commonly in women with **cirrhosis of the liver** than in normal women (SPEERT 1949), a fact that BREWER and FOLEY (1953) tried to disprove in their studies but could not. Presumably the damaged liver is unable to metabolize estrogen which then accumulates and overstimulates, unopposed by progesterone. GREENE (1941) reported endometrial carcinoma in rabbits that had damaged livers; he attributed the tumors to the reduced metabolism of estrogen.

The ovarian changes just described may result in an excessive or unopposed action of estrogen produced endogenously. We should like to compare with them the action of **exogenous estrogen.** A great many investigators have reported the development of an endometrial carcinoma after several years of estrogen therapy, in some instances after observing the development of all stages of hyperplasia that usually precede such a carcinoma (CORSCADEN and GUSBERG

1947; NOVAK and RUTLEDGE 1948; SPEERT 1948 [in 12.5% of his cases]; RIEHM and STOLL 1952; JENSEN and ØSTERGAARD 1954; KOFLER 1954; GUSBERG and HALL 1961; BOUTSELIS et al. 1963; LAUFER 1968; CUTLER et al. 1972, and numerous reports of single cases). RIEHM and STOLL (1952) were impressed by the histological peculiarities of these carcinomas, such as their formation of epithelial papillae in widely branching glandular lumina, their multicentric development, and their relatively high grade of differentiation. GUSBERG and HALL (1961) considered the glands of the adenomatous hyperplasias and carcinomas that develop after estrogen therapy to be so characteristic, they referred to an "estrogen carcinoma". From a study of our own cases of estrogen-induced carcinomas, we have been able to confirm all these histological peculiarities. The frequent occurrence of nodules of squamous epithelium in precancerous adenomatous hyperplasia is equivalent to the high percentage of adenoacanthomas that develop among "estrogen carcinomas" (cf. also ROBBOY and BRADLEY 1979). Ultrastructurally, the endometrial cells of postmenopausal women receiving estrogen resemble those of adenocarcinoma in at least three features: accumulation of lipid droplets, irregular nuclei, and perinuclear whorls of microfibrils (AYCOCK and JOLLIE 1979).

Large series of patient collectives studied in the United States have disclosed that postmenopausal patients treated with estrogen have a six-fold greater risk for developing an endometrial carcinoma; those treated for more than 5 years have a 15-fold greater risk (ANTUNES et al. 1979). In their studies SMITH et al. (1975), ZIEL and FINKLE (1975), BJERSING (1977), GREENWALD et al. (1977), HOOGERLAND et al. (1978) reached similar results. Following long-term use of conjugated estrogens, the risk of endometrial carcinoma remained significantly elevated even after estrogen-free intervals of over 10 years (SHAPIRO et al. 1985). Giving gestagen with the estrogen does not increase the risk, but may have a protective effect (GAMBRELL 1977; GREENBLATT et al. 1982). Not only the duration of treatment but also the dosage prescribed is important for the development of carcinoma (GRAY et al. 1977). The results of another study revealed that of 94 postmenopausal women developing endometrial carcinoma, 70% had received estrogens. In contrast, only 23% of a control group of women of the same age without carcinomas had received estrogens (ZIEL and FINKLE 1976). With sharp reduction in the dosage of estrogen the risk for endometrial carcinoma notably decreased (JICK et al. 1979). Many recent studies have been conducted with nearly identical results; their citation exceeds the design set for this monograph.

Several groups of investigators (LYON 1975; SILVERBERG and MAROWSKI 1975; KELLEY et al. 1976; COHEN and DEPPE 1977; REEVES and KAUFMANN 1977; SILVERBERG et al. 1977) have reported an increase in adenomatous hyperplasia and endometrial carcinoma in young women receiving oral contraceptives with predominant estrogen effect. The increase is explained by the relative estrogen predominance during persistent artificial anovulation.

TWOMBLY et al. (1961) noted that their lean patients treated with estrogen quickly excreted it, whereas their obese patients retained the hormone. They attributed the higher incidence of carcinoma in the obese women to that retention. – In addition, a great many investigators have reported on precancerous adenomatous hyperplasias of the endometrium developing after estrogen therapy (GEIST et al. 1941; KISTNER et al. 1956; BLOOMFIELD 1957; DOUGLAS and WEED 1959; GUSBERG and KAPLAN 1963). – Although the majority of the authors believed the endometrial carcinoma was related to the estrogen therapy, a few remained unconvinced of that relationship (LARSON 1954; DIBBELT et al. 1962). These differences are due in part to geographical factors. In the United States estrogen has been prescribed during the climacterium and even for young women for a much longer time than in the Federal Republic of Germany. Consequently, in the larger series of American patients treated with estrogen the relationship – estrogen: endometrial carcinoma – became apparent sooner. Furthermore, the duration of estrogen therapy proved to be much more important than the amount of the single doses (CORSCADEN and GUSBERG 1947; MÜHLBOCK 1959, 1963; JENSEN 1963), since most of the carcinomas developed after prolonged therapy with low doses of estrogen.

After estrogen therapy is discontinued a high-grade adenomatous hyperplasia may completely regress spontaneously (NOVAK and RUTLEDGE 1948; OSTERGAARD 1974), whereas adenomatous hyperplasia due to excessive endogenous estrogen will require prolonged therapy with high doses of gestagens before it regresses. KISTNER (1959) reported that progesterone therapy successfully caused two adenocarcinomas in situ to disappear.

A certain percentage of patients with endometrial carcinoma may give a history of having received **X-irradiation** many years before, usually for benign uterine leiomyomata or endometrial hyperplasias (NORRIS and BEHNEY 1936; COSTOLOW 1941; SCHEFFEY 1942; CORSCADEN et al. 1946; SMITH and BOWDEN 1948; HERTIG and SOMMERS 1949; SPEERT and PEIGHTAL 1949; MONTGOMERY et al. 1952; BARR and CHARTERIS 1955; TURNBULL 1956; PENTECOST and BRACK 1959; REICHER and PHILLIPS 1961; DIBBELT et al. 1962; BOUTSELIS et al. 1963; WALL et al. 1967), or for cervical carcinoma (RODRIGUEZ and HART 1982). When the patients with endometrial carcinoma of all these authors were grouped and analyzed, 7.2% were found to have had X-ray therapy to the pelvis, a percentage not significantly greater than that of control patients without carcinomas.

DIBBELT et al., found among their patients with carcinoma that 7.9% had had previous X-ray therapy of the small pelvis, whereas in their series of control patients 5.8% had received such therapy. Several other investigators were equally as cautious in relating X-ray therapy with the subsequent development of carcinoma (KOCH 1949; COPELAND et al. 1957; HOFMANN 1960; HUBER 1960; NIELSEN 1960; KEPP 1961; BRINKLEY et al. 1963; SHUTE 1963). By X-irradiating the ovaries of animals, HUSSY and WALLART (1915) produced follicular degeneration and hyperplasia of the theca cells with a definitely increased estrogen activity. FURTH and BUTTERWORTH (1936) were the first to describe the development of granulosa cell tumors in mice by irradiating their ovaries with X-rays.

Women who have had their ovaries removed rarely develop endometrial carcinoma. Nevertheless, in the literature there are 28 case studies of castrated women in whom endometrial carcinomas ultimately developed (MEYER 1923: one; SMITH 1941: three; RANDALL et al. 1951: four; CIANFRANI 1955: eight; BROMBERG et al. 1959: one; HENRIKSEN 1960: two; HOFMEISTER and VONDRAK 1970: nine), and I have observed another myself. According to the clinical records, at least four of these patients developed their carcinoma after many years of estrogen replacement therapy. In the other patients reported, estrogen was most probably compensatorily produced by the adrenal cortices, as has been frequently assumed in women after the menopause (NOVAK and RICHARDson 1941; RANDALL et al. 1957; SCULLY 1953; SMITH et al. 1959) and as has been demonstrated biochemically (HUSSLEIN 1950; KASE and COHN 1967). NISSEN-MEYER and SVERDRUP (1961) detected large amounts of estrogen in the urine of castrated women. Since oophorectomy will bring about a hypersecretion of LH, thus leading to a compensatory formation of estrogen, the development of an endometrial carcinoma in castrated women speaks for a relationship between carcinoma and hyperestrogenism rather than against it. Further, endometrial carcinomas developing after unilateral oophorectomy are becoming more common, particularly in women under 40 years of age (KEMPSON and POKORNY 1968). WILKINSON et al. (1973) reported on a patient with ovarian dysgenesis (Turner's syndrome) who received stilbestrol therapy for 9 years and developed an adenocarcinoma of the endometrium. In a search of the literature they found the reports of four similar cases and therefore interpreted the apparently interrelated train of events as an iatrogenic model for the induction of endometrial carcinoma. MCCARTY et al. (1978) cited 13 comparable cases and described one of their own patients, who developed an endometrial carcinoma after 31 years of estrogen therapy. VAN CAMPENHOUT et al. (1980) collected 18 similar cases.

Biochemical measurements of urine have indicated that women with corpus carcinomas have **persistently increased levels of estrogen** (PINCUS and GRAUBARD 1940), also in blood plasma (ALEEM et al. 1976). In addition, the vaginal epithelium of a high percentage of postmenopausal women with corpus carcinoma shows a distinct estrogen effect (HERRELL 1939; AYRE and BAULD 1946; LIMBURG 1951; NOVAK and MOHLER 1953; WIED 1953; LIU 1955; BERG and DURFEE 1958; STOLL and PECORARI 1962; CHANG and CRAIG 1963; CHARLES et al. 1965; RITCHIE 1965; CREPET and NUOVO 1967; DE WAARD and OETTLE 1967). According to HERTIG (1957), women with senile vaginitis never develop a corpus carcinoma. Some authors (e.g., CRAMER and WILDNER 1953) were unable to detect an increased level of estrogen in patients with endometrial carcinoma. Other investigators have reported an increase in the LH secretion in their patients with corpus carcinoma (SHERMAN and WOOLF 1959; VARGA and HENRIKSEN 1963), or an increase in androgens (WITTLINGER et al. 1975). These discrepancies, however, are only apparent. We know that androgenic substances are readily metabolized into estrogenic substances. HAUSKNECHT and GUSBERG (1973) found a significantly higher conversion rate of Δ^4-androstenedione to estrone in patients with endometrial cancer than in normal postmenopausal patients. Hence, the notable postmenopausal estrogen is probably estrone, and androstenedione its steroid precursor. In addition, androgens have been shown to activate the transfer of the estrogen receptor to the nucleus (ROCHEFORT et al. 1972). The concentration of estrogen receptor in differentiated endometrial carcinoma is very high as compared with that in normal endometrium (cf. p. 273).

It seems only logical to relate the endometrial *foam cells* with the persistently elevated levels of estrogen. Earlier workers who saw and described these cells were uncertain about their origin; they could never demonstrate evidence of a hypercholesterolemia or an inflammatory process. Many endometrial carcinomas with foam cells developed in patients who had received estrogen therapy for years; in one patient an ovary had once been removed. I have in my collection of endometrial carcinomas one tumor whose entire stroma had undergone change into foam cells; the patient had been treated with stilbestrol for 20 years. EPSTEIN (1976) noted that the foam cells developing in prostatic carcinomas after estrogen therapy resembled those arising in the endometrium. Since the stromal cells of the endometrial carcinoma electron-microscopically reveal an extensive well-developed ergastoplasm (WESSEL 1965), they are without doubt functionally active. TSENG et al. (1984) found two to five times higher values of estrogen synthesized in the medium of incubated tissue from endometrial adenocarcinoma as compared with normal endometrium. BLACK et al. (1941) found fat droplets in almost all stromal cells of the endometrium of a castrated patient treated with estrogen for 6 years. The normal endometrium of the menstrual cycle is free of such accumulations of fat. In contrast, the greatest number of foam cells (in over 50% of the cases) are found in adenomatous hyperplasias and fewer (30%) in glandular-cystic hyperplasias. Accordingly, it seemed logical to assume that the foam cells represented a reaction of the endometrial stroma to an unremittingly high, unopposed estrogen, be its source endogenous or exogenous. Previous studies suggested the foam cells contained cholesterol, which is known to be a precursor or by-product of estrogen synthesis (INHOFFEN 1940; WERBIN and LEROY 1954; DORFMAN 1957). The endometrial stromal cells are known to be subtle indicators of hormonal stimuli. The transformation of the stromal cells into foam cells resembles their change into decidual cells. Both of these processes of conversion first take place in the same regions of the stroma: in the superficial and well-vascularized regions. The one change excludes the other, however. When decidual cells and endometrial granulocytes develop, no foam cells appear; when the foam cells develop, no decidual cells or granulocytes form. The number of foam cells diminishes as the malignancy advances. Even in an early carcinoma decrease from the adenomatous hyperplasia is evident. Of the carcinomas, the adenoacanthoma contains the most foam cells (see Fig. 135).

Table 19 provides a survey of the endocrine disturbances associated with endometrial hyperplasias and carcinoma and relates these disturbances with the duration of endogenous or exogenous hyperestrogenism. I took into account only the glandular-cystic hyperplasias occurring after the menopause, since it is only these that are important as potential precursors of carcinoma (NOVAK 1956). As compared with the controls, the carcinoma and all forms of hyperplasia disclose very similar incidences of endocrine disturbances and hyperestrogenism. If the percentages for the various sources of hyperestrogenism listed under carcinoma are added, one obtains almost 100%, indicating that in the great majority of endometrial carcinomas an unopposed estrogen effect is to be expected. Consequently, it seems more likely that under the same hormonal stimulus a sequence proceeds from the glandular-cystic hyperplasia to adenomatous hyperplasia and ultimately to carcinoma; these pathological conditions should be looked upon as merely various ways in which the same persistent hormonal disturbance can express itself (see GORE and HERTIG 1966; GUSBERG 1967).

Some authors (HOFFBAUER 1931; MOSS 1946; THIESSEN 1952; WAY 1954; SOMMERS and MEISSNER 1957; GARNET 1958; PRINTER 1963; WYNDER et al. 1966) have tried to relate the hyperestrogenism seen with endometrial carcinoma and

Table 19. Relationships between endocrine abnormalities or endogenous and exogenous estrogen and endometrial carcinoma and its precursors

	Average age (years)	Nulliparae (%)	Obese patients (%)	Diabetic patients (%)	Patients with ovarian changes			Patients given therapy	
					Feminizing tumors (%)	Stromal hyperplasia (%)	Stein-Leventhal (%)	Estrogen (%)	X-irradiation (%)
Glandular-cystic hyperplasia[a]	After the menopause	36.0	52.0	16.0	10–92	60.0		21.5	
Adenomatous hyperplasia[b]	45–50	34.5	41.6	3.7	4.0			16.0	
Adenocarcinoma in situ[c]	49	33.0	54.0		5.0	42.5		6.3	15.6
Adenocarcinoma[d]	57.5	33.9	46.0	10.9	Total: 1.7 Postmenopausal: 2.9	72.2	Total: 4.1 Premenopausal: 21.2	13.2	7.2
Control patients	Equivalent	15.4	25.9	2.6	0.6	39.2	0.07		5.8

[a] After KOTTMEIER (1947), DHOM (1952), NOVAK (1956), FROMM (1959) (286 cases).
[b] After GARNET (1958), GUSBERG and KAPLAN (1963) (203 cases).
[c] After HERTIG et al. (1949) (64 cases).
[d] Compiled from the literature, numbering about 12000 cases (see DALLENBACH-HELLWEG 1964; further references: BENJAMIN and ROMNEY 1964; COUREY and GRAHAM 1964; TWEEDDALE et al. 1964; CHARLES 1965; LYNCH et al. 1966; WYNDER et al. 1966; WALL et al. 1967; DUNN et al. 1968; GEISLER and GIBBS 1968; PFLEIDERER 1968).

the associated endocrine disorders to a **disturbance of the pituitary gland,** providing thereby a single explanation for all the signs and symptoms. It is certainly conceivable, for example, that a disturbance in the secretion of LH would depress ovulation and thus stimulate a secretion of estrogen. Often the adrenals are also functionally abnormal, as evidenced by hypersecretion of the cortex (KAISER 1969). It seems so difficult to decide, however, what is primary and what is secondary in this complex endocrine disorder that one must be careful about postulating such dysfunction of the pituitary. Hyperestrogenism, on the other hand, seems to be a fundamental factor in the induction of endometrial carcinoma. "The overall effect of several risk factors may be to alter the intracellular levels of estrogen" (JAMES et al. 1982). The height of the estrogen level is much less important, however, than the constancy of its secretion. Certainly constitutional factors dispose to unopposed production of endogenous estrogen as well as to diabetes mellitus, hypertension, and obesity. An endocrine disturbance due to constitutional factors explains the frequently inherited disposition for endometrial carcinoma (LYNCH et al. 1966, 1967). According to BULLOUGH (1955) estrogen increases the permeability of the cell membrane for glucose.

On the other hand, in obesity estrogen seems to be stored in adipose tissue (TWOMBLY et al. 1967). Especially after the menopause and with obesity more estrogen is formed from androgen, as the conversion rate of androstendione into esterone increases (SCHINDLER 1977; SIITERI 1978). When patients in the postmenopause develop a bloody discharge while on estrogen therapy, a curettage discloses in a high percentage of them a precancerous or carcinomatous endometrium (BARTER et al. 1968).

The foregoing considerations lead us to the difficult and much-discussed question about **the importance of estrogen for the development of endometrial carcinoma.** The action of estrogen on the endometrium is fundamentally to induce regeneration to restore the tissue lost with menstruation. During a normal menstrual cycle that action is held in check by progesterone (which causes differentiation) and relaxin (which causes dissolution of the connective tissue); regeneration is maintained within physiological bounds. A persistent stimulation by unopposed estrogen over many years or even decades may, on the other hand, through the unremitting proliferation of the endometrium, greatly facilitate a spontaneous mutation or one caused by a carcinogen (BAUER 1963), especially in a genetically susceptible patient. As HAMPERL pointed out (1956), carcinogens act best in proliferating tissues. BÜCHNER (1961) spoke of the increase of accidental mutation accompanying an intensified doubling of the DNA. Accordingly, estrogen was regarded as a limited carcinogen which acts only on specific organs (BUTENANDT 1949, 1952; DONTENWILL 1961, 1965, 1966; WAGNER et al. 1967) or as a syncarcinogen (BAUER 1963; KRUSCHWITZ 1967). The aphorism by IGLESIAS (1965): "either I do differentiate and I die, or I do not differentiate and I kill", seems to apply especially well to the endometrial cells still under hormonal control. May estrogens alone under certain circumstances act as carcinogens? Although that question in general remains unanswered, at least for synthetic estrogens (stilbestrol) it seems they can, as the vaginal carcinomas and a recent report of an endometrial adenocarcinoma (BARTER et al. 1986) they induce (prenatally) in young women prove. It is well known that estrogens can induce benign and malignant tumors in experimental animals (for compilation refer to TAYLOR 1938; GARDNER 1939; ALLEN 1942; TAYLOR 1944; LIPSCHÜTZ 1950; GARDNER et al. 1959; TAKI and IIJIMA 1963; DALLENBACH 1971). We should also recall that estrogens directly influence the synthesis of DNA and the process of mitosis. Consequently, we need to ask whether estrogens might not possess a limited carcinogenic effect modified by circumstances, such as the lack of an opposing effect from progesterone. Otherwise, one will have to assume that ubiquitous carcinogens exist that can act on the endometrium but need estrogen stimulation (a cocarcinogen) to become fixed. For the patient such a cocarcinogenic action of estrogen would be just as important as a possible carcinogenic action. This discussion emphasizes once again how imperative it is that we learn how estrogen acts on its target cell.

That the effect of estrogen depends on genetic disposition explains why the individual response to a persistent secretion of unopposed estrogen is so diverse (BÜNGELER and DONTENWILL 1959). In women, the type and degree of proliferation caused by estrogenic overstimulation varies from patient to patient. Papillary growths or squamous metaplasia may develop (STOHR 1942), and in some women even myomata or diffuse myometrial hyperplasia or adenomyosis may occur. Only a few of these changes may arise or they may all appear together. The type of gland (for example, glands with papillae, or those lined either by tall cylindrical cells or by low cuboidal cells, or with foci of squamous metaplasia, and so forth) that evolves at the onset of the a patient's hyperplasia will persist through all subsequent stages and usually will still be seen in the carcinoma if that ultimately develops (GRUNER 1942; BEHRENS 1956). The histological picture of the endometrium is perhaps the most precise indicator for evaluating the intensity of estrogen effect; it surpasses by far the information obtained by biochemical determinations of either urine or blood. Figure 139 provides a schematic summary of the importance of estrogen in the development of endometrial carcinoma.

Glandular-cystic hyperplasia is the first response of the endometrium to an unopposed secretion of estrogen. Since the action of estrogen before the menopause can be blocked by the occasional secretion of progesterone, hyperplasia seldom progresses during that time. Depending on the levels of the two hormones, the histological picture may vary, either remaining unchanged or exhibiting variable secretory changes, proliferations of cystic glands, or regression. On the basis of our present knowledge it seems logical to classify glandular-cystic hyperplasia as a *facultative precancerous state* (Table 20). The same holds true

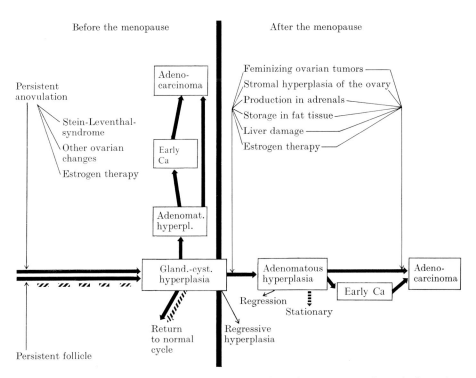

Fig. 139. Development of endometrial carcinoma from its precursors through the action of estrogen. *Heavy black arrow*, estrogen; *broken arrow* before the menopause, progesterone

Table 20. Evaluation of significance of endometrial carcinoma precursors

I. Precancerous lesions in the endometrium:

   a) Facultative:
   Irregular proliferation
   Circumscribed and diffuse glandular-cystic hyperplasias

   b) Relative obligatory:
   Adenomatous polyps
   Circumscribed adenomatous hyperplasias
   Juvenile adenomatous hyperplasias
   Diffuse adenomatous hyperplasias
   True stromal hyperplasia (rare)

II. Early carcinoma of the endometrium

---

for circumscribed hyperplasias and proliferating polyps, as well as for irregular proliferations, since these may at times skip a glandular-cystic stage and progress directly into an adenomatous hyperplasia.

The *adenomatous hyperplasia* is the first histological sign of a persistent unopposed effect of estrogen. It usually develops slowly from the glandular-cystic hyperplasia over a few years if the estrogen stimulus continues unabated; through the unremitting secretion of estrogen the glands are continuously driven to proliferate more and more. Usually the progression to adenomatous hyperplasia first comes about after the menopause; if it occurs before the menopause then during a protracted period of anovulation or estrogen substitution therapy. The level at which estrogen secretion continues determines what happens to the adenomatous hyperplasia. If the secretion of estrogen wanes, then the hyperplasia may regress. If the estrogen secretion remains high and the endometrium is left untreated, then the glands of the adenomatous hyperplasia continue to proliferate and within a few years become carcinomatous. Consequently, we should look upon adenomatous hyperplasia as an *obligatory precancerous state,* depending, however, on certain circumstances. The adenomatous hyperplasias that regress are almost always those induced by exogenous estrogens, whereby it may be possible to stop estrogen therapy and further stimulation in time. With endogenous hyperestrogenism, however, the state of hyperplasia is usually refractory if left untreated. We should also include in this group the localized forms of adenomatous hyperplasia and adenomatous polyps, although these may at times be spontaneously shed and totally discharged. The same pertains for juvenile adenomatous hyperplasia: if spontaneous ovulations fail to occur and if left ignored and untreated, it will inevitably progress to carcinoma.

The advance to irreversibility in this progression is morphologically detectable in only some of the cases, when foci of severe cytological atypia precede the development of an *early invasive carcinoma.* The decrease in cytoplasmic RNA observed in such regions is equivalent to that frequently described in early carcinomas of other locations (EMMELOT and BENEDETTI 1960; BERNHARD 1961; BÜCHNER et al. 1963). On the other hand, the acceleration in growth rate at the onset of malignancy may occur without any changes in cellular structure and thus elude histological detection (as for example, in the carcinoma of the prostate; HAMPERL 1952, 1957). Such concealed transition explains why it is often so difficult to distinguish an adenomatous hyperplasia from a beginning adenocarcinoma. Since adenomatous hyperplasia may prove difficult to evaluate histologically, it is advisable to gather information on the source and degree of the estrogen stimulation and on associated clinical signs and symptoms. In some cases of adenomatous hyperplasia the presence of foam cells in the endometrial stroma will be of prognostic importance, since they indicate that the estrogen stimulus has been intense for a long time.

An endometrial carcinoma may still be under the influence of estrogen, but it need not be. The repeated observation that some patients with endometrial carcinoma do not have elevated levels of estrogen (RAURAMO et al. 1964) can be explained by a decline in estrogen secretion after the carcinoma has developed. It can also be explained by the possibility that the cells of the endometrial carcinoma, an estrogen target tissue, have a much greater affinity for estrogen than do the carrier proteins of the plasma. Thereby, the endometrial carcinoma would take up, metabolize, or store in foam cells most of the estrogen available. During the preinvasive phase of endometrial carcinoma the plasma levels of estrogen are always high (ALEEM et al. 1976). When the endometrial carcinoma begins to grow autonomously, the high level of estrogenic stimulation may either persist or decrease. If the level remains high, then the adjacent non-carcinogenic endometrium continues to be hyperplastic. If the level decreases, the adjacent non-carcinogenic endometrium becomes atrophic, giving the false impression that the carcinoma had arisen in an atrophic endometrium (see Fig. 140).

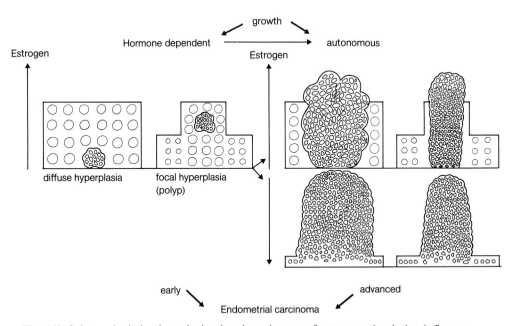

Fig. 140. Schema depicting how the level and persistence of estrogen stimulation influence the endometrium surrounding early endometrial carcinomas and later advanced stages

ζ) Progesterone Treatment of Endometrial Carcinoma

The demonstration that precancerous and carcinomatous growths may be hormone dependent and that gestagens inhibit mitoses (KAISER 1959; NORDQUIST 1964) and induce regression of endometrial carcinoma (VARGA and HENRIKSEN 1961) led to the clinical use of progesterone for treating adenomatous hyperplasia and inoperable carcinoma of the endometrium (THIESSEN 1956; KISTNER 1959; KISTNER and SMITH 1960; KELLEY and BAKER 1961, 1965; KISTNER et al. 1965; KISTNER 1982; DALLENBACH-HELLWEG et al. 1986). KOTTMEIER (1962) was able to improve the condition of nine out of 11 women suffering from corpus carcinoma with pulmonary metastases by giving them 0.2 mg of progesterone daily (later 150 mg per week). In four patients the pulmonary metastases disappeared. BERGSJÖ (1965), FRICK (1965) and MUSSEY and MALKASIAN (1966) treated their patients, who also had metastases from their endometrial cancers, with considerably larger doses of progesterone (from 200 mg three times a week to 1.5–2 g a week) and induced secretory changes in the tumors. In 25% of these patients the pulmonary metastases regressed. INGERSOLL (1965) also observed a regression of pulmonary and hepatic metastases in 25% of his patients with stage 4 endometrial carcinoma. In other series totalling about 400 patients who had received progesterone therapy for their endometrial carcinomas, usually as hydroxyprogesterone caproate (Delalutin), or medroxyprogesterone acetate (Depo-Provera), clinical improvement with regression of the primary tumor and metastases (especially the pulmonary and osseous) was reported in about one-third of the patients after 1–3 or more months of treatment (WENTZ 1964; ANDERSON 1965; KELLEY and BAKER 1965; BONTE et al. 1966; VARGA and HENRIKSEN 1965; SHERMAN 1966; WATERMAN and BENSON 1967; KENNEDY 1968; PECK and BOYES 1969; REIFENSTEIN 1971; PIVER et al. 1980). The longer the interval between primary gestagen therapy and recurrence, the better the response to the drug, a significant correlation because of the many diverse factors involved.

Patients responding survived four times as long as the non-responders. The degree of tumor differentiation proved important: about 50% of well-differentiated adenocarcinomas responded to gestagen therapy (BOQUOI and KREUZER 1973) whereas only about 15% of poorly differentiated did (KOHORN 1976). MARTZ (1968) recommended giving 500 mg Proluton twice a week for the treatment of pulmonary metastases but 2–5 g a week for metastases in the small pelvis and bones. Since there are no serious side-effects with the larger doses, these can be administered without concern.

We recommend treating patients with adenocarcinomas in stages 3 and 4 with continuous gestagen at a dose of 2 g per week for as long as they live. Patients with tumors in stage 1 should receive that treatment for 1 year. If the patient cannot be operated upon and her adenocarcinoma is well differentiated, one may consider therapy with gestagens alone. The success of that therapy can be followed with periodic curettages but must be maintained until the endometrium becomes atrophic. If treatment is discontinued prematurely, for example at the stage of arrested secretion, the tumor cells may recover their growth potentialities. Preoperative therapy with gestagens is also a possibility to be contemplated, especially when considerable time is required to prepare the patient for her operation. Basically, any gestagen preparation may be used.

Because of their greater gestagen potency, the 19-nortestosterone derivatives are more efficacious than those of progesterone (GAMBRELL 1977, 1978). The advantage of medroxyprogesterone acetate (MPA), however, is that it has no androgenic or estrogenic side effects.

It has been known from experience for some time, that well-differentiated endometrial carcinomas respond much better to gestagen therapy than do the poorly differentiated carcinomas. The modern immunohistochemical and biochemical techniques for measuring *estrogen and progesterone receptors* (see p. 16) have confirmed that experience and explained why it is true. The higher the degree of differentiation of a carcinoma, the more estrogen and progesterone receptors its cells produce (EVANS and HÄHNEL 1977; POLLOW et al. 1975; POLLOW and BOQUOI 1976; KAUPPILA et al. 1982; CHARPIN et al. 1986; GEISINGER et al. 1986) whereas at the same time the content of progesterone receptors may be high (MCCARTY et al. 1979; EHRLICH et al. 1981) or low (TSENG et al. 1977). Therapy with progesterone inactivates the estrogen and progesterone receptors (BJERSING 1977; RODRIQUEZ et al. 1979; VIHKO et al. 1980). To prevent the decrease in progesterone receptors, tamoxifen is added to the progesterone therapy as it blocks estrogen-promoted growth and increases the progesterone receptor concentration at the same time. The more poorly differentiated the carcinoma becomes, the more the nuclear receptors for progesterone decrease (YOUNG et al. 1976). Carcinomas without receptors are refractory to hormone therapy. From their studies MCCARTY et al. (1979) point out that the histological grading of endometrial carcinoma correlates with its levels of both estrogen and progesterone receptors, which are often considerably above those seen in normally cycling endometria. Receptor analysis may therefore provide the best criterion for selecting therapy for endometrial carcinoma, and may refine the prognostic value of histological grading.

Histophotometric measurements of carcinomatous tissues or normal tissues cultured in vitro revealed a distinct decrease in the synthesis of DNA and RNA after treatment with progesterone (NORDQUIST 1969, 1970; HUSTIN 1975, 1976; SIMON and HÖLZEL 1979; FERENCZY 1980). Their sets of chromosomes also became diploid and euploid. Ultrastructurally, large areas of heterochromatin reappeared (BARNI et al. 1981). These results mean that progesterone acts directly on the DNA synthesis of cells of endometrial carcinoma. At the same time, progesterone may exert its antiestrogenic effect by preventing estrogen from binding to its receptor. After gestagen therapy, the numerous nuclear inclusions, cytoplasmic vacuoles and lysosomes with disrupted membranes seen in electron-microscopic studies signify cellular injury (SIRTORI 1969). Three weeks after starting progesterone therapy the activity of alkaline phosphatase histochemically decreases (MOE 1972), whereas in only mature carcinomas the activity of 17β-hydroxysteroid-dehydrogenase rises sharply (POLLOW et al. 1975), paralleling the increase in content of progesterone receptors (POLLOW and BOQUOI 1976).

The histological changes produced in well-differentiated endometrial carcinomas by gestagen therapy resemble those that develop during a normal secretory phase. As early as three days after starting therapy secretory vacuoles appear in the glandular cells of the carcinoma (Fig. 141), the pseudostratified arrange-

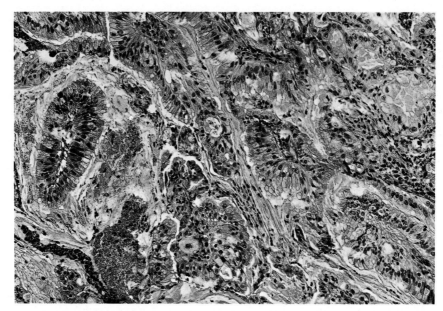

Fig. 141. Adenocarcinoma after several weeks of treatment with gestagens. Secretory change of the glandular epithelium; vacuoles forming in the basal parts of the cells; the nuclei have become rounded

ment of their nuclei recedes, and the number of mitoses decreases. As therapy continues, the production of glycogen and mucus by the glandular epithelium increases (cf. JOHN et al. 1974) in well-differentiated adenocarcinomas, whereas it remains unchanged in poorly differentiated tumors treated with progesterone (*Fukuma* et al. 1983). Finally, and characteristic of progesterone therapy, are the changes that develop in the non-carcinomatous endometrium (cf. p. 161 ff.). – The intrauterine administration of synthetic gestagens has the same effect on the carcinoma cells, as studies of uteri removed after such therapy proved (KISTNER et al. 1965; HUSTIN 1970).

Besides these histologically and biochemically detectable effects of progesterone directly on the endometrial carcinoma (HACKL 1968), progesterone most probably exerts an inhibitory action on the hypophysis since it depresses the secretion of LH.

Treatment with *clomiphene* (200 mg daily for 7 months) led to similar favorable results (WALL et al. 1964, 1965). This can be explained by the antiestrogenic action of clomiphene (see p. 186 ff.).

The resistance of poorly differentiated carcinomas to progesterone therapy might develop because the cells of the carcinoma have lost their dependency on estrogen long before, after which time the secretion of estrogen by the patient might have ceased. Since estrogen is needed to stimulate the target cells to produce progesterone receptors (see p. 50), progesterone therapy may be effectual in these patients if preceded by estrogen or if both hormones are given together (see also COLLINS 1972).

The analysis we have just made of the problems involved in the pathogenesis of endometrial carcinoma enables us to understand how rational gestagen therapy is for all forms of estrogen-induced hyperplasias after the menopause, and how such therapy serves as a prophylaxis against the development of endometrial carcinoma (see also KAISER 1969). Even in the precancerous hyperplasias, gestagen therapy must be continued over many months, until complete fibrous atrophy of the endometrium has been produced to avoid recurrences (see also EICHNER and ABELLERA 1971). According to GUSBERG (1976) all risk patients should be considered here, in whom an adenomatous hyperplasia might be detected early in a suction biopsy performed as an outpatient procedure.

For alleviating climacteric complaints many authors advocate treating with estrogens and gestagens together (WHITEHEAD et al. 1977; GAMBRELL 1978; HAMMOND et al. 1979). Of all patients receiving estrogen alone (1.25 mg daily) 94% developed endometrial hyperplasia, whereas when 10 mg medroxyprogesterone were added daily during the 4th week, only 6% developed the hyperplasia (cited from GAMBRELL 1977). With thymidine labeling, a suppression of DNA synthesis in glandular nuclei of the endometrium was observed following such combined therapy (FRIEDRICH and MEYER 1982). As the best prophylaxis to prevent the development of endometrial carcinoma, GAMBRELL (1978) recommends giving all postmenopausal women a test dose of gestagen, whether they are taking estrogens or not. If the patient experiences a withdrawal bleeding then that means she has a hyperproliferative endometrium and should be treated further cyclically with gestagens until the bleeding ceases. If the patient experiences no withdrawal bleeding, her endometrium is either refractory, resting or atrophic, and an endometrial carcinoma cannot develop. In their 4 year study, GAMBRELL et al. (1980) found that their postmenopausal patients treated with estrogen and progesterone had a significantly lower incidence of endometrial carcinoma than their patients receiving estrogens alone or even untreated patients. Their results are easier to understand when we recall that about 25% of all postmenopausal women continue to produce fairly high levels of estrogen after their menopause.

After **X-ray therapy** the endometrial carcinoma may lose its glandular character. The secretions become inspissated and giant cells may form (SHEEHAN and SCHMITZ 1950). In contrast to their response to gestagen therapy, the well-differentiated adenocarcinomas are usually resistant to irradiation, whereas the poorly differentiated or undifferentiated types respond to it fairly well. It is therefore very important to correctly classify the carcinoma as to histological type, since the treatment of choice depends on its proper classification.

c) Sarcoma of the Endometrium

The sarcomas that develop in the uterus almost always involve the endometrium, either primarily or secondarily, and depending on their sites of origin, may be divided into three groups: the endometrial sarcoma, the endometrial mixed mesenchymal tumor, and the leiomyosarcoma. In general the ratio of uterine sarcomas to uterine carcinomas (endometrial and cervical) is about 1:50. The sarcomas account for 2.04%–6.33% of all malignant tumors of the uterus (RANDALL 1943; WEISBROT and JANOVSKI 1963). The leiomyosarcoma is about three times more common than the endometrial sarcoma (BOUTSELIS and ULLERY 1962; BÖHM and STECH 1966; BARTSICH et al. 1968; KAHANPÄÄ 1986). Generally, the sarcomas appear in the fifth decade of life (RANDALL 1943; NORRIS and TAYLOR 1966; WILDNER and KLEIN 1967); the patients with leiomyosarcoma are somewhat younger than those with the other types of sarcoma.

The **endometrial stromal sarcoma (high-grade stromal sarcoma)** almost always *develops* from a stromal hyperplasia, which is equally as rare (see p. 134) and histologically similar except it does not invade. Thus, stromal hyperplasia may be referred to as a "sarcoma in situ". It may prove difficult to differentiate stromal hyperplasia from stromal sarcoma (SYMMONDS et al. 1957). Only a few investigators have assumed that a sarcoma could develop from a glandular-cystic hyperplasia (HUGHESDON and COCKS 1955), in which the stroma had presumably undergone intense circumscribed hyperplasia. The association of a uterine sarcoma with a pregnancy has been described several times (STUTZER 1947; BRUCE and DICK 1956; TAYLOR 1958). The tumor may simulate a placenta praevia. It usually arises from the stromal cells of the fundic endometrium, grows into the uterine cavity as a soft, polypoid or lobulated and knobby mass. At times it may enlarge the uterus to the size of a 6-month pregnancy. On the other hand, the endometrial stromal sarcoma invades the myometrium and its vessels early (in 75% of the cases), and may extend through the serosa to involve either directly or by the pelvic veins the neighboring organs and tissues. The surface of the freshly sectioned tumor is yellow, flecked by numerous small hemorrhages and cyst-like clefts. Necrotic portions may be discharged vaginally.

Histologically the *homologous type* of stromal sarcoma (Fig. 142) is most frequently observed. It can be differentiated from the *polymorphic type* (Fig. 143). Under low magnification the most striking feature is the disproportion between glands and stroma (Fig. 142a). The glands are unusually sparse and often absent in large regions of the stroma, but in other parts may be pushed together in small, irregular groups. Under higher magnification the hypercellularity of the stroma is readily apparent, the densely packed uniform cells possessing large nuclei, some of which are hypochromatic or undergoing mitosis (Fig. 142b). Usually, more than ten mitoses per 10 HPF can be counted (NORRIS and TAYLOR 1966). The cells are normally fusiform but when transected they appear round. Ultrastructurally they resemble stromal cells of the early proliferative phase (KOMOROWSKI et al. 1970; AKHTAR et al. 1975); their cytoplasm may be either scanty or abundant, depending upon their degree of differentiation, but generally appears immature, containing only a sparsely developed rough endoplasmic reticulum (BÖCKER and STEGNER 1975). Reticulum stains often reveal that each cell is enmeshed in a net of fibers, whereas the reticulum network may be poorly developed in some areas. Occasional cell clusters may be separated by focal hyaline deposits. Other intercellular substances are lacking. Small capillaries are abundant. – A distinction from the undifferentiated type of the malignant Müllerian mixed tumor may occasionally be difficult, particularly in tumors with very high mitotic rates (EVANS 1982). In such cases, immu-

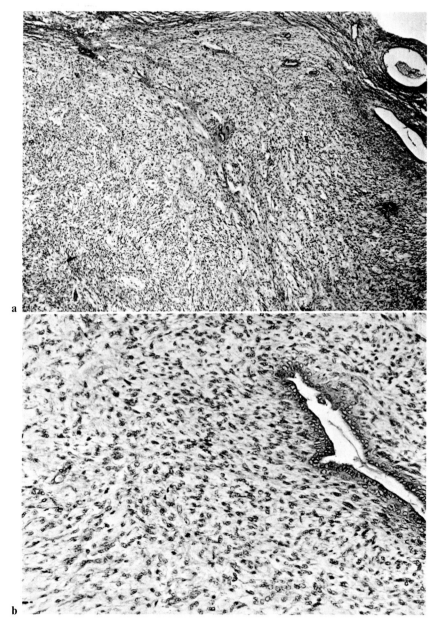

Fig. 142 a–d. Homologous endometrial stromal sarcoma infiltrating the myometrium. **a** Low magnification; **b** higher magnification. **c** and **d** (see p. 278) Polypoid surface of an endometrial stromal sarcoma. Curettings may contain only such small polypoid portions of the tumor. At low magnification (**c**) it may be mistaken for an edematous polyp. At high magnification (**d**) the sarcomatous character of the abnormal stromal cells can readily be recognized

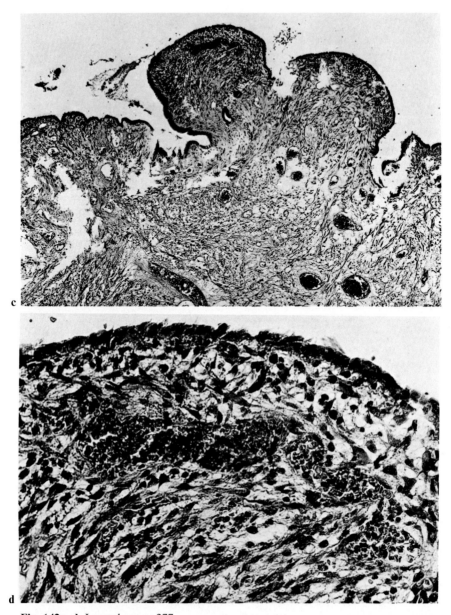

Fig. 142c, d. Legend see p. 277

nohistochemical studies of the intermediate filament composition of the tumor cells are of considerable help in the differential diagnosis: The tumor cells of high-grade as well as of low-grade stromal sarcomas do not react with desmin or cytokeratin antibodies, but stain exclusively with antibodies to vimentin, like normal endometrial stromal cells, whereas the areas of epithelial differentiation in poorly differentiated malignant Müllerian mixed tumors are decorated

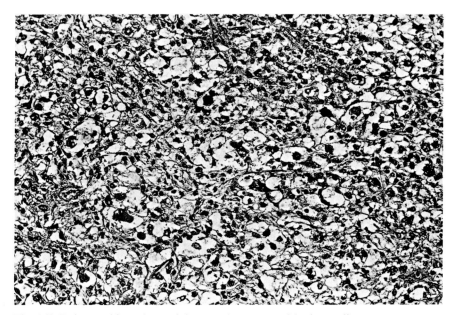

Fig. 143. Polymorphic endometrial stromal sarcoma with giant cells

with cytokeratin antibodies (LIFSCHITZ-MERCER et al. 1987). – Generally in the homologous type, the uniformity of the tumor cells is striking (*uniform pattern*). Some homologous stromal sarcomas show a *plexiform pattern* in which the cellular arrangement is not uniform, but condensed in branching cords which may resemble sex cords of a gonadal stroma in some areas (CLEMENT and SCULLY 1976; TANG et al. 1979; FEKETE and VELLIOS 1984).

The *polymorphic type* shows a great variation in nuclear size, shape and chromatin density; giant cells containing multiple nuclei or large bizarre forms are then often present (Fig. 143).

Only rarely do these neoplastic stromal cells differentiate along the two lines open to normal stromal cells. For example, BÖHM and STECH (1966) observed decidual-like changes in the sarcomatous cells, and KAZZAZ (1975) described a granulocytic sarcoma in a 69-year-old woman. The pleomorphic cells of her tumor had round, hyperchromatic nuclei and in their cytoplasm disclosed strongly birefringent, phloxinophilic granules. Histochemically, these cells corresponded to endometrial granulocytes. Independently, BÖCKER (1980) published electron-microscopic studies of neoplastic endometrial granulocytes and suggested these represented a special form of differentiation of endometrial stromal sarcoma. Another special form is the rare *clear cell stromal sarcoma* which is often misinterpreted as clear cell adenocarcinoma or clear cell leiomyoma. The recognition is possible by the absence of cytokeratin reactivity (as in adenocarcinoma) and by the failure to stain with desmin antibodies (as in leiomyoma) (LIFSCHITZ-MERCER et al. 1987). In addition, groups of endometrial foam cells may be detected among the tumor cells.

The nuclear polymorphism may be so slight that one has difficulty in recognizing the sarcomatous stromal cells as such and in not confusing them with hormonally stimulated stromal cells (OBER and JASON 1953). In such cases a beginning endometrial stromal sarcoma is often either easily overlooked or is erroneously diagnosed. An abnormally cellular, sarcoma-like stroma is no proof of sarcoma as long as the glands are evenly distributed. On the other hand, if abnormal stromal cells are found penetrating the myometrium, as they often do early, then that invasive growth alone makes it easier to recognize the tumor.

Endometrial stromal sarcoma often shows early local recurrences (KAHANPÄÄ 1986). It *metastasizes,* not only out into the peritoneal cavity but also by way of the blood vessels and lymphatics into the liver and lungs (WHEELOCK and STRAND 1953); metastases to the bones (FARROW et al. 1968) or heart (STEELE et al. 1968) are rare.

According to most authors the *prognosis* is extremely poor (see KOSS et al. 1965; WHITE et al. 1965; GÜNTHER 1967); MCDONALD et al. (1940) as well as BOUTSELIS and ULLERY (1962) state that even with radical surgery only about 20% of the patients survive more than 5–6 years. NORRIS and TAYLOR (1966), on the other hand, give somewhat higher survival rates. According to most clinical follow-up studies, the extension of the tumor at the time of diagnosis appears to be the most important prognostic factor: if the tumor extends beyond the inner half of the myometrium, survival chances are minimal to zero (WHEELOCK et al. 1985, and many other series).

The **low-grade stromal sarcoma (endolymphatic stromal myosis)** presents the same cellular structure as the homologous type of the high-grade stromal sarcoma (ZALOUDEK and NORRIS 1982). It may prove exceedingly difficult to differentiate between the two types (RUPPERT 1949; HUNTER et al. 1956; LAFFARGUE et al. 1966; GOLDMAN and GANS 1967). The cells composing the low-grade sarcoma differ from those of the homologous type of the high-grade sarcoma only, but not reliably, in their less-pronounced mitotic activity (YOONESSI and HART 1977), which is usually below nine mitoses per 10 HPF.

Characteristic of low-grade stromal sarcoma is an early and extensive invasion of the lymphatic vascular spaces of the myometrium and penetration into tissue clefts of the myometrium without destruction and necrosis. Whereas most of these low-grade stromal sarcomas have a uniform pattern, a plexiform arrangement is occasionally seen (CLEMENT and SCULLY 1976). The 5-year survival rate of patients with low-grade stromal sarcoma is higher than in patients with high-grade sarcoma (JENSEN et al. 1966; SAKSELA et al. 1974; DALLENBACH-HELLWEG 1980; according to EBERL et al. 1980 77% as compared with 41% in the high-grade sarcoma). The average age of these patients tends to be lower (below 50 years) than of those with high-grade endometrial sarcomas (EVANS 1982). Distant metastases are rare and occur only at a late stage.

Early radical hysterectomy remains the *treatment* of choice in all endometrial stromal sarcomas. Adjuvant chemotherapy has proved to be superior to radiation therapy, which did not improve survival rates. Since at least some low-grade as well as high-grade endometrial stromal sarcomas are hormone responsive, therapy with medroxyprogesterone acetate has been beneficial and has prolonged survival rates considerably (KAHANPÄÄ 1986). Such progestagen therapy seems all the more reasonable in view of a recent report of six endometrial sarcomas complicating ovarian thecomas, polycystic ovarian disease, or following estrogen therapy over 16 and 18 years, respectively, thereby suggesting an increased risk of endometrial sarcomas with endogenous or exogenous unopposed estrogen stimulation (PRESS and SCULLY 1985). Consequently, the content of estrogen and progesterone receptors should be determined in all stromal sarcomas.

The **malignant mixed mesenchymal tumors** (AARO et al. 1966; NORRIS et al. 1966; RACHMANINOFF and CLIMIE 1966; the "heterologous sarcoma" of OBER and TOVELL 1959) contain two or more types of sarcomatous tissues; for example, rhabdomyoblasts and chondroblasts. Some believe these mixed tumors represent a "malignant metaplasia" of modified endometrial stromal cells (ALZNAUER 1955). It seems just as logical to assume the cells of these mixed sarcomas originate from the so-called Müllerian epithelium, a tissue which undergoes mesenchymal differentiation during embryonal development, leaving its cellular descendants with partial potentialities for further differentiation (see Table 21). Occasionally the metastases from these mixed tumors consist of only one type of sarcomatous tissue. OBER (1959) regards the prognosis for these heterologous sarcomas to be even worse than that for the homologous endometrial stromal sarcoma.

Other rare types of sarcoma that may occur or develop from the mixed forms are *lymphosarcoma* (SCHLAGENHAUFER 1912; WALTHER 1934; BLAUSTEIN et al. 1962; BURROWS et al. 1964; FOX and MORE 1965; WRIGHT 1973; CHORLTON et al. 1974), which is thought to arise from the lymphoid follicles of the endometrium, and which has to be differentiated from severe chronic endometritis (see p. 205); *myelogenous* sarcoma (KAPADIA et al. 1978), as a local manifestation of a myelogenous leukemia (chloroma); *plasmocytoma* (ANDERSON 1949); malignant histiocytic tumor (BELLOMI and GAMOLETTI 1981); malignant *hemangioendothelioma* (ULESKO-STROGANOWA 1925; COHEN et al. 1949) or *angiosarcoma* (ONGKASUWAN et al. 1982); malignant hemangiopericytoma (BUSCEMA et al. 1987; see p. 224); *chondrosarcoma* (GEBHARD 1903; KOFINAS et al. 1984); and *rhabdomyosarcoma* (R. MEYER 1930; DONKERS et al. 1972; SIEGAL et al. 1983). These tumors are readily recognized by their characteristic cell types which may show various degrees of differentiation and consequently, pleomorphism; they are all extremely rare. The classification of angiosarcoma into endotheliomas, peritheliomas and so forth seems questionable since so few of these tumors have been described.

Leiomyosarcomas arising in the myometrium may infiltrate the endometrium secondarily. These tumors are densely cellular and characteristically composed of atypical muscle cells in various stages of differentiation. Among almost fully developed smooth muscle cells one finds shorter spindle cells with few myofibrils and distinctly pleomorphic nuclei. R. MEYER (1930) named such a tumor "sarcoma myocellulare". Ultrastructurally, the cells of these tumors are either poorly differentiated and elongated with numerous polyribosomes and meager Golgi bodies, or are myoblastic with typical myofilaments, or fibroblastic, rich in rough endoplasmic reticulum (BÖCKER and STEGNER 1975). The nuclei are generally large and hyperchromatic, mitoses abound. Since their number serves as

Table 21. Malignant mixed tumors, sarcomas and carcinomas of the uterine mucosa

Cell of origin	Designation	Interpretation
Müllerian epithelium (pluripotent)	1. Malignant mixed Müllerian tumor	1. Heterologous combination tumor (R. MEYER 1930)
	2. Sarcoma botryoides	2. Juvenile form of the heterologous combination tumor (STERNBERG et al. (1954)
	3. Carcinosarcoma 4. Müllerian adenosarcoma 5. Carcinofibroma	3.–5. Homologous combination tumor (R. MEYER 1930)
Müllerian epithelium with mesenchymal differentiation (partially pluripotent)	Malignant mixed mesenchymal tumors (chondro-, osteo-, rhabdomyosarcoma, etc.)	Pure heterologous tumor (OBER and TOVELL 1959)
Müllerian epithelium with epithelial differentiation (partially pluripotent)	Malignant mixed epithelial tumors (mucinous, mucoepidermoid adenocarcinomas, clear cell, serous papillary, squamous carcinoma)	Pure heterologous tumor
Epithelial and stromal cells of the endometrium (fixed potentialities)	Carcinosarcoma	Composition tumor (R. MEYER 1930)
Epithelial and stromal cells of the endometrium separate (fixed potentialities)	Carcinoma and sarcoma	Collision tumor (R. MEYER 1930)
Stromal cells of the endometrium (fixed potentialities)	Endometrial stromal sarcoma (low and high grade)	Pure homologous tumor (OBER and TOVELL 1959)
Epithelial cells of the endometrium (fixed potentialities)	Adenocarcinoma, adenoacanthoma, adenosquamous carcinoma	Pure homologous tumor

↓ Loss of potentialities

an important criterion for evaluating the invasive potential of the tumor, several portions of tumor should be examined histologically. Those parts with the most mitoses are then used for trying to evaluate the biological behavior of the tumor. In rare instances, a leiomyosarcoma of the endometrium may develop directly by neoplastic metaplasia of the endometrial stromal cells (BIRD and WILLIS 1965; BÖCKER 1980). The close relationship between neoplastic myogenic and stromal cells may explain the difficulty in immunocytochemical differentiation, since both actin and myosin, as in leiomyosarcomas, may rarely be present in stromal sarcomas as well (MARSHALL and BRAYE 1985). Besides the pure homogeneous leiomyosarcomas, *fibroleiomyosarcomas* may arise with fibroblastic cells predominating (LAFFARGUE et al. 1966).

Occasionally during treatment of a glandular-cystic hyperplasia with progesterone the endometrial stroma undergoes a *pseudosarcomatous proliferation,* its cells developing large, pleomorphic and hyperchromatic nuclei and its glands atrophying (DOCKERTY et al. 1959; CRUZ-AQUINO et al. 1967). Such endometrial changes should not be mistaken for an endometrial stromal sarcoma. They can be distinguished from that tumor by their lack of mitoses. In rare instances, however, an endometrial sarcoma may develop following treatment with some of the synthetic gestagens (cf. p. 178). On the other hand, progesterone therapy may induce regression of a stromal sarcoma and its pulmonary metastases (PELLILLO 1968).

d) Malignant Mixed Mesodermal Tumors

In addition to the malignant mixed mesenchymal tumors arising from the endometrial stroma or from Müllerian epithelium with its inherent mesenchymal potentialities, other malignant tumors may develop that have epithelial as well as mesenchymal components. Consequently, we call these "carcinosarcomas", or "malignant mixed mesodermal tumors". They constitute about 60% of all uterine sarcomas (SALAZAR et al. 1978). Under that heading R. MEYER (1930) distinguished between the combination tumors, the composition tumors, and the collision tumors. *Combination tumors* are those in which both epithelial and stromal cells arise from the same pluripotential stem cells, as for example, the carcinosarcomas that develop directly from the epithelial-like cells of the Müllerian duct (see Table 21). Since the sarcomatous and carcinomatous components of the *composition-tumors* probably also arise from mesenchymal and epithelial tissues of the endometrium, albeit from differentiated and more mature cells, it would seem logical to group the composition tumors with the combination tumors. The sarcomatous cells of these composition tumors, as might be expected from their reduced potentialities to differentiate further, are homogeneous. Those of the combination tumors, however, may vary greatly because of the pluripotentialities of the undifferentiated Müllerian epithelium from which they arise; they may, for example, contain both myxomatous and chondromatous parts (SCHRÖDER and HILLEJAHN 1920; ROEMER 1941; MOEGEN 1951; BERGER and DIETRICH 1957; TAYLOR 1958; CARTER and MCDONALD 1960; HOFFMEISTER and HANSCHKE 1960, and others). Consequently, these heterologous combination tumors have been renamed "malignant mixed Müllerian tumors" (STERNBERG et al. 1954; JOPP and KRONE 1962) or as "Mülleroblastome" (MARTIN et al. 1956).

Collision tumors may develop, according to R. MEYER, from the growing-together of a carcinoma and a sarcoma, each of which originates separately in various ways: (a) a malignant change of the epithelial cells and stromal cells may be induced at the same time by the same stimulus (JOPP 1965); (b) the carcinoma may provoke an abnormal hyperplasia of the stroma which in turn leads to development of the sarcoma (HARVEY and HAMILTON 1935; HINZ 1952); (c) the sarcoma may stimulate the development of the carcinoma (SEHRT 1905). Sarcomatous polyps that are invaded by adenocarcinomatous cells either at the surface or at the base (ALBRECHT 1928) also belong to the collision tumors. Both components, however, many remain separated (BREITER 1938; BAHARI et al. 1986).

When the growth of a tumor is well advanced, it may be very difficult, if not impossible, to distinguish a collision tumor from a true combination tumor or a composition tumor. If a mixed tumor is suspected, it is important to take samples of tissue from different parts to insure that the histological study is complete. Such thorough studies may reveal that a tumor presumed to be a pure carcinoma or sarcoma is instead a mixed tumor. Such a disclosure is important for the therapy and prognosis. Recent studies indicate that mixed tumors are more common than previously assumed. Every large polyp with a smooth surface might be a mixed tumor and should be studied histologically (TAYLOR 1958). On the other hand, we should separate the mixed tumors from poorly differentiated adenocarcinomas whose peripheral portions appear sarcomatous (the "carcinoma pseudosarcomatodes" of E. KAUFMANN) or whose stroma assumes a sarcoma-like appearance, a change thought to be caused by abnormal metabolic processes of the tumor cells (MARIANI et al. 1957). In this respect, cytokeratin markers, which are positive in most endometrial adenocarcinomas but negative in stromal sarcomas, may be helpful (MARSHALL and BRAYER 1985).

The **carcinosarcomas** of the endometrium, comprising the homologous combination tumors and the composition tumors, account for about 1.2% of the corpus carcinomas (BRÄUNIG and LOHE 1968). The average age of the patients, as calculated from larger statistics, is 62 years (NORRIS et al. 1966) or 61.3 years (BARTSICH et al. 1967). The youngest reported with such a tumor was a girl $14^1/_2$ years old (LANCET and LIBAN 1970). About 50% are nullipara. A *previous X-ray irradiation* (2000–8000 R 1–18 years before, with an average of 16.4 years) to the small pelvis seems to be etiologically important in the development of the tumor. BARTSICH et al. (1967) obtained a history of such therapy in 37% of their patients with carcinosarcoma; BOUTSELIS and ULLERY (1962) found it in 17%; NORRIS and TAYLOR (1965, 1966) reported that 12% of all their patients with a uterine sarcoma and 13% of their patients with carcinosarcomas had received previous X-ray therapy. SPEERT and PEIGHTAL (1949), HILL and MILLER (1951), SYMMONDS and DOCKERTY (1955), VELLIOS et al. (1963), O'CONNOR (1964), PILLERON and DURAND (1968), THOMAS et al. (1969), DOSS et al. (1984), and many others also disclosed that a high percentage of their patients with carcinosarcoma had previously been given X-ray therapy. Some hold that prior therapy with estrogen may be of etiological importance (KARPAS and SPEER 1957; PRESS and SCULLY 1985).

Grossly, the carcinosarcomas almost always bulge into the uterine cavity as soft, pedunculated polyps; they may even protrude from the outer cervical os. On section the tumors appear gray-yellow. They invade the myometrium and lymphatic channels early, soon reach the structures of the small pelvis (adnexae, bladder, and rectum), then spread throughout the peritoneum, into the vagina, and metastasize to the paraaortic, paraesophageal and paratracheal lymph nodes, and hence to the liver and lungs.

Most investigators report that the *prognosis* is very poor (OBER 1959). The average length of survival after the first clinical symptoms appear varies from 6 to 12 months (HILL and MILLER 1951; STERNBERG et al. 1954; TAYLOR 1958, 1972; BRÄUNIG and LOHE 1968). HALL and NELMS (1953) as well as BARTSICH et al. (1967) never saw a patient survive 5 years and 77% of the patients lived less than 2 years. In the series reported by NORRIS and TAYLOR (1966), 70% of the patients died between 1 month and 5 years after therapy was started. WILLIAMSON and CHRISTOPHERSON (1972) observed a 5 year survival rate of only 20.5%. Women with homologous mixed tumors, however, survive longer than the women with heterologous mixed Müllerian tumors (OBER 1959; KRUPP et al. 1961). Thus, it is important to differentiate histologically between these two types. The extent of tumor growth at the time of operation is especially important for evaluating the prognosis (CHUANG et al. 1970). In the series of MORTEL et al. (1974), the 5-year survival was 60% when the tumor was limited just to the uterus, compared with 32% for the overall series. The age of the patient is also important: premenopausal patients have a slightly better prognosis than those postmenopausal.

Histologically, the homologous carcinosarcomas (homologous combination and composition tumors of R. MEYER) consist of tubules or cords of carcinoma cells usually in various stages of maturity intimately surrounded by the sarcomatous stroma. The carcinomatous gland-like structures may exist either as small acini or as large follicles. Their lining epithelial cells, which often contain PAS-positive substances, may form papillae. Occasionally foci of squamous metaplasia are seen with well-developed pearls of keratinized cells. In short, the carcinomatous component may reveal all the variations of an adenocarcinoma. The sarcomatous cells are all spindle-shaped like those of endometrial stromal sarcomas (in composition tumors), or they may become pleomorphic and large, just as those of endometrial stromal sarcomas may, and occasionally show myoblastic differentiation (in combination tumors) (Fig. 144d).

On the other hand, in the **malignant mixed Müllerian tumors** (the heterologous combination tumors) the sarcomatous components may be extremely pleomorphic. Next to poorly differentiated mesenchymal cells one often finds bizarre forms of chondrocytes and osteoblasts, of muscle cells with cross-striations (Fig. 144c), of fat cells (MORTEL et al. 1970) and of ganglion cells (RUFFOLO et al. 1969); myxomatous transformation also occurs. Electron-microscopically, all developmental stages from primitive mesenchymal cells to differentiating rhabdomyoblasts and chondroblasts as well as epithelial cells can be identified, providing further evidence for the hypothesis that these tumors arise from pluripotential Müllerian epithelium (SILVERBERG 1971; BORAM et al. 1972; BÖCKER and STEGNER 1975; ISHIKAWA et al. 1979). Immunohistochemical staining with epithelial markers may detect antigen-containing cells in mesenchymal portions of the tumor, suggesting an early stage of epithelial differentiation in mesenchymal cells of the malignant stroma (RAMADAN and GOUDIE 1986). The carcinomatous portions of these heterologous mixed tumors differentiate along all lines possible for the Müllerian epithelium. They may form not only papillary struc-

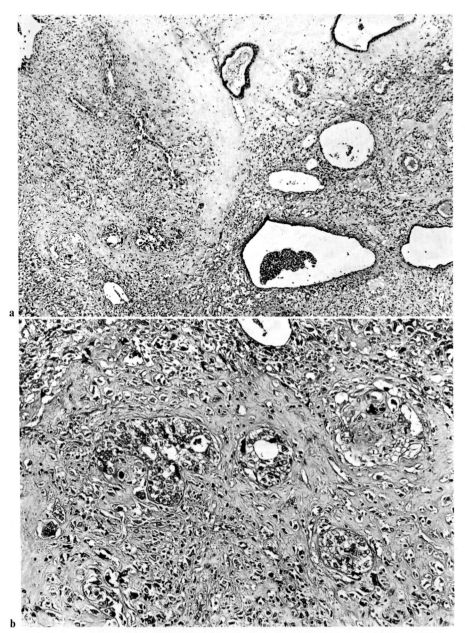

Fig. 144a–d. Malignant mixed Müllerian tumor with heterologous sarcomatous and carcinomatous components. **a** Low magnification; **b** higher magnification. **c** Rhabdomyblasts with cross striation within the sarcomatous stroma. **d** Carcinosarcoma, also derived from pluripotent Müllerian epithelium (cf. Table 21), is a homologous combination tumor.

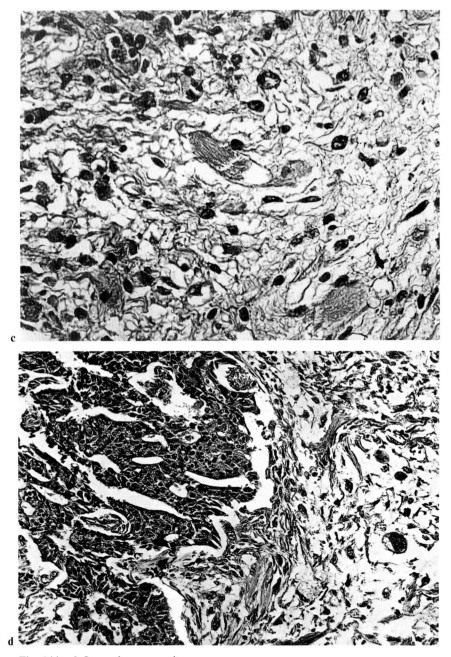

Fig. 144c, d. Legend see opposite page

tures but also mucus-secreting endometrial glands, or may contain fallopian tube epithelium or psammoma bodies (KRUPP et al. 1961; LAUCHLAN 1968). Their capacity to differentiate is limited, however, to only those forms that normally develop from the Müllerian epithelium. These tumors differ therefore from the teratomas (STERNBERG et al. 1954). Those tumors showing chondroblastic differentiation have a slightly better prognosis than those containing rhabdomyoblasts (NORRIS et al. 1966; BÖCKER and STEGNER 1974). Occasionally mixed Müllerian tumors may arise within a polyp. If still limited to it when first detected the prognosis may be favorable (BARWICK and LIVOLSI 1979). Those arising from a papillary adenofibroma retain their characteristic histological structure (cf. p. 224) occasionally with accumulations of clear cells surrounding cleft-like spaces. They likewise have slightly better survival rates.

The metastases of these mixed Müllerian tumors may consist of both carcinomatous and sarcomatous elements, or of only one of these components; the purely carcinomatous metastases are more common than those of only sarcomatous elements (HERTIG and GORE 1960; BARTSICH et al. 1967).

The tumors arising after previous radiotherapy are generally heterologous and develop in the younger women (VARELA-DURAN et al. 1980).

The *sarcoma botryoides* of children, which arises from the cervical mucosa, is analogous to the malignant mixed Müllerian tumor that develops from the adult endometrium. As STERNBERG et al. (1954) explained, the reason these two tumors correspond is that the endocervical stroma of children is like adult endometrium. Later, with sexual maturity, the endocervical stroma changes. Since the sarcoma botryoides resembles both grossly and microscopically the malignant mixed Müllerian tumors and differs from them only in its site of origin, it may be grouped with them. It grows from the cervix in polypoid, grape-like clusters, and may be composed of sarcomatous parts of diverse character containing cords and gland-like structures of carcinomatous cells. The prognosis of the sarcoma botryoides is the same as that of the malignant mixed Müllerian tumors. When it arises in the cervix, it often invades the endometrium secondarily. It may also arise in the vagina in children, for the vaginal stroma at such an age resembles that of the endometrium.

The papillary adenofibroma, representing a benign variant of the malignant Müllerian mixed tumor (cf. p. 224) may undergo various types and degrees of malignant change (see Fig. 145): in the *Müllerian adenosarcoma,* the malignant change is limited to the mesenchymal component, the epithelial component is histologically and biologically benign. The general structure of the glands and their endometrial-type adenomatous appearance closely resemble those of the benign cystadenofibroma. Some glandular spaces may be cystically dilated and contain mucin. The mesenchymal component is, however, more cellular

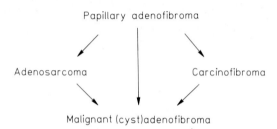

Fig. 145. Possible ways for papillary adenofibroma to undergo malignant transformation

and composed of small sarcomatous fibroblasts or stromal cells with mild atypia and moderate mitotic activity (more than four mitoses per 10 HPF; CLEMENT and SCULLY 1974; KATZENSTEIN et al. 1977; FOX et al. 1979; ZALOUDEK and NORRIS 1981, 1982). Characteristic are round concentric hypercellular foci forming perivascular nodules or periglandular cuffs (Fig. 146b, c) (GLOOR 1979; CZERNOBILSKY et al. 1983). The sarcomatous cells may also be heterologous, with rhabdomyoblasts and chondroblasts mixed in among the stromal cells, but all are of low-grade malignancy (ROTH et al. 1976), rendering thereby a

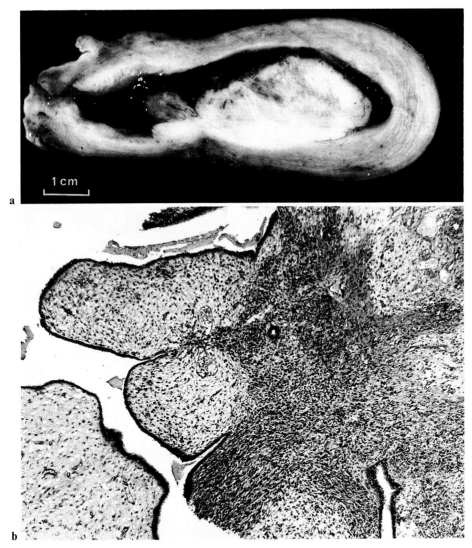

Fig. 146a–c. Müllerian adenosarcoma of the endometrium. **a** Gross tumor protruding into the enlarged uterine cavity with shallow infiltration and pushing borders toward the myometrium. **b** Low magnification: finger-like projections of sarcomatous stroma and sparse slit-like glandular remnants. **c** (see p. 290)

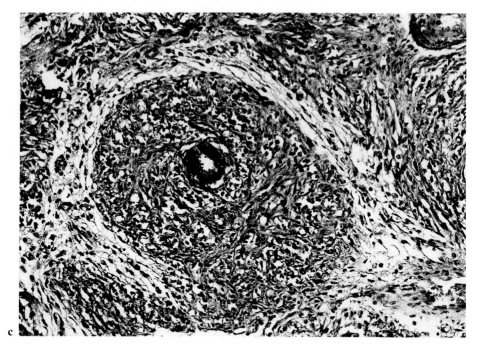

Fig. 146c. Higher magnification: concentric periglandular condensation of sarcomatous stromal cells

more favorable prognosis (VALDEZ 1979). If these tumors contain larger rhabdomyosarcomatous areas they must be distinguished from malignant mixed Müllerian tumors because these have a different prognosis and require a different type of therapy. An important criterion in this differential diagnosis is the absence of carcinomatous cells and the presence of benign glands as integral parts of the adenosarcoma. For the same reason, the diagnosis of adenosarcoma must exclude stromal sarcomas with trapped normal endometrial glands, particularly if the tumor shows an unusually rapid progression (OKAGAKI et al. 1979). The sarcomatous stroma may occasionally, as in endometrial stromal sarcoma, contain foci with sex cord-like differentiation (HIRSCHFIELD et al. 1986) or groups of foam cells (CZERNOBILSKY et al. 1983). Whereas the papillary adenofibroma of the endometrium may resemble an ovarian or mammary adenofibroma, so may the adenosarcoma resemble cystosarcoma phyllodes of the breast (CLEMENT and SCULLY 1974). Most adenosarcomas occur in the early postmenopause, but some also in adolescense. Adenosarcomas do invade the myometrium, but only at a late stage (Fig. 146a). They have a recurrence rate of 40% following hysterectomy.

In rare instances, a *carcinofibroma* develops from an adenofibroma. Here the epithelial component is malignant, but the mesenchymal component is benign (ÖSTÖR and FORTUNE 1980; THOMPSON and HUSEMYER 1981). The epithelial component consists of carcinomatous glands, which may be cystically dilated or microalveolar and which may form branching intraluminal epithelial papillae or nodules of squamous metaplasia. The lining epithelium is atypical and resembles that of adenocarcinomas. The surrounding stroma of fibroblasts corresponds to that of benign cystadenofibromas. The tumor may invade the myometrium like an adenocarcinoma. It can be differentiated from adenocarcinomas with a desmoplastic stromal reaction by its widely spaced carcinomatous glands.

Recently, two malignant primitive *neuroectodermal tumors* of the endometrium have been observed in a 12-year-old and in a 57-year-old patient (HENDRICKSON and SCHEITHAUER 1986). They contained only poorly differentiated neuroectoderm and primitive stroma. They were considered to be of either teratomatous origin with one-sided differentiation, or of mesodermal derivation with heterologous metaplasia.

One *endodermal sinus tumor* arising in the endometrium has been reported in the literature (PILERI et al. 1980). The tumor developed in a 28-year-old woman. Histologically a pseudo-papillary pattern with Schiller-Duval bodies was seen and α-fetoprotein was detected immunohistochemically. The tumor proved fatal. As possible sites of origin of the tumor were displaced germinal cells or an abnormal ovum.

e) Metastatic Tumors

The carcinomas that metastasize to the endometrium most commonly originate in either the cervix, or ovaries, or fallopian tubes. They usually reach the endometrium by way of lymphatic channels; their spread by way of the fallopian tube (for ovarian carcinomas) or blood vessels is rare.

MITANI et al. (1964) found the endometrium to be involved in 25% of the *portio and cervix carcinomas* operated on, even in eight of 57 patients with stage 1 carcinoma. Even an endocervical carcinoma in situ may spread to the endometrium and involve endometrial glands (SALM 1969; KANBOUR and STOCK 1978; WILKINSON et al. 1980). It is important to recognize when the endometrium is invaded since that involvement makes the survival rate worse (PEREZ et al. 1975). The prognosis was somewhat better when spread of the tumor was limited to the endometrium than when it also involved the myometrium. Since in most patients the cervical tumor is evident clinically, no diagnostic problems arise in recognizing the metastatic carcinoma when separate curettings are taken from cervix and endometrium (Fig. 147).

When either the papillary adenocarcinoma of the ovary, the most common *ovarian carcinoma* (NEUMANN 1927), or the rare *adenocarcinoma of the fallopian tube* (OLESEN and ALBECK 1949) metastasizes to the endometrium, the site of origin of the primary tumor may not always be obvious. In curettings these tumors are usually misdiagnosed as primary endometrial carcinomas because histologically they resemble one another so closely. Such cases become clarified only after the surgical specimen is examined. On occasions the tumor in the curettings reveals a special type of differentiation that points to the site of origin of the tumor (for example, psammoma bodies). When these bodies are found in a papillary adenocarcinoma, they most probably indicate that the primary tumor has arisen in the ovary. If they are seen in an adenocarcinoma with small acini, then a primary carcinoma of the rectum should be considered.

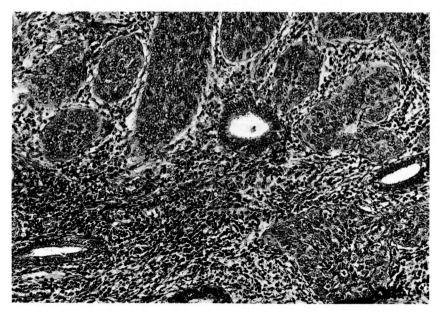

Fig. 147. Extension of a epidermoid carcinoma of the cervix into the endometrium

The extremely rare primary psammocarcinomas of the uterus (see p. 251) are solid, and usually free of glandular structures.

In the differential diagnosis several questions should be raised: is the tumor really a metastasis from a carcinoma of the adnexae, or it is a second primary tumor, or does the adnexal tumor represent a metastasis from a primary endometrial carcinoma? In 79% of the cases these questions can be answered (KOTTMEIER 1953). If, however, the tumors at both the endometrial and adnexal sites appear histologically similar and have reached about the same size, then these questions may prove difficult to settle (KAYSER 1959; WOODRUFF and JULIAN 1969). When a radical hysterectomy is performed, it may be possible to draw conclusions from the anatomy of the tumor spread. When the mucosa of an organ (here the fallopian tube or uterus) is the primary seat of a tumor, or an ovarian cystadenoma undergoes malignant transformation, the changes are so characteristic there is no problem in saying where the tumor arose. Likewise, small ovaries with bilateral multinodular tumor spread associated with a deep myometrial invasion of an endometrial carcinoma can be safely diagnosed as ovarian metastases of a primary endometrial carcinoma. Histological criteria, on the other hand, may not prove as reliable. For example, the endometrioid carcinoma of the ovary looks microscopically just like an endometrial carcinoma. That should not surprise us, since both the ovary and endometrium originate from the Müllerian duct. In a series of 34 simultaneous carcinomas involving the endometrium and ovary, 12 were classified as 2 independent neoplasms, 22 as metastases (ULBRIGHT and ROTH 1985). Since well-differentiated endometrial adenocarcinomas very seldom metastasize to the ovary and vice versa (in about 4%, HERTIG and GORE 1960), a simultaneous ovarian carcinoma usually

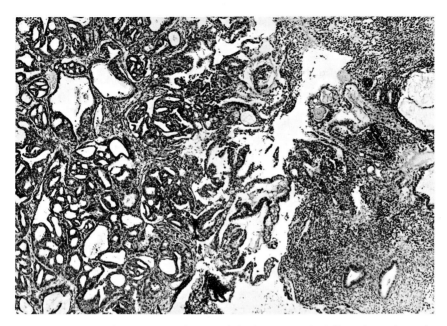

Fig. 148. Metastasis of an adenocarcinoma of the breast (*at the left*) to the endometrium. Such a metastasis can usually be distinguished from a primary endometrial adenocarcinoma by its discrete and sharp localization, and by its type of glandular structure, characteristic of the breast but not of the endometrium

represents a second primary tumor. On the other hand, endometrial carcinomas with ectopic Müllerian differentiation, like serous papillary carcinomas, tend to metastasize early to the ovaries (EIFEL et al. 1982; personal observations). In general, two primary carcinomas of endometrium and ovary are associated with a much more favorable prognosis than one primary carcinoma of either site with metastases to the other organ.

In contrast, metastases to the endometrium from distant primary carcinomas are rare, having been reported mostly as single observations. Metastatic carcinomas of the endometrium after resection of a *breast carcinoma* (ESCH 1929; SZEGVARY et al. 1963; KLAER and HOLM-JENSEN 1972) have become more frequent (KUMAR and HART 1982; KUMAR and SCHNEIDER 1983). They can be recognized and safely diagnosed as such when the endometrial tumor retains the typical solid, microalveolar or scirrhous qualities of the primary breast tumor (see Fig. 148). Difficulties in diagnosing metastases arise when the endometrial tumor is a well-differentiated adenocarcinoma. What is more likely in these cases is that after one target organ for estrogen (breast) is removed, another primary tumor (endometrial carcinoma) arises in a second target organ (endometrium). WEINGOLD and BOLTUCH (1961) found an isolated metastasis from a breast carcinoma in a leiomyoma of the myometrium; the endometrium was not involved.

RATNER and SCHNEIDERMAN (1948) reported on the spread of *renal cell carcinoma* to the uterus, and OBIDITSCH-MAYER (1951) on uterine metastases from *bile duct carcinomas.* Metastases from *carcinoma of the stomach,* a very common tumor in Japan, have been observed in the uterus (STEMMERMANN 1961); three times in the endometrium and five times in the endocervix. POST et al. (1966) described the *metastasis of a primary carcinoid of the ileum and appendix* to the uterus; MAZUR et al. (1984), described endometrial metastases from four primary carcinomas of colon, appendix, and stomach; KUMAR and HART (1982) described metastases of primary tumors of the colon, stomach, pancreas, gallbladder, lung, urinary bladder, and thyroid, most of which, however, involved the myometrium only. Other investigators have observed single cases in which an *adenocarcinoma of the bronchus* metastasized to the endometrium. Metastases of a malignant melanoma have been found in the endometrium in rare instances (BAUER et al. 1984). – A *leukemic infiltration* of the endometrium may be expected with a generalized chronic leukemia (MCDONALD and WAUGH 1939; cf. KAPADIA et al. 1978). A polymorphic cellular endometrial infiltrate containing Reed-Sternberg cells has been described in a patient with Hodgkin's disease (HUNG and KURTZ 1985).

f) Primary Carcinomas of the Ecto- and Endocervix as Components of Curettings

Since the endometrial curette must pass through the endocervical canal, with a complete curettage one can always expect to find some fragments of endo- and ectocervical mucosa in the curettings. If a carcinoma is suspected clinically it is advisable to scrape the endocervical canal first and collect these curettings separately before scraping the uterine cavity. With such a procedure the tumor can be localized. Even when the curettings are not collected separately, in the majority of cases it is possible to say from the histological studies where the tumor arises. In considering now only the *carcinomas* of the uterus (the sarcomas and carcinosarcomas, which spread throughout the uterus early, have already been discussed) the possible types that may occur are shown in Table 22.

The less a uterine tumor differentiates, the less it resembles the tissue from which it arises, and the greater the difficulty in classifying the tumor or in

Table 22. Histological type and predominant site of origin of carcinomas of the uterus

Histological type	Predominant site of origin

1. Keratinizing squamous cell carcinoma
2. Non-keratinizing epidermoid carcinoma
3. Mucoepidermoid carcinoma
  a) solid-cystic variety
  b) glandular variety
4. Clear cell carcinoma
5. Mucinous adenocarcinoma
	Ecto- and endocervix

6. Adenocarcinoma, endometrial type 7. Adenoacanthoma 8. Adenosquamous carcinoma 9. Serous papillary carcinoma	Endometrium

stating where it arises. Most of the types of tumor that occur commonly, however, can be classified (DALLENBACH-HELLWEG and BRÄHLER 1960).

Desquamated lamellae of *a keratinizing or non-keratinizing squamous cell carcinoma* most probably come from the portio, or depending on the extent of tumor growth and the age of the patient (or displacement of the squamocolumnar junction), they may originate from the endocervical canal. If the curettings contain only single lamellae of atypical epithelial cells (Fig. 149) so that their relation to the stroma cannot be determined, then a carcinoma in situ may also be present. To clarify such cases a conization of the cervix is necessary. It is very rare to find a carcinoma in situ or even an invasive carcinoma arising on the surface of a cervical polyp (FETTIG and SIEVERS 1966).

The pure *adenocarcinoma* of the cervical mucosa differs from the adenocarcinoma of the endometrium principally in that it produces more mucus and of a different kind (see p. 249), and its epithelial cells usually form single rows without papillae (Fig. 150). The mixed tumors, which characteristically originate from partially potent cells located at the union of squamous epithelium with columnar epithelium, exhibit various degrees of maturation: the *mucoepidermoid carcinoma* differentiates in two directions – in that taken by the portio epithelium, and in that by the endocervical epithelium. Thus, we find this tumor composed of strands of keratinizing carcinoma cells admixed with either glandular or solid-cystic formations that produce mucus (as in Fig. 128). In contrast to the rare clear cell carcinomas of the endometrium, the *clear cell carcinomas* of the endocervix fail to produce glandular structures (Fig. 151); because these tumors are poorly differentiated it is difficult to classify them. They produce only scanty amounts of mucus or glycogen. Structurally their cells resemble

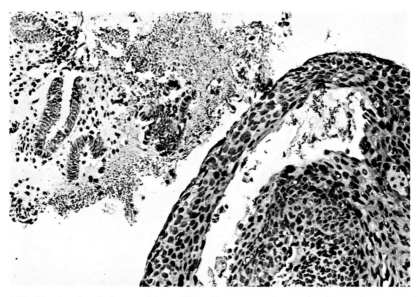

Fig. 149. Sheets of cells in curettings either from a carcinoma in situ or from marginal portions of a carcinoma

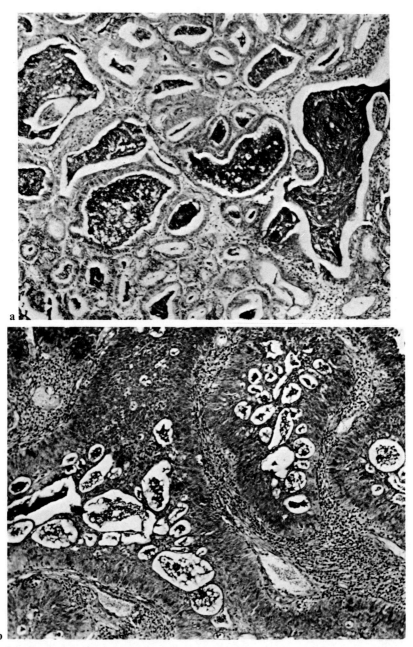

Fig. 150a, b. Mucin-secreting adenocarcinoma of the endocervical mucosa; **a** mature; **b** immature

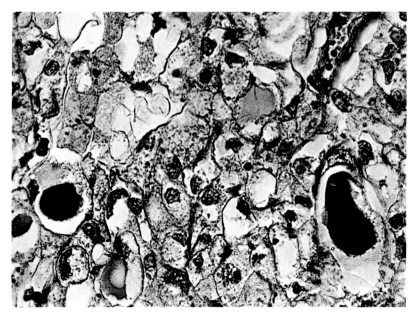

Fig. 151. Clear cell carcinoma of the cervical mucosa

modified precursors of the cervical epithelium. On the other hand, mucinous, mucoepidermoid and clear cell carcinomas may arise from foci of analogous metaplasias in the endometrium. These endometrial tumors may be indistinguishable from corresponding carcinomas originating in the endocervix.

As is to be expected, all types of *intermediary forms* may be found between pure squamous cell carcinomas, pure adenocarcinomas, and the mixed tumors. The beginning transitions may appear as unicellular formations of mucus or keratin in either solid tumors or gland-producing tumors. When we give such transitional forms a name, we should hold to the principal: *a potiori fit denominatio*, "what predominates determines the name". With that attitude in mind, it is possible from most curettings to state with fair accuracy where the tumor most likely arises. A definitive answer, however, can be obtained only from the resected uterus if the tumor has not already destroyed anatomical landmarks.

D. The Diagnosis of Normal and Pathologic Pregnancy from Curettings

1. The Early Intrauterine Pregnancy and Its Disturbances

a) Therapeutic Abortion (Induced Abortion)

If for clinical or socioeconomic reasons it becomes necessary to interrupt an early pregnancy, a curettage usually yields so much amnion, immature placenta, and abundant decidual tissue that no difficulties in diagnosis arise. Although these tissues are generally normal, they are of value for us, serving as ideal standards which we need for comparison in evaluating and diagnosing tissues from diseased pregnancies. Histological, cytological and cytogenetic studies of the embryo lie within the province of research workers who concern themselves ordinarily with specific problems, for example, chromosomal abnormalities, inherited deficiencies of cellular enzymes. Then too, study of the embryo in the daily routine of gynecological pathology is seldom required, since a primary injury of the fetus causing abortion almost always reveals itself by failure of the fetal vessels in the placental villi to develop.

By using the well-known stages of development of placental villi as our guidelines, we can determine with fair accuracy the age of gestation of a therapeutic abortion merely by examining the *placental tissue.* On the 13th day of gestation the primary villi begin to form from the syncytium, which developed from the cytotrophoblasts[1] after these came in contact with maternal blood on the 9th day. From the 15th day on fetal mesoderm begins to penetrate the solid primary villi, converting them into the secondary villi. On about the 20th day capillaries sprout forth in the mesodermal cores, forming the tertiary villi (Fig. 152). The initial erythrocytes in these vessels are nucleated, but by the onset of the 9th week of pregnancy the first anuclear erythrocytes are normally seen. By the 12th week of pregnancy, virtually all fetal erythrocytes are anucleated. From the stage of the secondary villi on, two distinct layers of trophoblasts envelope the villi. With progressive differentiation, however, the inner layer of cytotrophoblasts gradually regresses, leaving the outer layer of syncytiotrophoblasts broader and thus more conspicuous. By the end of pregnancy only a few scattered cytotrophoblasts remain. Also, the layer of syncytiotrophoblasts becomes thinner with time. The villous stroma about the blood vessels diminishes as these enlarge and dilate. In that way the distance separating

---

[1] In accord with modern usage we refer to the cells of the inner layer of the trophoblast as "cytotrophoblasts" or "cytotrophoblastic cells", and those of the outer syncytial layer as the "syncytiotrophoblasts" ("syncytiotrophoblastic cells"), acknowledging, however, as HERTIG does (1968), that the term "trophoblasts" is often misused.

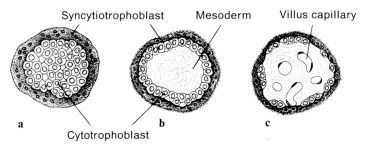

Fig. 152a–c. Normal stages in the development of placental villi, as seen in cross-section
a primary, **b** secondary, **c** tertiary villus

fetal and maternal blood becomes less and less, adapting to the growing nutritional demands of the embryo. In addition, through growth and subdivision into finer branchings the surface area of the villi is greatly increased. The Hofbauer cells found in moderate numbers in early pregnancy gradually disappear as pregnancy advances. It is not unusual to find, even in what is regarded as a normal early pregnancy, that a few villi have undergone hydropic degeneration. They are seen in about 20% of therapeutic abortions (JURKOVIC and MUZELAK 1970), most commonly in the chorion laeve (FUJIKURA et al. 1971). On the other hand, a therapeutic abortion may be induced before abnormal products of conception are expulsed spontaneously. Consequently, a small percentage (3%–6%) of therapeutic abortions show abnormalities in placental-fetal development.

The *decidua* first begins to develop around the blastocyst a few days after implantation. The histological changes that distinguish the predecidual from the decidual stage, however, begin to manifest themselves by the 9th day after ovulation (that is, 2 days after implantation). The decidual cells continue to increase in size; their pale nuclei with prominent nucleoli enlarge, thereby increasing their surface area. Other decidual cells accomplish the same by developing double nuclei. The abundant cytoplasm denotes increased amounts of RNA, glycogen, and various enzymes, particularly carbonic anhydrase and 3β-steroid dehydrogenase, which indicates that the decidual cells actively participate in the metabolism of steroids. Correlating with that is the increase in the smooth endoplasmic reticulum, a change that reaches its maximum at about the 40th day of gestation. The endoplasmic reticulum is sparsely granular; its differentiation is maximal by the 40th day of pregnancy. The margins of the cells are now sharp and distinct, enveloped by fine reticular fibers. Contacts or gap-like junctions join processes that sprout from the same cell (LAWN et al. 1971). As the decidual change progresses, the cells come closer together, establishing contacts with one another and an epithelioid arrangement, actively adapting to the demands imposed by the rapidly growing placenta and fetus (LIEBIG and STEGNER 1977). Ultrastructurally, the metabolic activity of the decidual cells appears to be maximal by the 70th day of pregnancy and begins to decline after the 100th day (WYNN 1974). The number of endometrial granulocytes has by then greatly increased. Their nuclei become lobulated, enlarging their surface area. Their intracytoplasmic granules increase in size and number. The glands, which start to produce glycogen again, remain highly active until the 8th week of gestation. Thereafter they begin to involute. A most striking change is the abundance of dilated, thin-walled vessels in the stroma, some of which reveal the typical endothelial proliferations induced by relaxin (see p. 39f. and Fig. 10). That these cells piling up and filling parts of the vascular lumina are in fact proliferated endothelial cells and not, as some authors believed, invading trophoblasts, has recently been verified by immunhistochemical studies: the intravascular cells were negative for HCG, but were found to be positive with factor VIII-related antigen for endothelial cells (TUTTLE et al. 1985). The high fibrinolytic activity found at the time of implantation decreases; instead, the ground substances of the decidua become rich in acid mucopolysaccharides (SCHMIDT-MATTHIESEN 1968; see also p. 36). Ultrastructurally, the dense extracellular material surrounding the mature human decidual cell resembles the basement membrane of the epithelium (WYNN 1974).

By the 17th day of gestation the decidua has reached its greatest height, measuring about 1 cm. Later when the decidua basalis, capsularis and parietalis separate, and because the blastocyst and placenta grow so rapidly, the destructive and remodeling processes that normally evolve in the decidua may be accompanied by small necroses and focal infiltrates of polymorphonuclear leukocytes. Localized aggregates of endometrial granulocytes with their lobulated nuclei should not be mistaken, however, for inflammatory cells. It is relatively easy to differentiate the two kinds of cells, not only by using special stains but also by showing that where leukocytes are aggregated the tissue is undergoing necrosis and lysis. Where intact endometrial granulocytes congregate, one never finds such destruction of tissue. It is important to realize that small resorptive necroses normally occur in healthy pregnancies (therapeutic abortions). Accordingly, a diagnosis of septic abortion should be made only when extensive inflammation and necrosis are found.

The *solutions injected* into the amnion **to induce abortion** (saline, rivanol, prostaglandins) cause degenerative changes in the villi and decidua, stasis of blood in the intervillous spaces, and thrombosis and hemorrhage in the decidua basalis and marginalis. After saline solutions the fetal membranes may become edematous and the subchorial tissues necrotic (HONORE 1976; PURI et al. 1976). After curetting the endometrial cavity, bleeding is better stanched than after a normal delivery, since the curette produces a profuse exudation of fibrin, which rapidly coats the wound. The spiral arteries become plugged with aggregates of platelets and fibrin. Endothelial proliferations, decidual cells and the trophoblast involute (SLUNSKY 1976).

b) Spontaneous Abortion

α) Causes

Attempts to compare the frequency of spontaneous abortion with that of criminal abortion are fraught with immediate failure. The very clandestine nature of criminal abortion precludes any gathering of data about it. On the other hand, the functional or morphological anomalies that cause spontaneous abortion may escape histological search. If malformations are detected, they may prove important in evaluating the prognoses of future pregnancies for the patient. Contrary to earlier opinions, one can find recognizable remnants of chorionic villi in curettings from 75% of the women suffering spontaneous abortion (THOMSEN 1955). All "blighted" or abortive ova disclose disturbances in the development not only of the embryonic anlage but also of the chorionic villi, particularly their differentiation into tertiary villi at the proper time. THOMSEN (1955) was able to demonstrate such disturbed development in 61% of all spontaneous abortions, but only in 3% of proven criminal abortions. These statistics should encourage every pathologist to look for possible abnormalities especially in the placenta, in every specimen of abortion submitted.

Factors acting during the first trimester to cause abortion of the conceptus may be fetal (genetic) or maternal. Since the abortions occurring during the second trimester are often caused by gross placental disturbances (for example, circumvallate), they are outside the domain of this monograph and I shall not discuss them further.

HERTIG and SHELDON (1943) and HERTIG and LIVINGSTONE (1944) estimated from a large series of patients in Boston that 25% of all pregnancies ended with abortion; of these 25%, about a half occurred spontaneously. In turn, about 62% of that half (30%–70% according to other authors) was due to blighted or pathological ova (with early death or absence of the embryo, hypoplasia of the trophoblasts, hydropic change or fibrosis of the chorionic villi); 38% were due to maternal factors (anomalies of the uterus, basal hematoma, or bacterial infections). About 4% of all spontaneous abortions were habitual. In the majority of these the embryo was defective; repeated abortions by the same patient disclosed the same defect (WALL and HERTIG 1948).

Spontaneous abortions resulting from blighted (pathological) ova sharply increase in the older age groups (McMAHON et al. 1954). This is particularly true for abortions with demonstrable *chromosomal anomalies* (KERR and RASHAD 1966, also for earlier literature; GROPP 1967; JACOBSON and BARTER 1967). Chromosome anomalies arising from faulty gametogenesis or gene mutation are found in 27%–60% of all spontaneous abortions (BOWEN and LEE 1969; GÖCKE et al. 1985). They are particularly frequent in recurrent abortions (LUCAS et al. 1972; ROTT et al. 1972) and in virtually 50% of anatomically abnormal embryos and fetuses (SINGH and CARR 1967); they occur in only 3.3% of therapeutic abortions (LARSON and TITUS 1970) and in 0.5% of live-born infants. According to newer studies (YAMAMOTO et al. 1975; TSUJI and NAKANO 1978), however, chromosomal abnormalities were identified in 6.8% of induced abortions. Approximately 50% of all chromosomal anomalies analyzed in larger series are trisomies, 20%–25% monosomies, 15% triploidies, 5% tetraploidies, and 5% structural anomalies. The trisomies increase as the mothers became older; the monosomies are indipendent of age. In abortions with abnormal chromosomes the period of gestation is significantly shorter and the embryonic development less advanced than in abortions with normal chromosomes (PHILIPPE and BOUE 1969; MIKAMO 1970). Polyploid sets are commonly associated with missed abortions in which the chorionic villi reveal hydropic swelling. In ten such abortions, CARR (1969) was able to demonstrate triploidy in nine and tetraploidy in one. By using the method developed by BARR et al. for determining nuclear sex chromatin BOHLE et al. (1957) and HIENZ and STOLL (1962) were able to show that during the 3rd–4th month of pregnancy the mortality of male fetuses exceeded that of the female fetuses. From comprehensive studies HERTIG (1967) concluded that 50% of all ova fertilized after a delayed ovulation (on the 15th day of the cycle or later) aborted, whereas when ovulation took place before the 14th day, then 92.3% of the fertilized ova developed normally. Delayed ovulation induces intrafollicular overripeness of the ovum. That may lead to disturbances in both meiotic metaphases because of degeneration of spindle fibers and loss in the polarization of chromosomes (MIKAMO 1970). According to new estimates, half of all fertilized ova die before they begin to implant because of chromosomal abnormalities (KNÖRR and KNÖRR-GÄRTNER 1977).

Other generally exogenous causes of chromosomal damage are: *vitamin deficiencies, X-irradiation, hypoxemia* as well as *deficiency or overdosage of endogenous or exogenous sex hormones* (GROSSER 1948; MEY 1961). Observations by CARR (1970) support that idea. He compared 54 abortuses from women who conceived within 6 months after discontinuing hormonal contraception with 227 unselected abortions. Chromosomal anomalies were present in 48% of the postcontraceptive group but were found only in 22% of the unselected group. Of the abortuses of the postcontraceptive group, 30% revealed polyploidy as compared with only 5% of the control group. Ninety-five percent of all blastocysts that implanted during use of chlormadinone proved to be malformed with hydropic, avascular villi and atrophic trophoblastic cells (KÜHNE et al. 1972). Histological and embryological studies revealed that after stopping antifertility agents the frequency of disturbances of early embryogenesis doubles (POLAND 1970). Our own studies support these statistics. We saw hydropic swelling of avascular chorionic villi with atrophy of the trophoblast about twice as often as in unselected abortions (see Fig. 153), and we found that the composition of the agent taken determined more the degree of damage than did the length of time since discontinuing the agent (DALLENBACH-HELLWEG 1978). The contradictory results of other authors (BOUE et al. 1975; LAURITSEN 1975; KLINGER et al. 1976) no doubt depend upon the differences in composition of the antifertility agents used or upon the differences in the ages of the patients studied: for example, in the collective reported by LAURITSEN, after discontinuing the agents, young women developed chromosomal anomalies almost twice as often as the older women, although spontaneous anomalies are known to occur more often in the older. Other reports suggest that inducers of ovulation also increase chromosomal anomalies (BOUE and BOUE 1973).

In addition, an *abnormally developed endometrium* may disturb implantation of the blastocyst, as for example, an irregularly proliferating or a deficient secretory endometrium. In our curettings of abortions after discontinuing oral contraceptives, we have found a deficient secretory phase in about 50% of the specimens (see Fig. 153). Here, the decreased height of the endometrium will only allow a shallow implantation. In addition, since decidual cells will not develop, the blastocyst will not be anchored in place. If the fertilized ovum implants improperly, such as in shallow or polypoid implantation, abortion

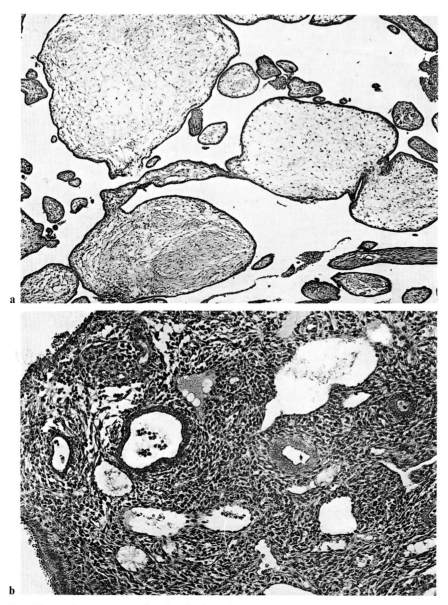

Fig. 153a, b. Spontaneous abortion in the 4th month, after discontinuing oral contraceptives which had been taken continuously for 6 years. **a** Malformed avascular hydropic villi (molar degeneration). **b** The associated endometrium is irregularly and deficiently developed

may result (KRONE 1961). GRUENEWALD (1965) suggested that a premature shedding of the decidua might cause abortion. Such a decidual detachment would be possible if too much or uninhibited relaxin were released from endometrial granulocytes. Secondary disturbances of implantation, such as bacterial infections, may also cause abortions that are clinically recognized. On the other hand, since blighted ova are often discarded shortly after fertilization and make no attempts to implant, they go unnoticed and are never registered as spontaneous abortions. For that reason disturbances of implantation assume a subordinate theme in this chapter and, because of their signs and symptoms, are classed and discussed under the causes of infertility.

β) Microscopic Changes

After LANGHANS (1901), HITSCHMANN (1904) also concerned himself with the microscopic diagnosis of abortion just before he undertook a study of the menstrual cycle. The detachment in abortion, unlike that of a normal menstruation or pregnancy, usually develops from necrosis in the upper layer of the decidua. The placenta and decidua almost always involute completely. The degree and extent of their involution are dependent on how long the initiating hemorrhage lasted and on the cause of the abortion. If the embryo dies first then involution is protracted, and therefore may assume extreme forms. With bacterial infections the decidua is particularly subject to rapid necrosis, thereafter the placenta. By carefully studying all structures it is often quite possible to conclude what the etiology of the abortion was.

The *glands* of the **decidua** may react in various ways, depending upon whether the embryo perished first, or secondarily after destruction (usually by infection) of the placenta. If the embryo dies first, the placenta may survive for long periods, producing its hormones, particularly gonadotropin, until it is dis-

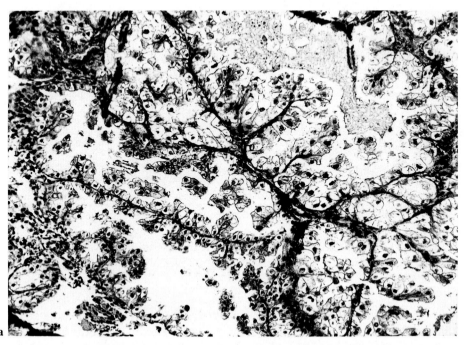

Fig. 154a, b. Arias-Stella phenomenon. **a** Low magnification; **b** high magnification. This phenomenon must be differentiated from a clear cell adenocarcinoma (cf. Fig. 129)

charged (CASSMER 1959). Since the dead fetus is unable to properly assimilate and metabolize gonadotropin, the hormone accumulates in the maternal circulation and decidua (ZONDEK 1947). In the decidua gonadotropin apparently overstimulates the glandular epithelial cells, causing their nuclei to enlarge, the chro-

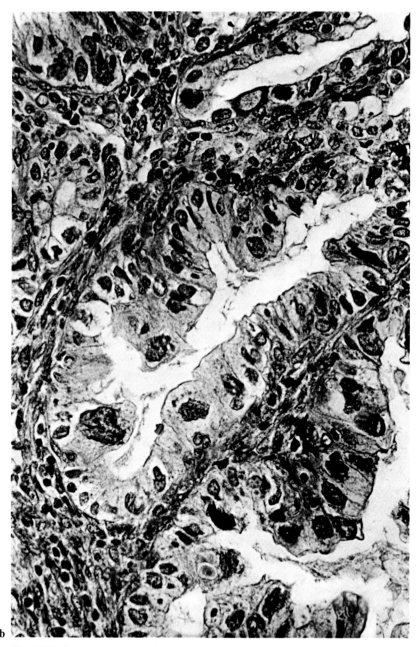

Fig. 154b. Legend see opposite page

matin to increase greatly, and their cytoplasm to swell and become unusually clear (Fig. 154). This phenomenon, first mentioned by DEELMAN (1933), then by OVERBECK (1953), was more precisely described by ARIAS-STELLA in 1954. It can be produced in the female rat by injecting it with gonadotropin (ARIAS-STELLA 1955; DALLENBACH 1966, see also for review of literature) or in women with clomiphene (BERNHARDT et al. 1966). The phenomenon indicates a hormonal hyperstimulation, not an involution as some authors maintain. In animal experiments after the hormone is discontinued for a few days the cellular changes disappear. Histochemical studies of the abundant, clear cytoplasm have to date revealed only PAS-positive granules (OVERBECK 1959) which were susceptible to digestion by diastase (BESWICK and GREGORY 1971). Electron-microscopic studies (DE BRUX and ANCLA 1964; TRASHER and RICHART 1972), however, suggest the glandular epithelial cells actively secrete and have a high protein metabolism. Microspectrophotometric measurements of their nuclear DNA always yield polyploid values but never aneuploid (SACHS 1968; WAGNER and RICHART 1968). The nuclei of some glandular epithelial cells, however, may be degenerated instead of hyperactive, indicating the phenomenon is waning. Occasionally we see signs of hyperactivity and involution together, a reason, perhaps, why opinions about the cause diverge (FIENBERG and LLOYD 1974). Occasionally, nuclear pseudoinclusions consisting of invaginations of cytoplasm may mimic a herpetic endometritis with associated cytological atypia (DARDI et al. 1982). A similar herpes-like nuclear clearing may be observed in close association with the Arias-Stella reaction (MAZUR et al. 1983). Ultrastructural studies show that this clearing is due to replacement of normal chromatin by a network of fine filaments rather than herpes virus DNA. If one examines the histological preparations carefully enough, one can find an Arias-Stella phenomenon in about 50% of all abortions (and possibly the cause of the abortion as well). The reaction may also occur in the endocervical glands where it should not be mistaken for a carcinoma (CORE 1979). If an Arias-Stella phenomenon is lacking, then the decidual and endometrial glands are often collapsed, having prominent star-like shapes similar to those of irregular shedding (see Fig. 78), which at times may also be caused by death of the fetus and placental tissues. In these instances we assume both die at the same time, and all hormones of pregnancy rapidly decrease.

If no bacterial infection occurs to provoke an intense infiltration of inflammatory cells, then the *decidual cells* always involute very slowly. They gradually shrink, their cell margins pulling away from one another to leave wide spaces between them. A well-developed network of collagenous fibers or vast "lakes" of homogenous protein-rich matrix are left behind. The cytoplasm of the decidual cells becomes homogeneous, staining intensely. The nucleus condenses, appearing pyknotic. As a characteristic feature of their slow involution, the devidual cells form in their cytoplasm so-called collagen inclusions (HAMPERL 1958), which become visible only with stains for connective tissue (Fig. 155; Color Plate IIc). As electron-microscopic studies have proved, however, these are not true inclusions but rather deep indentures of the cell membrane filled with pericellular fibrils of collagen (WESSEL 1959). They represent a disturbance of collagen formation at the cell membrane, and are associated with the shrink-

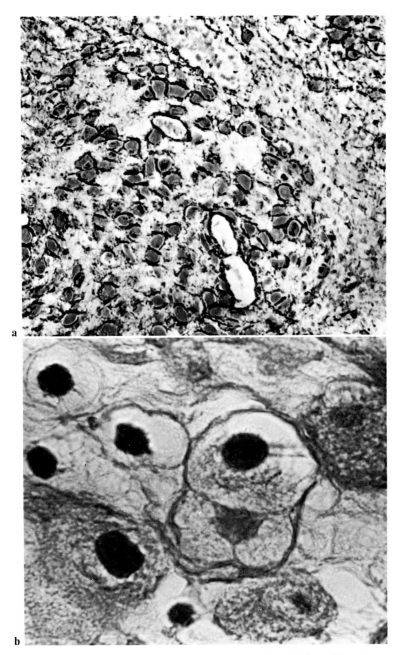

Fig. 155a, b. Collagen inclusions in slowly regressing decidual cells. **a** Silver impregnation after GOMORI: the reticular fibers surrounding the decidual cells are thickened. The inclusions in the cells are black. **b** Masson trichrome stain. Plume-shaped inclusion in the lower part of the middle cell

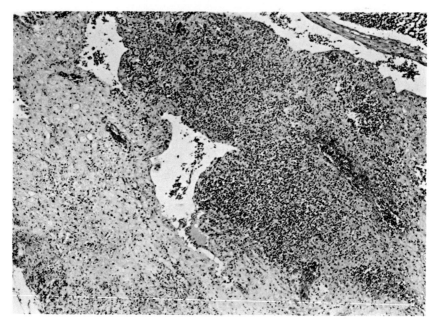

Fig. 156. Focal necrosis of the decidua (*at the right*) with heavy infiltrates of polymorphonuclear leukocytes

age of the cell and its loss of turgor (DALLENBACH-HELLWEG 1961). Thus, we find them most commonly in decidua of blighted ova as well as in the intrauterine decidua of extrauterine pregnancies (see p. 329). At times these collagen inclusions may be the only diagnostic clue that an abortion had occurred a while before.

In contrast, with intense inflammation the decidual cells, until then intact, undergo rapid necrosis and enzymatic lysis; the network of connective tissue disintegrates, and the reticulum fibers dissolve away (Fig. 156). Occasionally one finds portions of necrotic decidua adjoining portions that are in the process of slowly shrinking, usually when the decidual remnants become secondarily infected long after the fetus has died (*endometritis post abortum*). The inflammations causing an early abortion are usually non-specific, with a few exceptions such as listeriosis, mycoplasma, or viruses (see p. 208 f.). Specific infections generally lead to stillbirth in the third trimester. In 34 women with repeated abortions, RAPPAPORT et al. (1960) were able to culture listeria from the cervical secretion in 25. CRAMER and WADULLA (1950) recovered leptospira in a few abortions. In addition, toxoplasmosis appears to be a rare cause for abortion (SHARF et al. 1973; see also p. 210). In rapid involution as well as in slow, protracted involution the widely dilated, thin-walled *vessels* of the decidua are usually filled with blood. Occasionally one finds pronounced endothelial proliferation (Fig. 157).

If the portions of decidua come from regions where chorion has invaded (decidua basalis), then one will find *trophoblasts* with one or more nuclei. These cells also involute but in general survive longer than the surrounding decidual

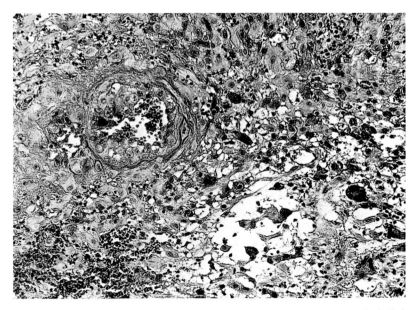

Fig. 157. Chorionic invasion of trophoblastic cells into the decidua. Endothelial cells lining maternal arteriole are proliferating. Note the differences between the two types of cells

cells. When no placental tissue is found in the histologic sections, then the discovery of such trophoblasts amid remnants of decidua may be decisive in differentiating an intrauterine pregnancy from an extrauterine (Fig. 158).

The **placental villi** found in the curettings of spontaneous abortions due to *maternal causes* are usually regular in shape and well preserved, although the decidua is shrunken or necrotic. Occasionally, however, the villi are necrotic or hyalinized. In these instances they lose their sheath of trophoblastic cells, and are embedded in coagulated blood or fibrin. Only with the aid of connective tissue stains (for example, van Gieson; Fig. 159) can they be distinguished from the "sea" of fibrin that engulfs them ("ghost villi"). Between these two extremes one often finds all transitions of rapid or gradual degeneration of villi. One must take care in differentiating these regressive changes of normally structured villi from those of villi, which are primarily maldeveloped. Such a distinction is possible, however, only if the villi are not necrotic and are present in sufficient numbers, since occasionally, even when development proceeds regularly, a few villi may appear abnormal. If after normal development the maternal circulation fails, then the trophoblastic syncytium degenerates first. If, on the other hand, the fetal circulation fails, then the regressive changes first appear in the blood vessels and stroma of the villi. Nonetheless, these structures remain recognizable as such until complete necrosis sets in. Regressive changes of normally structured villi include degeneration of the syncytial trophoblast, readily distinguishable by its eosinophilia. The vessels of the villous stroma obliterate, the surrounding stroma becomes fibrous (Fig. 160), hyalinized, or edematous. As these changes progress, the stromal cells and blood vessels gradually disappear. The ground

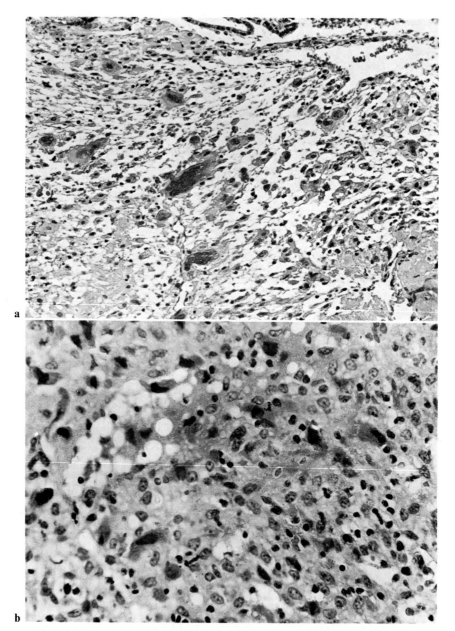

Fig. 158a, b. Chorionic invasion of the decidua. **a** Multinucleated syncytiotrophoblasts; **b** cytotrophoblasts with single nuclei

substance may undergo fibrinoid or mucoid degeneration, as its metachromasia with toluidine blue or mucus stains demonstrates so well.

In abortions due to maternal causes, fibrin may also be precipitated. As GRAY (1956) suggested, the fibrinoid or hyaline degeneration of the villous

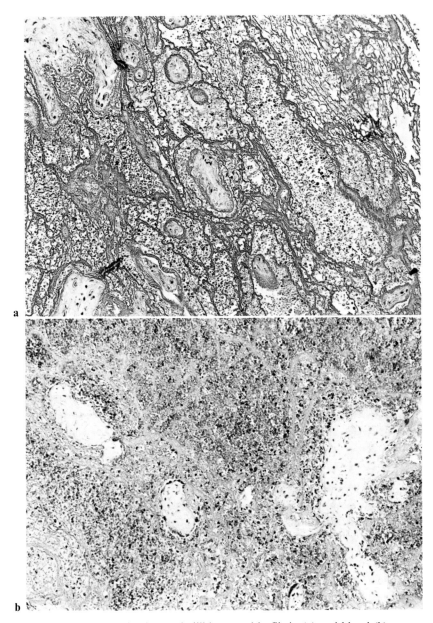

Fig. 159a, b. Necrotic placental villi immured in fibrin (a) and blood (b)

stroma might be related to an incompatibility between mother and fetus. In addition, one may find nucleated erythrocytes in the capillaries of the villi later than normal, indicating enhanced fetal erythropoesis to compensate for insufficient maternal circulation (GERDES and SCHULTE 1966).

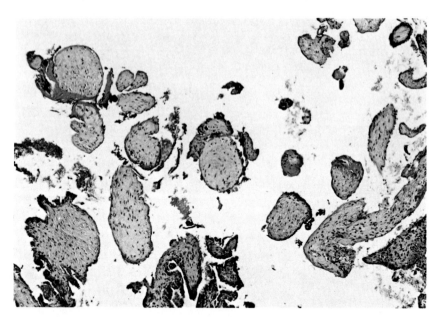

Fig. 160. Fibrosis of villi of a spontaneous abortion during the 3rd month

Maternal infections occasionally leave characteristic changes in placental villi. For example, traces of rubella infection (German measels) can be recognized by proliferation, degeneration, necrosis, and shedding of endothelial cells of the allantoic vessels in the chronionic plate and stem villi. Occasionally, endoangiopathia obliterans develops in the terminal villi.

Primary malformation of the villi is characterized by definite changes, which vary in their severity depending upon the age of the pregnancy (or length of survival of the placenta) and upon the underlying cause. If the villi fail to become vascularized through defective growth or death of the embryo, they do not degenerate but instead develop abnormally. Sooner or later, the villi swell through hydropic change, ultimately reaching sizes much greater than normal. As HERTIG (1968) emphasizes, the swelling is not a true degeneration but rather the result of the immature trophoblast continuing to take up fluid. By necessity, the fluid accumulates in the loose stroma of the villi since these lack blood vessels for carrying the fluid away: "mole-like degeneration" of the villi in embryonal abortion, according to VOGEL (1969). Usually, as the villi swell, the trophoblasts covering them become atrophic, the nuclei of the syncytiotrophoblasts pyknotic. Langhans' cells are always absent (Fig. 161). Acid mucopolysaccharides may be deposited within the villous stroma (EMMERICH 1967). Branching syncytial knots may develop as a result of arrested villous ramification. Such changes develop very rarely in villi of normal structure (ABACI and ATERMAN 1968; NAYAK 1968).

The hydropic villi of blighted ova differ histologically from those of partial or complete hydatidiform moles in two respects, which we use as diagnostic criteria. First, although the villi of a blighted ovum are swollen and their mesen-

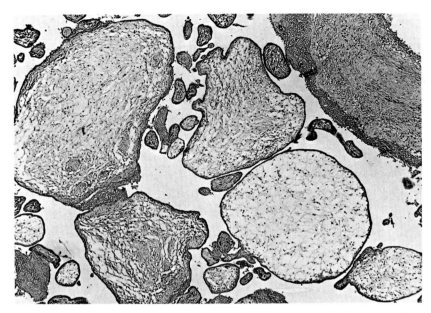

Fig. 161. Hydropic swelling of villi of a spontaneous abortion during the 2nd month with a trisomy 13 karyotype, extremely flattened trophoblastic epithelium

chymal fibers loosely dispersed by the edema, they never contain large central cystic spaces as do the villi of hydatidiform moles (see Fig. 163b). Secondly, the trophoblasts ensheathing the villi of blighted ova are atrophic or degenerating. In contrast, the trophoblastic cells of molar villi are more or less hyperplastic, and occasionally even anaplastic. Some authors (HERTIG and EDMONDS 1940; HUBER et al. 1957) postulated that when a blighted ovum fails to abort, and is retained and survives, it eventually becomes a true hydatidiform mole. Proof of that theory is, however, still lacking. According to HÖRMANN and LEMTIS (1965), a blighted ovum is usually aborted between the 11th and 13th week; a hydatidiform mole is usually expelled after the 16th week. Curettings repeated from the same patient have shown, however, that a hydatidiform mole may be discharged as early as the 6th–8th week of pregnancy, at which time the villi are only slightly enlarged, with no or very little edema and discrete trophoblastic proliferation. Remnants of that same mole curetted later will show fully developed proliferating hydatidiform villi and trophoblast. The differential diagnosis between an early stage of hydatidiform mole and a molar degeneration of villi accompanying a blighted ovum must, therefore, be made carefully. No attempts should be made to correlate the number of Hofbauer cells with a malformation since the function of these cells remains unknown. As ECKMAN and CARROW (1962) noted, in all forms of abortion the structural changes may vary strikingly from villus to villus, the differences depending qualitatively and quantitatively on how long the products of conception are retained.

To evaluate chromosomal anomalies, histological study of the placental villi may prove especially informative and certainly is easier to perform than the cytogenetic methods (PHILIPPE 1973; BREUKER et al. 1978). Recent observations

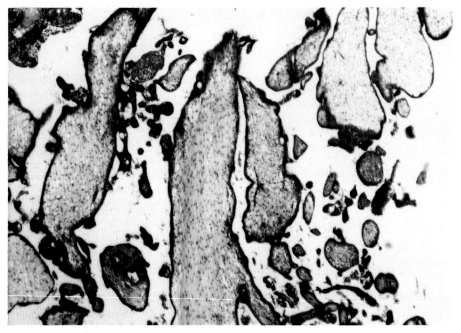

Fig. 162. Placental villi of a spontaneous abortion with a monosomy X karyotype. Excessive branching of syncytial knots

correlating cytogenetic and histological findings have revealed that the most common chromosomal anomalies are often associated with characteristic morphological changes in the embryo and placenta (MÜNTEFERING et al. 1982; GÖCKE et al. 1985).

In *trisomies* the amniotic sac is usually small and the embryo barely visible. Owing to the arrested ramification, the chorionic villi are reduced in number, are plump, avascular and slightly hydropic. The trophoblast is flattened, single- or, occasionally, double-layered (Fig. 161).

In *monosomies*, the embryo is often autolyzed. The umbilical cord is shortened. The chorionic villi differ greatly in their diameters and are irregular in shape. The villous stroma is cellular and contains only a few and poorly developed vessels. The trophoblast often forms branching syncytial knots (Fig. 162).

In about 80% of the *triploidies* the triploid karyotype (69 XYY, XXY, or XXX) consists of 23 X maternal and 46 YY, 46 YX or 46 XX paternal chromosomes from two sperms that have penetrated the ovum. This aberration results in the development of a *partial hydatidiform mole,* in which the vesicular villi may be apparent grossly. In contrast to the complete hydatidiform mole, however, an embryo is present but malformed. Only 15%–20% of the triploids are digynic arising by a single sperm fertilizing a diploid egg. These have non-molar placentas and better survival chances.

c) Partial Hydatidiform Mole

On microscopic examination, approximately half of the villi are greatly enlarged. They show arrested branching with invaginations, scalloping of the villous outlines (Fig. 163), and at times form pseudocysts with trophoblastic inclusions

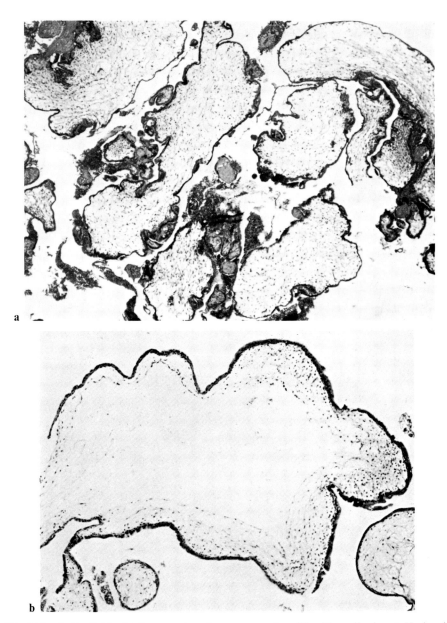

Fig. 163a, b. Partial hydatiform mole. **a** Large avascular villi with scalloping. **b** Hydropic swelling and scalloping of villi with central, cystic spaces lined by endothelial-like cells

in the villous mesenchyme (Fig. 164b). Excessive villous edema results in central cistern formation. The villous trophoblast is partially atrophic, but shows focal hyperproliferation and branching usually of the syncytial layer only (Fig. 164a).

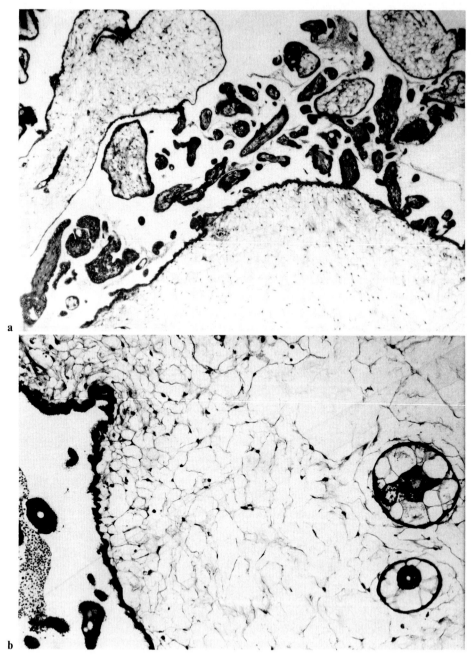

Fig. 164a, b. Partial hydatidiform mole with greatly enlarged placental villi between small villi. Proliferation of syncytial trophoblast (**a**) and trophoblastic inclusions (**b**)

These edematous villi are intermingled with normal villi. Both types of villi may contain fetal blood vessels with red blood cells which may still be nucleated by the 16th week of gestation. In addition, very early as well as late stages of partial moles (before the 8th week and after the 16th week of gestation) tend to have fewer and smaller cisterns that can easily be overlooked (SZULMAN and BUCHSBAUM 1987).

The partial hydatidiform mole must be differentiated, because of its better prognosis, from the complete mole, which shows a generalized villous edema resulting in large cisterns and an extensive hyperplasia of the syncytio- and cytotrophoblast. An embryo is always absent. Measurements of the DNA content of the nuclei of the villous stromal cells reveal equivalent polyploid levels in partial moles, whereas in complete hydatidiform moles, diploid levels are found. HCG titers in patients with complete moles are much higher and remain elevated longer than those of patients with partial moles. Patients with partial moles have a slightly higher average age than those with complete moles (CZERNOBILSKY et al. 1982). In summary, almost all of the characteristic features of the complete mole can be found in partial moles as well, but to a minor degree (SZULMAN and SURTI 1982, 1984). Furthermore, despite the differences in their karyotypes, genetic relationships between the two exist: triploidies, associated with partial moles have, like the true moles, a diploid set of chromosomes from the father but an additional haploid set from the mother. Recent experiments have led to the assumption that maternal and paternal haploid sets are not functionally equivalent: apparently the genes of the maternal chromosomes contribute to the early development of the embryo, those of the paternal chromosomes to the development of the trophoblast (SZULMAN, personal communication). Paternal sets only (as in the complete mole) result in early death of the embryo and excessive overgrowth of the trophoblast; predominance of paternal sets (2:1), as in the partial mole, result in a maldeveloped embryo and less extensive proliferation of the trophoblast. Maternal sets cause only fetal malformations owing to an underdeveloped trophoblast. In contrast to the complete moles, partial moles show no propensity for malignant change (SZULMAN and SURTI 1978, 1982; CZERNOBILSKY et al. 1982; OHAMA et al. 1986), and only rare cases of persistent partial moles have been observed (MOSTOUFI-ZADEH et al. 1987). A possible explanation could be that the presence of a maternal haploid set in the triploidy protects against uncontrolled trophoblastic growth and the evolution of cancer.

d) Complete Hydatidiform Mole, Invasive Mole, and Choriocarcinoma

In most instances, a complete mole develops when an "empty egg" (egg without the maternal haploid set) is fertilized by a single sperm with a 23 X set of chromosomes that duplicate, resulting in a diploid karyotype of 46 XX. A 46 YY ovum fertilized by a sperm with a 23 Y set would be non-viable (VASSILAKOS 1977; SZULMAN and SURTI 1978). The rare moles with a karyotype of XY are heterozygous and result from ova fertilized by two sperms, one containing the X and the other the Y chromosome. Whereas in the partial hydatidiform mole the hydropic swelling evolves in only one part of the placenta bordering normal villi, and the trophoblast is only slightly proliferated, in contrast, in the complete hydatidiform mole the vesicular swelling and villous degeneration develop diffusely and rapidly. Both cyto- and syncytiotrophoblasts proliferate excessively. The embryo is absent, leaving the villi with no means by which they can rid themselves of the abundant fluid passed into them by the trophoblasts. As fluid accumulates, the villi swell, ultimately ballooning up to grape-like vesicles. The concomitant proliferation of the trophoblasts may be attributed to a stimulating effect of maternal blood on these cells. They resemble the immature trophoblasts that invade to form the solid anlage of the primordial chorionic villi.

As early as 1895 MARCHAND [and soon thereafter LANGHANS (1901)], thoroughly described these histological changes in the hydatidiform mole. Initially the ground substance of the villi becomes water logged and homogeneous. The mesenchymal connective tissues gradually disappear and the blood vessels fail to develop. With time the villi swell to enormous sizes. Through coalescence of small vacuoles of edema fluid large cisterns form, expanding to compress the surrounding mesenchymal cells so flat these seem to line the cysts like endothelial cells (see Fig. 165a). Both layers of the trophoblastic cells covering the villi, but especially the syncytiotrophoblasts, possess enlarged pleomorphic nuclei and proliferate intensely, usually as irregular nodules or as club-shaped masses (Fig. 165b). Accordingly, the titer of gonadotropin is markedly elevated (as compared with other moles or malformations, KAESER 1949), and an Arias-Stella phenomenon may be demonstrated (see ROACH et al. 1960; WYNN and HARRIS 1967). Vacuoles, varying from small to large and clustered together, often appear in the syncytiotrophoblasts. Their vacuolated state resembles the formation of lacunae during early chorial invasion when the primordial villi develop. The trophoblastic cells proliferate most at the placental site of attachment. The surrounding decidua often reveals an invasion by chorionic elements that may extend down to the myometrium, a condition once referred to as "syncytial endometritis". This invasion, however, does not differ from that occurring during normal placentation.

It may be quite difficult to *predict from histological sections* how a hydatidiform mole will behave biologically or what its *prognosis* will be. It is advisable to take samples of tissue from different regions, particularly where portions of decidua or blood clot are found (HERTIG and MANSELL 1956). The potentially malignant quality of the trophoblastic cells is especially difficult to judge, since these cells are normally invasive. The degree of trophoblastic proliferation, a criterion often used for the histological grading of hydatidiform moles, is of little value in evaluating prognosis. Statistics indicate that more patients with a grade 1 mole (with little to no hyperplasia of the trophoblast) later develop a choriocarcinoma than do patients with a grade 2 (moderate hyperplasia) or grade 3 (intense hyperplasia with anaplasia) mole (ELSTON and BAGSHAWE 1972). Consequently, in the clinical follow-up of patients who had a hydatidiform mole it is important that their gonadotropin levels be determined. Electronmicroscopically some moles resemble choriocarcinomas, e.g., the cells of the trophoblast are poorly differentiated. When these changes progress, they may herald the development of a choriocarcinoma. About 50% of all choriocarcino-

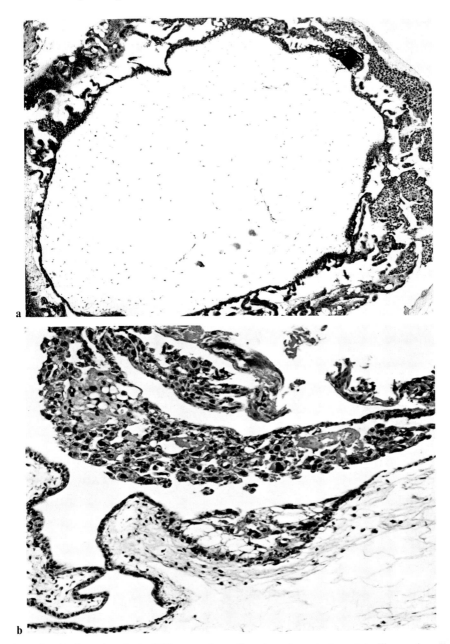

Fig. 165a, b. Complete hydatidiform mole: **a** Greatly enlarged placental villus and excessive proliferation of cyto- and syncytiotrophoblast. **b** Higher magnification of intense trophoblastic proliferation

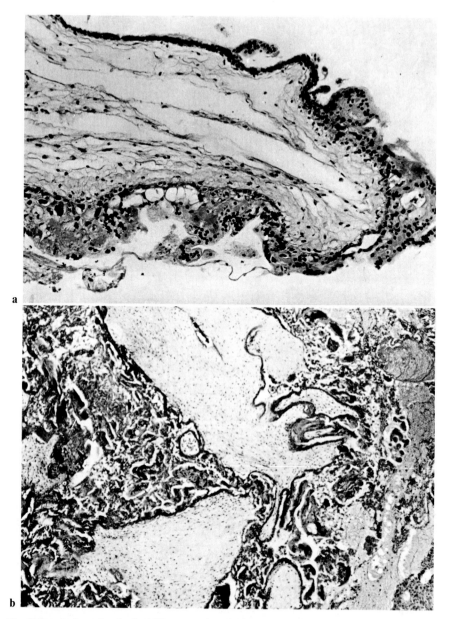

Fig. 166a, b. Invasive hydatidiform mole, with pronounced proliferation of the trophoblastic epithelium. **a** High magnification; **b** survey view

mas arise from hydatidiform moles. On the other hand, in European populations, only about 2% of hydatidiform moles are followed by choriocarcinoma (RINGERTZ 1970).

If such sheets of clumps of cells invade the myometrium or villi, and free trophoblastic cells are found growing within a myometrial blood vessel, then it seems justifiable to diagnose an **invasive mole**. The main difference is in the quantity of proliferation; the trophoblastic cells still resemble those of a benign hydatidiform mole (Fig. 166). Although the entire myometrium may be invaded, the prognosis, nevertheless, is usually good. The diagnosis, however, can rarely be made from curettings; one usually needs the resected uterus to determine the extent of growth.

Choriocarcinoma in curettings generally consists of solid or plexiform cords or clumps of poorly differentiated trophoblast cells with hypertrophied irregular nuclei and with high growth potentialities, as suggested by their restless, disorderly appearance. Placental villi are usually absent. The cords of tumor, admixed with necrotic decidua and clotted blood, may be composed of only cytotrophoblasts or syncytiotrophoblasts. Occasionally the two intermingle with one another. The atypical cells that are always present are easier to detect among the cytotrophoblasts than among the syncytiotrophoblasts, which even normally exhibit great variation in size of cell or nucleus (Fig. 167). Cells of choriocarcinomas differ electron-microscopically from the normal trophoblast only by their deeply indented nuclear membrane, their large nuclear pores, their irregularly shaped mitochondria, their scanty endoplasmic reticulum, and their RNA granules lying free throughout the cytoplasm (LARSEN 1973; for previous literature, see there). The choriocarcinoma usually develops weeks after abortion at the site of placental attachment. From there it invades the myometrium and its vascular channels (Fig. 168). Consequently, the curettings frequently contain fragments of myometrium, which, in contrast to those of benign chorial invasion, are penetrated and compressed by hyperplastic rows of atypical, anaplastic

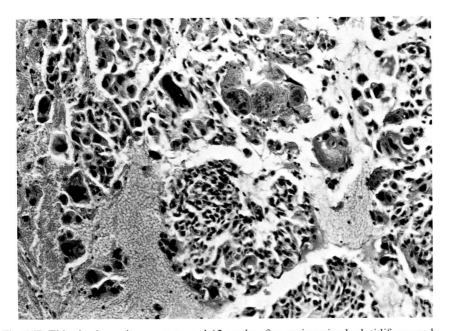

Fig. 167. This choriocarcinoma appeared 12 weeks after an invasive hydatidiform mole

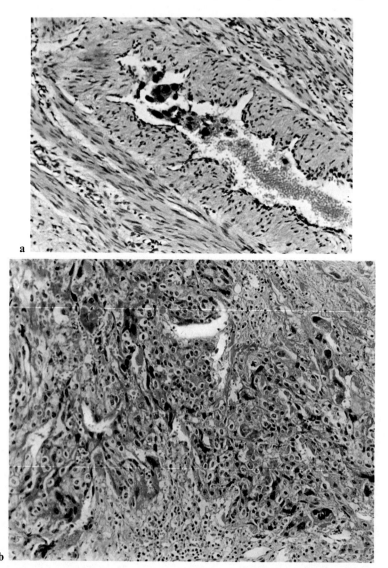

Fig. 168. Invasive growth with penetration (**a**) of a vessel and (**b**) of the myometrium

trophoblasts, causing necrosis and hemorrhage. The maternal tissues appear to be unable to mobilize any defense mechanisms (for example, immune cell response). Diagnosis of a frank choriocarcinoma seldom constitutes a problem. In an attempt to classify choriocarcinoma histologically, NISHIKAWA et al. (1985) found four criteria to be significant in determining high-grade malignancy: formation of tumor islands, massive proliferation of intermediate-type trophoblasts, perpendicular invasion into adjacent muscle, and cytological atypia at the invasion front. A common mistake is to over-evaluate a benign hydatidiform mole and diagnose it as a choriocarcinoma (NOVAK 1953; HERTIG 1968; BAG-

SHAWE 1969). Such a diagnosis is justified only when the histological sections reveal extensive necrosis of tissue in the absence of chorionic villi and when the biological behavior of the tumor suggests it is malignant (e.g., high levels of gonadotropins, clinical history of persistent bleeding, subinvolution of the uterus). At times the malignant chorial invasion may be exceedingly difficult to distinguish from a benign invasion (placental site reaction). An important criterion of benign invasion is the advance of individual cells along preformed clefts in the tissue without encroaching upon or injuring adjacent muscle cells. SCHOPPER and PLIESS (1949) drew attention to these differences and accordingly proposed that the clinically benign chorial invasion of the myometrium be called a *"chorionepitheliosis"* to separate it clearly from the choriocarcinoma. During delivery, groups of trophoblastic cells may lodge in the cervix or vagina and grow to produce nodules which give the false impression of a metastatic choriocarcinoma. These nodules of displaced trophoblast are referred to as "benign chorionepitheliosis externa". On the other hand, a choriocarcinoma may be so poorly differentiated that it does not produce gonadotropin; consequently, gonadotropin levels remain low and are of little diagnostic value in these tumors.

The prognosis of a true choriocarcinoma used to be very poor. The 5-year survival rate in RINGERTZ's series was 50%, but for those without a preceding mole only 14%. Newer chemotherapeutic regimes, especially those employing amethopterin (methotrexate), have proved highly effective in curing patients of the disease.

A rare special type of *gestational choriocarcinoma* has been observed developing during a seemingly normal pregnancy within the placenta and unrelated to hydatidiform mole. The primary tumors were only of microscopic size, arose from the villous cytotrophoblast and produced disseminated metastases that caused rapid death (BREWER and MAZUR 1981).

e) Placental Site Trophoblastic Tumor

KURMAN et al. (1976) first described this rare variant of the trophoblastic tumor, under the name "trophoblastic pseudotumor", as an exaggerated form of the placental site reaction with deep but reversible myometrial invasion and presumably a benign clinical course. Experience with a larger series of patients has shown, however, that this tumor is capable of malignant behavior (SCULLY and YOUNG 1981). Several cases of malignant metastasizing placental site trophoblastic tumors have been reported subsequently (GLOOR et al. 1983; ECKSTEIN et al. 1985; HOPKINS et al. 1985, see there for further references).

Grossly, the tumor is often well-circumscribed, yellowish, less friable and less hemorrhagic than choriocarcinoma. Microscopically, it consists of cells of only the intermediate trophoblast type, which closely resemble those of the basal plate. The tumor cells infiltrate the myometrium individually, in small rows, and surround blood vessels. Vascular invasion is much less frequent than in choriocarcinoma. The nuclei of the cells are diploid, in contrast with the aneuploid nuclei of choriocarcinoma. The β-HCG levels are lower than with choriocarcinoma. Despite these differences, the clinical behavior of these placental site trophoblastic tumors may be unpredictable. The mitotic rate appears to be the most reliable criterion for predicting prognosis (SCULLY and YOUNG 1981), since the malignant tumors showed more than four mitoses per 10 HPF, the benign ones fewer. Malignant placental site tumors respond much less favorably to chemotherapy than do choriocarcinomas, therefore hysterectomy is essential.

This rare and intriguing tumor must be differentiated from a normal placental site reaction. Such a differentiation may prove to be exceedingly difficult, however, especially when only curettings are available for examination. The distinction from an undifferentiated carcinoma is possible immunohistochemically with antibodies against HPL and β-HCG which react positively with most (HPL) or some (β-HCG) of the cells of the placental site tumor.

f) Late Endometrial Changes Following Intrauterine Abortion

If the embryo were **aborted** or expelled **months before,** then a retrospective explanation of why it did so may prove impossible. Usually in such cases the placental villi cannot be demonstrated. Fragments of *decidua* may also be lacking, or if present, they appear as completely hyalinized, nodular or garland-shaped remnants about spiral arterioles that are still large and conspicuous (Fig. 169). At times in these homogeneous, pale-staining regions of stroma one may discover barely recognizable remains of single decidual cells, enough evidence, however, to point to what kind of change has taken place. Now and then trophoblastic cells may remain visible in these regions for several months. Ultimately with complete hyalinization these portions of endometrial stroma resemble a small corpus albicans of the ovary. If these decidual remnants are absent, however, then only a presumptive diagnosis can be made of suspected previous abortion. Since that diagnosis carries implications that may be of utmost importance for the patient, yet about which the pathologist may know nothing, he should exercise great prudence in making it, and if possible confer with the patient's physician.

The *endometrium* about decidual remnants almost always shows an infiltration of inflammatory cells (endometritis post abortum), and is often still undergoing irregular shedding. At a later stage a new proliferative phase may predominate. Since that proliferation may at times proceed irregularly, either because decidual remnants act as mechanical irritants or because hormonal balance fails to become reestablished, histological pictures of hyperplasia (the so-called adaptation hyperplasia of VELTEN, personal communication) may evolve that resemble glandular-cystic hyperplasia (cf. p. 108). Hyaline deposits may appear in the stroma of this adaptation hyperplasia just as they do in other glandular-cystic hyperplasias (see p. 112). Although their causes are entirely different, these hyaline deposits of hyperplasias may be confused with hyalinized remnants of decidua. Consequently, in certain instances it may be difficult to distinguish a beginning or modified cystic hyperplasia with prominent hyaline deposits from hyalinized decidual remnants with an associated adaptation hyperplasia. If there had been an abortion, a diligent search will reveal characteristic stigmata

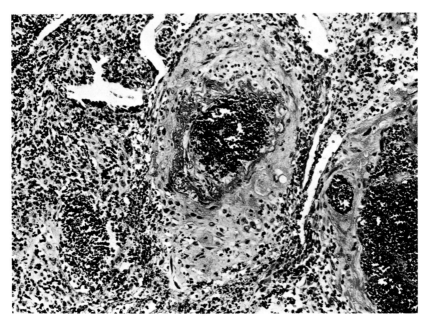

Fig. 169. Garland-like remnants of decidua near dilated stromal vessels several weeks after an intrauterine abortion. The surrounding endometrium is involuted and infiltrated with chronic inflammatory cells: endometritis post abortum

of the previous pregnancy: unaltered groups of hypertrophied spiral arterioles and at times single involved glands showing persistent secretory changes. Besides the infiltrates of inflammatory cells in the endometrial stroma, groups of hemosiderin-filled macrophages may be found that otherwise are rarely seen (HINZ and SOLTH 1959).

A curettage performed after an abortion often yields many fragments of tissue from the proliferated and papillary *endocervical mucosa*. Histologically, the fragments show the characteristic glandular hyperplasia, squamous metaplasia and vacuolization of the epithelial cells that develop with pregnancy (MEINRENKEN 1956; Fig. 170).

If, after abortion, portions of the placenta remain attached to the decidua or directly to the myometrium they prevent the endometrium from regenerating and usually cause protracted bleeding. The retention of placental tissue occurs more often in women who have injured their endometrium by antifertility agents or intrauterine devices than in women who have never used these agents (REYNIAK et al. 1975). As fibrin and coagulated blood accumulate about the retained tissues, a protuberant mass gradually develops, a so-called **placental polyp,** which may occasionally reach the size of a hen's egg and become quite firm. Eventually the polyp disintegrates at its attachment and is cast off with a lochial discharge. Its center usually consists of necrotic villi but also at times of fairly well-preserved villi and trophoblastic cells (Fig. 171). From histological studies we know such trophoblastic cells may survive for long periods. Placental polyps removed several years after the last pregnancy may still contain intact, viable-appearing

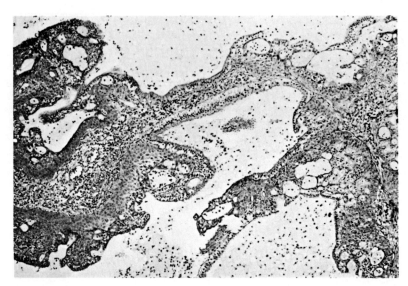

Fig. 170. Endocervicitis post abortum with extensive squamous metaplasia and reserve cell hyperplasia

trophoblasts. Villi, although hyalinized, kept their characteristic shape and structure and could be identified in a placental polyp retained for 21 years (SWAN and WOODRUFF 1969).

Several authors have reported finding portions of **cartilage and bone** in surgically removed uteri, and have postulated that these foreign tissues represented dystrophically calcified remnants of fetal tissue and bone from one or more abortions months to years before (DE BRUX et al. 1956; see here for earlier literature; ROBINSON 1964; NEWTON and ABELL 1972). Others were of the opinion that the cartilage and bone represented a reaction to the chronic inflammation associated with the abortions (GANEM et al. 1962; HSU 1975). In contrast, from the study of two such cases MEYER-FÜRST (1961) thought the osseouschondral tissues had resulted from previous hysterography. BANIECKI (1963) described plates of cartilage enclosed by normal endometrium. He regarded the cartilage as altered remnants of retained menstrual tissues, since he believed cartilaginous products of conception should be surrounded by an inflammatory reaction. Finally, ROTH and TAYLOR (1966) maintained that mature stromal cells were capable of cartilaginous metaplasia. In nine endometria containing cartilage they were able to exclude the possibility that fetal parts had been retained. They succeeded in demonstrating focal concentrations of acid mucopolysaccharides, which they interpreted as transitions in the formation of cartilage. They might have seen, however, a benign teratoma of the endometrium (see p. 225f.). In the differential diagnosis it is necessary to rule out a malignant mixed Müllerian tumor of the uterus that produces neoplastic bone and cartilage. – Several reports of **glial tissue** in the endometrium have stimulated various interpretations. ZETTERGREN (1956, 1973), URBANKE (1962), VANEK and LANE (1963), STOLZ et al. (1964), HANSKI (1971) and NIVEN and STANSFELD (1973) thought the glial tissue they found represented remnants of fetal tissue from a previous abortion, implanted in the uterus during curettage. Implanted glial

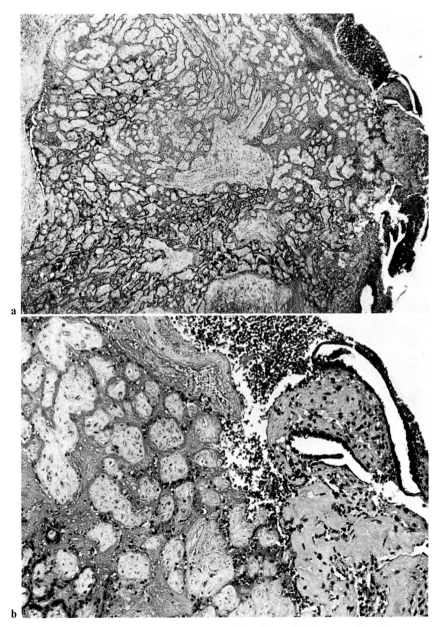

Fig. 171a, b. Placental polyp. **a** Low magnification; **b** higher magnification

tissue may remain active for a long period and may proliferate, perhaps because of its known low concentration of isoantigens (Fig. 172). HAMPERL et al. (1959) agreed that fetal glial tissue lodged in the endometrium most likely is able to grow independently; they also discussed the possibility, however, of pluripotent cells arising locally to grow autonomously like tumor cells, a hypothesis with which BAZALA (1966) concurs (cf. p. 224).

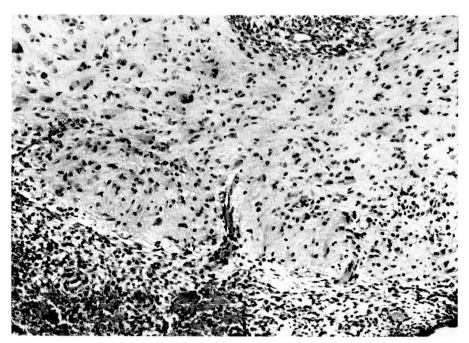

Fig. 172. Glial proliferation in the endometrium 15 months after an intrauterine abortion

2. The Endometrium Associated with Extrauterine Pregnancy

The decidua developing during an extrauterine pregnancy *with viable fetus* differs from that formed during a normal uterine pregnancy only by the absence of trophoblasts, chorionic villi and associated reactions in the adjacent stroma (formation of a hyaline-fibrinoid boundary) and blood vessels (dilatation prior to formation of intervillous spaces). Enlargement of the decidual blood vessels associated with an extrauterine pregnancy develops only at the onset and is never pronounced (SPEERT 1958).

After death of the fetus of an extrauterine pregnancy the decidua regresses. The regression, however, proceeds gradually, because the hormone-secreting chorionic villi in the wall of the fallopian tube insure that the corpus luteum involutes only very slowly. In addition, because the endometrial cavity contains no dead fetus, it remains free of any significant inflammation. Consequently, the decidua rarely is spontaneously expelled; instead it regresses and because the next ovulation may be greatly delayed (OVERBECK 1953), the endometrium may actually atrophy. With gradual and ultimate, severe shrinkage of the stroma, the *glands* collapse. These often exhibit the Arias-Stella phenomenon, their lining cells possessing swollen, clear cytoplasm and large, grotesque nuclei. Since the phenomenon generally develops focally, its incidence, as reported by different authors, varies, depending upon the precision and care exercised in examining the endometrial curettings. The *decidual cells* also shrink, eventually being no larger than the endometrial granulocytes, which seem to increase in number because the decidual cells become smaller. The granules of the endometrial granulocytes, however, do increase in size and number. An extremely dense network of reticulum fibers forms around the decidual cells. To demonstrate that network methods of silver impregnation are ideal. As the ground substance loses acid mucopolysaccharides, it becomes distinctly fibrous (OVERBECK 1962). Consequently, the groups of spiral arterioles that had failed to involute become more prominent than ever. While these changes progress, a few regions of the decidua begin to disintegrate and become necrotic. In contrast, other regions will have lost their decidual character because of severe shrinkage. Histologically as well as hormonally, the picture represents that of irregular shedding. If the decidual cells complete their retrogressive changes, becoming once again small and spindly, then the glands lined by large clear epithelial cells (Arias-Stella phenomenon) may be the only evidence of the foregoing pregnancy (FREDERIKSEN 1958). In other words, the regression of the stroma regularly precedes that of the glands.

Such changes may still be evident many weeks after the abortion. As a new follicle proceeds to maturity (about 1 month after onset of bleeding; according to BANIECKI 1953, no earlier than 6–7 weeks after death of the fetus) the endometrium begins to proliferate anew. During that process of regeneration the old portions of mucosa gradually become incorporated or replaced by the new tissues; the exact mechanisms involved in the replacement, however, escape detailed histological analysis. As the Arias-Stella phenomenon slowly abates, the epithelial cells of the glands flatten out; their cytoplasm becomes vacuolized and their polymorphic nuclei shrink. Although involution may be extreme, some glands continue to retain abnormal amounts of glycogen (CRAMER 1957). When these terminal changes of the glands finally disappear, and the new proliferation dominates the picture, it becomes impossible to even suspect that there had been a preceding pregnancy. The endometrium may then resemble that of an anovulatory cycle, although there may still be clinical signs of a previous extrauterine pregnancy.

The clinically important and therefore much-discussed question of whether it is possible from curettings *to differentiate between an extrauterine pregnancy and an intrauterine* cannot always be answered decisively, even when all available special histological methods are employed. A clear-cut decision is feasible only when one finds fetal tissues (chorionic villi or trophoblasts). If trophoblastic cells cannot be identified in routine histological sections, then immunohistological markers [antibodies against chorionic gonadotropins (HCG) or placental lactogens (HPL) or against cytokeratin] may help to reveal inconspicuous trophoblasts hidden within the fragmented curettings (ANGEL et al. 1985; SASAGAWA et al. 1986). If these are not found, even though new step-sections of the tissue have been examined, then the best one can do is to make a diagnosis of probable extrauterine pregnancy, basing that decision on the fact that the decidua of an extrauterine pregnancy involutes very slowly and rarely reveals inflammatory changes. Occasionally, however, a severe endometritis may accompany an acute salpingitis, which is the cause of the extrauterine pregnancy. That the involution is greatly retarded is indicated, first, by the increased numbers of collagen inclusions in the decidual cells; second, by the failure of the decidua to shed, thus allowing the decidual cells to shrink severely; and third, by the greatly delayed regeneration of the endometrium. In addition, the Arias-Stella phenomenon serves as evidence that the embryo has died and gonadotropin is still being produced by placental tissues, which may remain viable for a long time. These placental tissues more commonly belong to an extrauterine pregnancy than to an intrauterine (67% against 43.6%, according to OVERBECK 1962; see also BEATO et al. 1968). The differences here between the two types of pregnancy are quantitative, not qualitative. According to MEIN-RENKEN (1952) and HOMMA (1958) hyaline rings more often develop around the capillaries of the involuting compacta of intrauterine pregnancies than of extrauterine. They do develop, however, in the extrauterine pregnancies. On the other hand, the extrauterine implantations often lack the hemosiderin deposits and fibrinoid exudates found in the stroma of intrauterine pregnancies (HINZ and TERBRÜGGEN 1952). No histochemical reaction exists that accurately distinguishes between the endometria of intrauterine or extrauterine pregnancies (LEWIN 1960). Attempts to differentiate the two seem all the more futile when one considers that the changes occurring in the endometrium may vary greatly, depending upon the type, extent and time of disturbance befalling the extrauterine or intrauterine pregnancy (see ARRONET and STOLL 1950). For example, sudden rupture of the tube may cause the decidua to rapidly degenerate, or intrauterine abortion may be unusually prolonged. A review of 1000 tubal pregnancies from the literature (OVERBECK 1962) disclosed that curettage yielded decidua in only 43% (according to ROMNEY et al. 1950, in only 19%). Since almost any endometrial change may develop with an extrauterine pregnancy, even a glandular-cystic hyperplasia (KIEF and MUTH 1951) or so-called adaptation hyperplasia (VELTEN) or even an endometrial atrophy remaining refractory after therapy with antifertility agents, then one is not justified in reporting from the curettings alone that no extrauterine pregnancy exists merely because one finds no fetal tissues (see BRUNTSCH 1954). In problem cases the detection of fetal tissues may be of decisive importance (HOFMANN and LEGERLOTZ 1968). We help the attending gynecologist considerably in doubtful cases even when we report no more than "suspicion of intrauterine pregnancy" or "extrauterine pregnancy unlikely". He will be able to modify his care of the patient accordingly. After curettage, persistent bleeding indicates that an extrauterine pregnancy undoubtedly exists, the blood emanating from the site of placental implantation in the wall of the fallopian tube (BRUNTSCH 1954). In such instances the clinician is reponsible for the final diagnosis, not the pathologist.

Decidua without pregnancy. If one detects decidua in curettings but finds no fetal tissues, then the diagnosis of possible intrauterine or extrauterine pregnancy may be made, but only with reservations. In BOBEK's series of patients (1957) the suspicion of extrauterine pregnancy based on the presence of decidua alone proved correct in only 20% of cases. Just as the lack of decidua is poor evidence for proving the absence of an extrauterine pregnancy, so is the presence of decidua little proof that a pregnancy does exist. A large cyst of a corpus luteum or a persistent corpus luteum may induce a decidual change in the endometrium that is histologically identical with the decidua of a young intrauterine or extrauterine pregnancy (TE LINDE and HENDRIKSEN 1940; ISRAEL 1942;

Table 23. Source of decidua

	Intrauterine pregnancy	Ectopic pregnancy	Arrested secretion (hormonally induced)	IUCD (mechanically induced)
Last menstrual period	More than 4 weeks ago	More than 4 weeks ago	More than 4 weeks ago	*Less than* 4 weeks ago
Glands	High secretion, occ. Arias-Stella	High secretion, occ. Arias-Stella	*Atrophic*	High secretion, occ. Arias-Stella
Extent of decidualization	Complete	Complete	Complete	*Focal*
Inflammatory infiltration	Present	*None*	None	Present
Fetal elements	*Often present*	None	None	None

SPECHTER 1953). It may be that in such cases an overproduction of gonadotropin induces not only the cyst of the corpus luteum but also the decidual change of the endometrium. Other causes of decidual change in the absence of pregnancy are granulosa cell tumors and certain hormone-secreting carcinomas of the ovary (SPECHTER 1953). Therapy with gestagens (for example, for endometriosis) may also lead to the development of decidua, which, however, differs from that of pregnancy since it lacks secreting glands. If glands are present in this decidua, they are atrophic (*"starre Sekretion"* = "arrested secretion"). All these causes explain why from time to time we may observe an intrauterine decidua in old women (see p. 162 and Fig. 84). Decidual change may also be provoked by mechanical stimulation and closely resemble the deciduomas of rats and mice that are readily induced by trauma. Characteristic of the mechanically produced decidual change is its localized development; for example, its adjacency to a non-medicated intrauterine device (see p. 193). It is very important for the clinician to know what type of decidua is present and how it was induced. The differential diagnosis should therefore be given careful thought. Characteristics that may help in reaching a definitive diagnosis are listed in Table 23.

3. The Postpartum Endometrium

Within 10 days after delivery, the inner surface of the uterus is covered again by an unbroken layer of epithelial cells that grow out from the stumps of glands in the basalis. Within 3–5 weeks post partum the regeneration is completed. The blood vessels at the site of placental attachment become occluded by constricting, and by endothelial proliferation, thrombosis, and hyaline degeneration. As the underlying endometrium proliferates, these vessels and the surrounding remnants of decidua become sequestered from the uterine wall

(Fig. 173). After 6 weeks only deposits of hemosiderin are evident. After 3 months the site of placental attachment cannot usually be recognized; not even scar tissue remains. BÜTTNER (1911) reported, however, he was able to detect hyaline changes in the placental bed up to 1 year after delivery. If mothers do not breast-feed, the endometrium reaches an advanced proliferative phase by the 3rd postpartum week (VOKAER 1956). Breast-feeding, on the other hand, greatly retards the proliferation; the glandular epithelium becomes only moder-

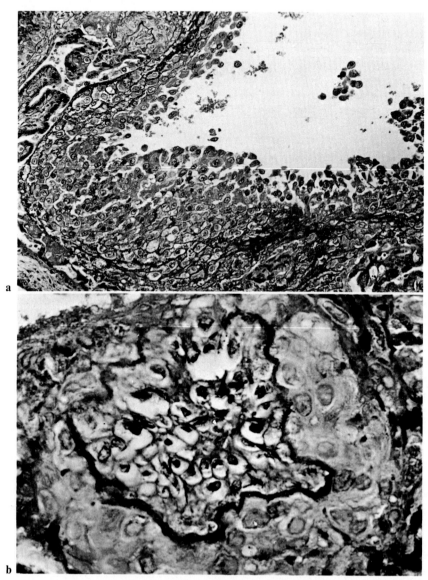

Fig. 173a, b. Endothelial proliferation within a thin-walled vessel at the site of separation of the placenta (**a**), and in the placental bed post partum (**b**)

ately high (GROSS et al. 1957). Generally, women who are not breast-feeding first ovulate in the 7th postpartum week. Women who breast-feed do not usually ovulate before the 13th week (SHARMAN 1967).

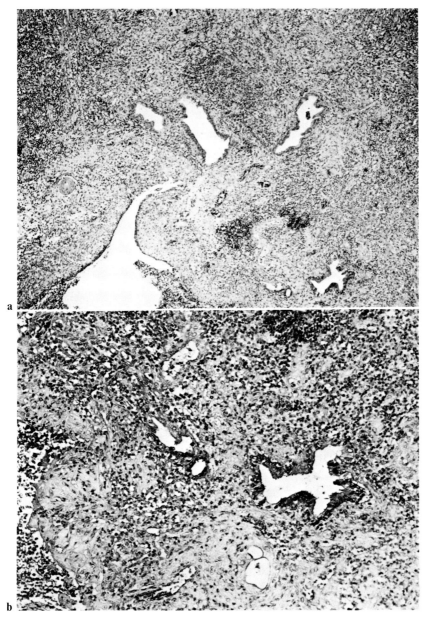

Fig. 174a, b. Endometritis post partum. Focal infiltrates of polymorphonuclear leukocytes, lymphocytes, and plasma cells with destruction of glands. The glands are still involuting and star-shaped. a Survey view; b higher magnification

Uterine hemorrhage during the postpartum period means that the endometrium is not involuting and regenerating as it should. Curettage often becomes necessary. In two-thirds of such cases the histological studies disclose that retained portions of placenta, decidua or fetal membranes are responsible for the defective involution (BACHMEYER and STOLL 1960). The condition is referred to as *"endometritis post partum"*. The remnants of retained tissue are almost always necrotic, the shape of a placental polyp, and encased in coagulated blood and fibrin, or surrounded by proliferating endometrium. The glands of the endometrium are irregularly dilated, lined by cells of variable height possessing elongated nuclei. The stroma is composed of small or spindle-shaped cells and focally infiltrated with inflammatory cells. These infiltrates migrate into and destroy the glandular epithelium and are particularly heavy around the focal necroses (Fig. 174). Frequently the curettings contain fragments of the superficial myometrium, which have become edematous and soft because of the neighboring inflamed endometrium. If severe inflammatory infiltrates are diffuse, even in the absence of necrotic tissue remnants, a chlamydial infection must be considered in the differential diagnosis (see p. 210). At times the myometrial fragments may also reveal inflammatory infiltrates or even well-preserved trophoblastic cells as remnants of the chorial invasion. The postpartum retention of placental or decidual tissue regularly leads to endometritis, which resolves to heal eventually only after the retained tissues are surgically removed. In contrast, the focal infiltration of leukocytes seen in remnants of placenta or decidua expelled from the uterus shortly after delivery does not mean endometri-

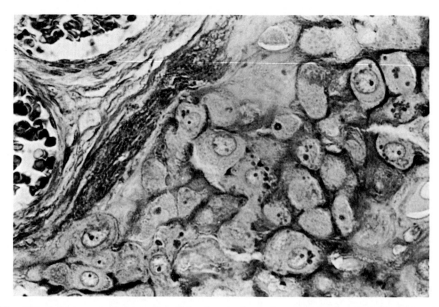

Fig. 175. Relaxin-containing cells of the basal plate of a mature placenta. The granules correspond to the paranuclear granules of the endometrial granulocytes. Phloxine-tartrazine stain

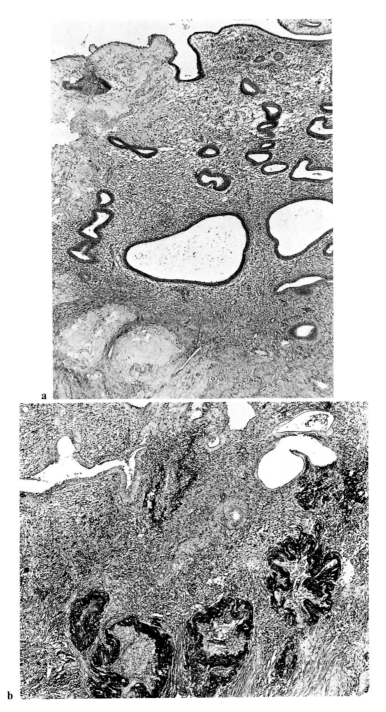

Fig. 176a, b. Postpartum "adaptation hyperplasia". **a** Hematoxylin-eosin stain; **b** PAS stain. The PAS stain reveals a garland-like ring of decidual remnants about blood vessels

tis. Rather it represents a physiological reaction to the processes involved in detachment of the placenta at the basal plate.

The curettings of about one-third of the patients experiencing postpartum bleeding (according to LESTER et al. 1956, as many as two-thirds) reveal no fragments of placental or decidual tissue, or inflammatory changes that might explain the bleeding. These endometria often do disclose, however, *pathological changes in the walls of blood vessels,* which are usually greatly dilated and congested with blood. Their walls, like many of the neighboring myometrial fibers, show hyaline degeneration; thus they are unable to contract. Their elastic fibers are destroyed. BACHMEYER and STOLL (1960) have suggested that proteolytic enzymes from the trophoblasts may initiate the hyalinization. Usually these enzymes cease to be active when Nitabuch's stria becomes established at the basal plate. If, however, trophoblasts invade the myometrium, then, because of their affinity for maternal vessels, they could cause the vessel wall to hyalinize prematurely, making it impossible for the vessel to contract effectively later. In addition, the normal, relaxin-induced endothelial proliferation, which usually progresses to occlude the lumen, may fail to develop. Apparently the basal trophoblastic cells (Fig. 175), which normally can function like endometrial granulocytes, fail to release their relaxin. That failure indicates the hormonal control of placental detachment is disturbed. Such dysfunction may also be a factor in causing postpartum bleeding. With the same mechanism we can explain partial uterine involution at the placental bed (BACHMEYER and STOLL 1960; OBER and GRADY 1961). Multiparae apparently experience partial involution most often; the condition becomes more common as the number of births increases (RUTHERFORD and HERTIG 1945), since the ability of the uterus to involute diminishes after each pregnancy.

Occasionally the first postpartum proliferation develops irregularly, its glands undergoing cystic dilatation. Such changes usually ensue when an estrogen stimulus persists, as with postpartum anovulatory cycles (DUBRAUSZKY 1950). This so-called *adaptation hyperplasia* (VELTEN) may also cause bleeding in the postpartum period (Fig. 176a). At times it may reach the severity of a glandular-cystic hyperplasia. If the patient's clinical history is not known but she is fairly young, then groups of prominent or involuting arterioles, enveloped occasionally by hyalinized remnants of decidua and found in a glandular-cystic hyperplasia (Fig. 176b), may provide an important clue to the right diagnosis. MEISSNER and SOMMERS (1950) described the changes of adaptation hyperplasia in diabetic women who had received estrogen and progesterone during their pregnancies.

In rare instances an irregular shedding due to a protracted fall in progesterone may result in a postpartum bleeding. An insufficient or persistent corpus luteum is then more likely the cause for the slow fall in progesterone than a newly fertilized ovum.

References

Aalders J, Abeler V, Kolstad P, Onsund M (1980) Postoperative external irradiation and prognostic parameters in stage I endometrial carcinoma. Obstet Gynecol 56:419

Aaro LA, Symmonds RE, Dockerty MB (1966) Sarcoma of the uterus. A clinical and pathologic study of 177 cases. Am J Obstet Gynecol 94:101

Abaci F, Aterman K (1968) Changes of the placenta and embryo in early spontaneous abortion. Am J Obstet Gynecol 102:252

Abraham AA (1978) Herpesvirus hominis endometritis in a young woman wearing an intrauterine contraceptive device. Am J Obstet Gynecol 131:340

Adler L (1926) Schleimhautpolypen des Uteruskörper. In: Halban-Seitz (ed) Biologie und Pathologie des Weibes, vol IV. Urban & Schwarzenberg, Berlin

Agrawal K, Fox H (1972) Subepithelial endometrial collagen. Am J Obstet Gynecol 114:172

Aguirre P, Scully RE, Wolfe HJ, De Lellis RA (1984) Endometrial carcinoma with argyrophil cells: a histochemical and immunohistochemical analysis. Hum Pathol 15:210

Aikawa M, Ng APB (1973) Mixed (adenosquamous) carcinoma of the endometrium. Cancer (Philad) 31:385

Akhtar M, Kim PY, Young I (1975) Ultrastructure of endometrial stromal sarcoma. Cancer (Philad) 35:406

Akinla O, Luukkainen T, Timonen H (1975) Important factors in the use-effectiveness of the copper-T-200 IUD. Contraception 12:697

Alberhasky RC, Connelly PJ, Christopherson WM (1982) Carcinoma of the endometrium. IV. Mixed adenosquamous carcinoma. A clinical-pathological study of 68 cases with long-term follow-up. Am J Clin Pathol 77:655

Albrecht H (1928) Pathologische Anatomie und Klinik des Uterussarkoms. In: Halban-Seitz (ed) Biologie und Pathologie des Weibes, vol IV. Urban & Schwarzenberg, Berlin

Aleem FA, Moukhtar MA, Hung HC, Romney SL (1976) Plasma estrogen in patients with endometrial hyperplasia and carcinoma. Cancer (Philad) 38:2101

Allen E (1942) Estrogenic hormones in the genesis of tumor and cancers. Endocrinology 30:942

Alznauer RL (1955) Mixed mesenchymal sarcoma of the corpus uteri. Arch Pathol 60:329

Ames S, Janovski NA (1963) Ovarian hilus cells and endometrial carcinoma with reference to radiation. Obstet Gynecol 22:68

Ancla M, de Brux J (1964) Etude au microscope électronique des artérioles spiralées de l'endomètre humain. Ann Anat Pathol 9:209

Ancla M, de Brux J (1965) Occurrence of intranuclear tubular structures in the human endometrium during the secretory phase and of annulate lamellae in hyperestrogenic states. Obstet Gynecol 26:23

Ancla M, Simon P, de Brux J, Robey M (1965) Modifications endométriales après administration prolongée de lynestrenol. Etude au microscope optique et électronique. Gynecol Obstét 64:231

Ancla M, de Brux J, Musset R, Bret JA (1967) Etude au microscope électronique de l'endomètre humain dans différentes conditions d'équilibre hormonal. Arch Pathol 15:136

Ancla M, de Brux J, Simon P (1967) Aneurysmal microthrombosis associated with intrauterine devices in the human endometrium. Lab Invest 17:61

Anderson DG (1965) Management of advanced endometrial adenocarcinoma with medroxyprogesterone acetate. Am J Obstet Gynecol 92:87

Anderson PE (1949) Extramedullary plasmocytomes. Acta Radiol (Stockh) 32:365

Andres AG, Feigel II, Djukowa II, Korotkowa TM (1949) Die Morphologie des Phosphorstoffwechsels in Gesundheit und Krankheit. 4. Mitt. Die Phosphatasen des weiblichen Endometriums in einzelnen Phasen des Cyclus, bei einigen pathologischen Zuständen und maligner Entartung. Arkh Patol 11:58 [Russian]. Ref. in: Ber Pathol 5:32 (1950)

Andrews WC (1961) Estrogens and endometrial carcinoma. Obstet Gynecol Surv 16:747

Angel E, Davis JR, Nagle RB (1985) Immunohistochemical demonstration of placental hormones in the diagnosis of uterine versus ectopic pregnancy. Am J Clin Pathol 84:705

Annos T, Thompson IE, Taymor ML (1980) Luteal phase deficiency and infertility: difficulties encountered in diagnosis and treatment. Obstet Gynecol 55:705

Ansari AH, Cowdrey CR (1974) Gravlee jet washer for endometrial dating. Fertil Steril 25:127

Ansari AH, Cowdrey CR (1974) Endometrial biopsy using Gravlee jet washer and suction curette. Int J Fertil 19:129

Anthony CL, Roddick JW (1962) Ovarian hilus cells and endometrial carcinoma. Am J Obstet Gynecol 83:1299

Antunes CMF, Stolley PD, Rosenshein NB et al. (1979) Endometrial cancer and estrogen use. Report of a large case-control study. N Engl J Med 300:9

Arias-Stella J (1954) Atypical endometrial changes associated with the presence of chorionic tissue. Arch Pathol 58:112

Arias Stella J (1955) Abnormal endometrial changes induced in the rat. The effects of chorionic hormone and estrogen. Arch Pathol 60:49

Armenia CS (1967) Sequential relationship between endometrial polyps and carcinoma of the endometrium. Obstet Gynecol 30:524

Armstrong EM, More IAR, McSeveney D, Carty M (1973) The giant mitochondrion – endoplasmic reticulum unit of human endometrial glandular cell. J Anat 116:375

Armstrong EM, More IAR, McSeveney D, Chatfield WR (1973) Reappraisal of the ultrastructure of the human endometrial glandular cell. J Obstet Gynaecol Br Cwlth 80:446

Arnold M (1968) Histochemie. Springer, Berlin Heidelberg New York

Arrata WS, Zarou GS (1963) Postmenopausal hematometra. Am J Obstet Gynecol 85:959

Arronet GH, Bergquist CA, Parekh MC et al. (1973) Evaluation of endometrial biopsy in the cycle of conception. Int J Fertil 18:220

Arronet G, Latour J (1957) Studies on the endometrial glycogen. J Clin Endocrinol 17:261

Arronet G, Stoll P (1950) Eine klinisch-histologische Studie zur Tubengravidität. Zentralbl Gynäkol 72:795

Artner J, Kratochwil A (1965) Über den Wirkungsmechanismus der Ovulationsunterdrückung durch Anovlar. Fortschr Geburtshilfe Gynäkol 21:171

Aschheim S (1915) Zur Histologie der Uterusschleimhaut. Über das Vorkommen von Fettsubstanzen. Z Geburtshilfe Gynäkol 77:485

Asherman JG (1948) Amenorrhoea traumatica (atretica) J Obstet Gynaecol Br Cwlth 55:23

Ashkenazy M, Lancet M, Borenstein R, Czernobilsky B (1983) Endometrial foam cells. Acta Obstet Gynecol Scand 62:193

Asplund J, Holmgren H (1947) On the occurrence of metachromatically granulated cells in the mucous membrane of the human uterus. Acta Anat (Basel) 3:312

Atkin NB, Richards BM, Ross AJ (1959) The deoxyribonucleic acid content of carcinoma of the uterus. An assessment of its possible significance in relation to histopathology and clinical course, based on data from 165 cases. Br J Cancer 8:773

Atkinson WB (1950) Studies on the effects of steroid sex hormones on alkaline phosphatase in the endometrium. In: Engle ET (ed) Menstruation and its disorders. Thomas, Springfield, p 3

Atkinson WB (1955) The histochemistry of normal and abnormal growth in the human endometrium. Tex Rep Biol Med 13:603

Atkinson WB, Engle ET (1947) Studies on endometrial alkaline phosphatase during

the human menstrual cycle and in the hormone-treated monkey. Endocrinology 40:327
Atkinson WB, Gusberg SB (1948) Histochemical studies on abnormal growth of human endometrium. I. Alkaline phosphatase in hyperplasia and adenocarcinoma. Cancer (Philad) 1:248
Atkinson WB, Engle ET, Gusberg SB, Buxton CL (1949) Histochemical studies on abnormal growth of human endometrium. II. Cytoplasmic ribonucleic acids in normal and pathological glandular epithelium. Cancer (Philad) 2:132
Atkinson WB, Gall EA, Gusberg SB (1952) Histochemical studies on abnormal growth of human endometrium. III. Deposition of glycogen in hyperplasia and adenocarcinoma. Cancer (Philad) 5:138
Attramadal A (1970) Cellular localization of ^{3}H-oestradiol in the hypothalamus. An autoradiographic study in male and female rats. Z Zellforsch 104:572
Augustin E (1952) Die Bedeutung des histologischen Glykogennachweises im Endometrium für die Beurteilung des cyclischen Geschehens im Ovar. Arch Gynäkol 181:341
Ausems EWMA, van der Kamp J-K, Baak JPA (1985) Nuclear morphometry in the determination of the prognosis of marked atypical endometrial hyperplasia. Int J Gynecol Pathol 4:180
Aycock NR, Jollie WP (1979) Ultrastructural effects of estrogen replacement on postmenopausal endometrium. Am J Obstet Gynecol 135:461
Aycock NR, Jollie WP, Dunn LJ (1979) An ultrastructural comparison of human endometrial adenocarcinoma with normal postmenopausal endometrium. Obstet Gynecol 53:565
Ayre JE, Bauld WAG (1946) Thiamine deficiency and high estrogen findings in uterine cancer and in menorrhagia. Science 103:441
Azadian-Boulanger G, Secchi J, Laraque F, et al. (1976) Action of a midcycle contraceptive (R2323) on the human endometrium. Am J Obstet Gynecol 125:1049
Azzopardi JG, Zayid I (1967) Synthetic progestogen-oestrogen therapy and uterine changes. J Clin Pathol 20:731
Baak JPA (1984) The use and disuse of morphometry in the diagnosis of endometrial hyperplasia and carcinoma. Pathol Res Pract 179:20
Baak JPA, Diegenbach PC (1977) Quantitative nuclear image analysis: differentiation between normal, hyperplastic and malignant appearing uterine glands in a paraffin section. Eur J Obstet Gynecol Reprod Biol 7:33
Bachmeyer H, Stoll P (1960) Blutung im Wochenbett. Dtsch Med Wochenschr 85:1798
Badib AO (1970) Biologic behavior of adenoacanthoma of endometrium. Am J Obstet Gynecol 106:205
Baggish MD, Woodruff JD (1967) The occurrence of squamous epithelium in the endometrium. Obstet Gynecol Surv 22:69
Bagshawe KD (1969) Choriocarcinoma – the clinical biology of the trophoblast and its tumours. Arnold, London
Bahari CM, Gorodeski IG, Avidor I (1986) Case report of two primary tumors: Müllerian adenosarcoma and endometrial adenocarcinoma. Isr J Med Sci 22:127
Bailar JC (1961) Uterine cancer in Connecticut: late deaths among 5-year survivors. JNCI 27:239
Baker JR (1946) The histochemical recognition of lipine. Q J Microsc Sci 87:441
Baker JR (1963) Cytological technique. The principles underlying routine methods. Methuen, London
Baker MC (1968) A chromosome study of seven near-diploid carcinomas of the corpus uteri. Br J Cancer 22:683
Balasch J, Vanrell JA, Duran M, Gonzales-Merlo J (1983) Luteal phase evaluation after clomiphene-chorionic-gonadotropin induced ovulation. Int J Fertil 28:104
Bamforth J (1956) Carcinoma of the body of the uterus and its relationship to endometrial hyperplasia. J Obstet Gynaecol Br Emp 63:415
Baniecki H (1928) Menorrhagien als Folge mangelhafter Abstoßung des Endometrium. Zentralbl Gynäkol 52:955
Baniecki H (1953) Das Schleimhautbild des Uterus vor und nach dem Eitod bei Tubargravidität. Verh Dtsch Ges Pathol 36:324

Baniecki H (1963) Die Bewertung von Knorpel-Knochenbefunden im Endometrium des Uterus. Verh Dtsch Ges Pathol 47:406

Bannatyne P, Russell P, Wills EJ (1983) Argyrophilia and endometrial carcinoma. Int J Gynecol Pathol 2:235

Barber HRK, Graber EA, O'Rourke JJ (1969) Are the pills safe? Thomas, Springfield

Barber KW, Dockerty MB, Pratt JH, Hunt BA (1962) Prognosis in endometrial carcinoma by modified Dukes typing. Surg Gynecol Obstet 114:155

Barbour EM (1961) Histochemical change in endometrium. Normal endometrium. J Obstet Gynaecol Br Cwlth 68:662

Barnett H (1965) Squamous cell carcinoma of the body of the uterus. J Clin Pathol 18:715

Barni S, Novelli G, Zanoio L, et al. (1981) Chromatin analysis in human endometrial adenocarcinoma before and after treatment with 6-methyl-17-hydroxyprogesterone acetate (MPA). Virchows Arch [B] 37:167

Baron DA, Esterly JR (1975) Histochemical demonstration of lysosomal hydrolase activity in endometrial mononuclear cells. I. Normal endometrium. II. Abnormal endometrium. Am J Obstet Gynecol 123:790

Barr W, Charteris AA (1955) The treatment of 850 cases of simple uterine haemorrhage by intrauterine application of radium. J Obstet Gynaecol Br Emp 62:187

Bartelmez GW (1931) The human uterine mucous membrane during menstruation. I Involution and variability. Am J Obstet Gynecol 21:623

Bartelmez GW (1933) Histological studies on the menstruating mucous membrane of the human uterus. Contrib Embryol Carnegie Inst 24:141

Bartelmez GW (1941) Menstruation. JAMA 116:702

Bartelmez GW (1957) The phases of the menstrual cycle and their interpretation in terms of the pregnancy cycle. Am J Obstet Gynecol 74:931

Barter JF, Austin JM, Shingleton HM (1986) Endometrial adenocarcinoma after in utero diethylstilbestrol exposure. Obstet Gynecol 67:84S

Barter RH, Brennan G, Newman W, Merrill KW (1968) The place of curettage in the diagnosis of carcinoma of the endometrium. Am J Obstet Gynecol 100:696

Bartsich EG, O'Leary JA, Moore JG (1967) Carcinosarcoma of the uterus. Obstet Gynecol 30:518

Bartsich EG, Bowe ET, Moore JG (1968) Leiomyosarcoma of the uterus. Obstet Gynecol 32:101

Barwick KW, Livolsi VA (1979) Heterologous mixed Müllerian tumor confined to an endometrial polyp. Obstet Gynecol 53:512

Bauer KH (1963) Das Krebsproblem. Springer, Berlin Heidelberg New York

Bauer RD, McCoy CP, Roberts DK, Fritz G (1984) Malignant melanoma metastatic to the endometrium. Obstet Gynecol 63:264

Baulieu EE (1979) Current approaches to steroid hormone cell interactions. In: Juxe K, Hökfelt T, Luft R (eds) Central regulation of the endocrine system. Plenum, New York, pp 239–260

Baulieu EE, Mortel R, Robel P (1980) Estrogen and progesterone receptors in human endometrium: regulatory and pathophysiological aspects, in press

Baxter JD, Funder JW (1979) Hormone receptors. N Engl J Med 301:1149

Bayard F, Damilano S, Robel P, Baulieu EE (1978) Cytoplasmic and nuclear estradiol and progesterone receptors in human endometrium. J Clin Endocrinol Metab 46:635

Bayer R (1965) Die Endometriumreaktion auf Chlormadinoazetat bei Frauen mit monophasischer und biphasischer Zyklussteuerung. I. Langzeitbehandlung mit Kleindosen. II. Langzeitbehandlung mit ansteigenden Dosen zwischen 10 mg und 30 mg Chlormadinoazetat, Z Geburtshilfe Gynäkol 164:47, 62

Bazala V (1966) Glioma uteri (gliosis endometrii.) Geburtshilfe Frauenheilkd 26:1511

Beato M, Castano-Almendral A, Beato W (1968) Der histologische Befund des Endometriums zur Differentialdiagnose der Extrauteringravidität. Geburtshilfe Frauenheilkd 28:355

Becker V (1950) Fremdkörperreaktionen des Endometrium nach intrauteriner Sulfonamid-Applikation. Geburtshilfe Frauenheilkd 10:597

Behrens H (1953) Die Variationsmöglichkeiten im Aufbau der Uterusschleimhaut in den einzelnen Phasen des mensuellen Zyklus. Thieme, Leipzig

Behrens H (1954) Das histologische Bild der glandulären Hyperplasie, unter besonderer Berücksichtigung der atypischen Erscheinungsformen. Arch Geschwulstforsch 7:101

Behrens H (1956) Histologische Studien am Endometrium als Grundlagen klinischer Diagnostik. Thieme, Leipzig, pp 61–112

Behrens H (1956) Endometritis tuberculosa und Endometriumsfunktion. Geburtshilfe Frauenheilkd 16:623

Behrens H (1958) Die Bedeutung der atypischen Hyperplasia endometrii für die Klinik. Geburtshilfe Frauenheilkd 18:645

Beier HM (1981) Hormonal control of implantation. Proc 2nd Innsbruck Winter Conference

Beilby JOW, Farrer-Brown G, Tarbit MH (1971) The microvasculature of common uterine abnormalities other than fibroids. J Obstet Gynaecol Br Cwlth 78:361

Bellomi A, Gamoletti R (1981) Malignant histiocytic tumor presenting as a primary uterine neoplasm. A cytochemical and electron microscopic study. J Pathol 134:233

Belt WD, Anderson LL, Cavazos LF, Melampy RM (1971) Cytoplasmic granules and relaxin levels in porcine corpora lutea. Endocrinology 89:1

Bengtsson LP, Ingemansson CA (1959) Amenorrhoea associated with retention of fertility. Acta Obstet Gynecol Scand 38:62

Benjamin F, Romney SL (1964) Disturbed carbohydrate metabolism in endometrial carcinoma. Cancer (Philad) 17:386

Berg JW, Durfee GR (1958) The cytological presentation of endometrial carcinoma. Cancer (Philad) 11:158

Berger J, Dietrich FM (1957) Maligner mesenchymaler Mischtumor des Uterus. Geburtshilfe Frauenheilkd 17:1136

Berger J, Mumprecht E (1959) Beurteilung ovarieller Funktionsphasen am Endometrium mit Hilfe histochemischer Reaktionen. Saure und alkalische Phosphatase, Phosphoamidase und Glycogenfärbung. Schweiz Med Wochenschr 89:433

Bergqvist A, Jeppsson S, Kullander S, Ljungberg O (1985) Human endometrium transplanted into nude mice. Histologic effects of various steroid hormones. Am J Pathol 119:336

Bergsjö P (1962) Carcinoma uteri et ovarii. Acta Obstet Gynecol Scand 41:405

Bergsjö P (1965) Progesterone and progestational compounds in the treatment of advanced endometrial carcinoma. Acta Endocrinol (Kbh) 49:412

Bernhard W (1961) Elektronenmikroskopischer Beitrag zum Studium der Kanzerisierung und der malignen Zustände der Zelle. Verh Dtsch Ges Pathol 45:8

Bernhardt RN, Bruns PD, Drose VE (1966) Atypical endometrium associated with ectopic pregnancy. Obstet Gynecol 28:849

Berry A (1966) A cytopathological and histopathological study of bilharziasis of the female genital tract. J Pathol Bacteriol 91:325

Besch W, Wolfmüller H, Raufelder W (1984) Beitrag zur Ichthyosis uteri mit und ohne maligne Neoplasie. Pathologe 5:148

Beswick IP, Gregory MM (1971) The Arias-Stella phenomenon and the diagnosis of pregnancy. J Obstet Gynaecol Br Cwlth 78:143

Bettendorf G, Breckwoldt M (1964) Klinisch-experimentelle Untersuchungen mit hypophysärem Human-Gonadotropin. Arch Gynäkol 199:423

Bettendorf G, Breckwoldt M, Czygon PJ (1965) Klinisch-experimentelle Untersuchungen mit Clomiphen. Geburtshilfe Frauenheilkd 25:673

Beutler HK, Dockerty MB, Randall LM (1963) Precancerous lesions of the endometrium. Am J Obstet Gynecol 86:433

Bezemer PD, Baak JPA, de With C (1977) Discriminant analysis, exemplified with quantitative features of endometrium. Eur J Obstet Gynecol Reprod Biol 7/3:209

Bhatia NN, Hoshiko MG (1982) Uterine osseous metaplasia. Obstet Gynecol 60:256

Bibbo M, Kluskens L, Azizi F, et al. (1982) Accuracy of 3 sampling technics for the diagnosis of endometrial cancer and hyperplasia. J Reprod Med 27:622

Bickenbach W, Paulikovics E (1944) Hemmung der Follikelreifung durch Progesteron bei der Frau. Zentralbl Gynäkol 68:153

Bigazzi M, Nardi E, Bruni P, Petrucci F (1980) Relaxin in human decidua. J Clin Endocrinol 51:939

Bilde T (1967) Ovarian stromal hyperplasia associated with hyperoestrogenism in a postmenopausal woman. Acta Obstet Gynecol Scand 46:429

Bird CC, Willis RA (1965) The production of smooth muscle by the endometrial stroma of the adult human uterus. J Pathol Bacteriol 90:75

Birkenfeld A, Beier HM, Schenker JG (1986a) The effect of clomiphene citrate on early embryonic development, endometrium and implantation. Hum Reprod 1:387

Birkenfeld A, Navot D, Levij IS, et al. (1986b) Advanced secretory changes in the proliferative human endometrial epithelium following clomiphene citrate treatment. Fertil Steril 45:462

Biskind GR, Biskind MS (1949) Experimental ovarian tumors in rats. Am J Clin Pathol 19:501

Biskind MS, Biskind GR (1944) Development of tumors in the rat ovary after transplantation into the spleen. Proc Soc Exp Biol 55:176

Biswas B, Finbow JAH (1975) Quantitative study of uterine curettage in the menstrual cycle. J Clin Pathol 28:905

Bitensky L, Cohen S (1965) The variation of endometrial acid phosphatase activity with the menstrual cycle. J Obstet Gynaecol Br Cwlth 72:769

Bjersing L (1977) Endometrial hyperplasia and carcinoma: Histopathology and hormonal factors. Acta Obstet Gynecol Scand 65:83

Black J, Heyns OS, Gillman J (1941) The value of basal fat in the human uterus as an indicator of optimum progesterone activity. J Clin Endocrinol 1:547

Blackwell P, Fraser I (1981) Superficial lymphatics in the functional zone of normal human endometrium. Microvasc Res 21:142

Blaustein A (1982) Morular metaplasia misdiagnosed as adenoacanthoma in young women with polycystic ovarian disease. Am J Surg Pathol 6:223

Blaustein A, Payan HM, Kish M (1962) Genital stromal changes induced by malignant lymphomata and leukemia. Obstet Gynecol 20:112

Blaustein A, Shenker L, Post RC (1968) The effects of oral contraceptives of the endometrium. Int J Fertil 13:466

Blaustein A, Bigelow B, Demopoulos RI (1978) Association of carcinoma of the breast with adenosquamous carcinoma of endometrium. Cancer (Philad) 42:326

Bloch J (1931) Über einen Fall von ausgedehnter Aktinomykose des weiblichen Genitale, der Lunge und der Pleura. Arch Gynäkol 145:219

Bloomfield A (1957) Two cases of excessive uterine hypertrophy following on prolonged oestrogen administration. J Obstet Gynaecol Br Emp 64:413

Blye RP (1973) The use of estrogens as postcoital contraceptive agents. Am J Obstet Gynecol 116:1044

Board JA, Borland DS (1964) Endometrial effects of mestranol-norethindrone sequential therapy for oral contraception. Obstet Gynecol 24:655

Bobeck S (1957) Endometrial reaction in ectopic pregnancy. Acta Obstet Gynecol Scand 36:499

Böcker W (1974) The fine structure of uterine sarcomas. Pathol Res Pract 169:140

Böcker W, Stegner H-E (1974) Zur Klinik und Pathologie der Uterussarkome. Arch Gynäkol 216:235

Böcker W, Stegner H-E (1975) Mixed müllerian tumors of the uterus. Ultrastructural studies on the differentiation of rhabdomyoblasts. Virchows Arch Pathol Anat [A] 863:337

Böcker W, Stegner H-E (1975) A light and microscopic study of endometrial sarcomas of the uterus. Virchows Arch Pathol Anat [A] 368:141

Böcker W, Strecker H (1975) Electron microscopy of uterine leiomyosarcomas. Virchows Arch Pathol Anat [A] 367:59

Bohle A, Stoll P, Vosgerau H (1957) Morphologische und statistische Untersuchungen über die intrauterine Absterbeordnung in der ersten Hälfte der Schwangerschaft. Klin Wochenschr 35:358

Böhm W, Stech D (1966) Zur Morphologie und Klinik der Uterusschleimhautsarkome. Geburtshilfe Frauenheilkd 26:1040

Böhm W, Seewald H-J, Voigt R, Süss C (1977) Infektionsrisiko und Komplikationen nach IUD-Applikation. Zentralbl Gynäkol 99:1484

Bohnen P (1927) Wie weit wird das Endometrium bei der Menstruation abgestoßen? Arch Gynäkol 129:459

Bokhman JV (1983) Two pathogenetic types of endometrial carcinoma. Gynecol Oncol 15:10

Bonney WA, Glasser SR, Noyes RW, Cooper CL (1966) Endometrial response to the intrauterine device. Am J Obstet Gynecol 96:101

Bonte JB, Drochmans A, Ide P (1966) 6α-Methyl-17α-hydroxy-progesterone acetate as a chemotherapeutic agent in adenocarcinoma of the uterus. Acta Obstet Gynecol Scand 45:121

Bontke E (1960) Histochimie de l'endomètre prémenstruel et gravide. In: Ferin, Gaudefroy (eds) Les fonctions de nidation utérine et leurs troubles. Masson, Paris, p 269

Boquoi E, Kreuzer G (1973) Histomorphologische Untersuchungen an Endometriumkarzinomen unter Gestagen-Therapie (Chlormadinoazetat). Geburtshilfe Frauenheilkd 33:697

Boram LH, Erlandson RA, Hajdu SI (1972) Mesodermal mixed tumor of the uterus. Cancer (Philad) 30:1295

Borell U (1966) Contraceptive methods, their safety, efficacy and acceptability. Acta Obstet Gynecol Scand [Suppl 1] 45:9–64

Borell U, Fernström I, Westman A (1953) Hormonal influence on the uterine arteries. Acta Obstet Gynecol Scand 32:271

Borell U, Nilsson O, Westman A (1959) The cyclical changes occurring in the epithelium lining the endometrial glands. An electron-microscopical study in the human being. Acta Obstet Gynecol Scand 38:364

Borglin NE (1962) Progestational activity of ethinyl-oestrenol in amenorrhoea. Acta Endocrinol (Kbh) 39:415

Boronow RC, Morrow CP, Creasman WT et al. (1984) Surgical staging in endometrial cancer: clinical-pathologic findings of a prospective study. Obstet Gynecol 63:825

Boschann HW, Kur S (1957) Über die Wirkung des 17-Äthinyl-19-Norestosteron-önanthats, eines neuen Gestagens mit Depotcharakter auf das menschliche Endometrium und das atrophische Vaginalepithel. Geburtshilfe Frauenheilkd 17:928

Botella-Llusia J (1967) Tuberculosis of the endometrium. Proc 5th World Congr Fertil Steril Stockholm 1966. Excerpta Medica, Amsterdam, p 514

Boué J, Boué A (1973) Les avortements spontanés humains. Études cytogénétiques et épidémiologiques. Rev Fr Gynécol 68:625

Boué J, Boué A, Lazar P (1975) In: Blandau (ed) The epidemiology of human spontaneous abortions with chromosomal anomalies, aging gametes. Karger, Basel

Boutselis JG, Ullery JC (1962) Sarcoma of the uterus. Obstet Gynecol 20:23

Boutselis JG, deNeef JC, Ullery JC, George OT (1963) Histochemical observations in the normal human endometrium. Obstet Gynecol 21:423

Böving BG (1964) Das Eindringen des Trophoblasten in das Uterusepithel. Klin Wochenschr 42:467

Bowen P, Lee CSN (1969) Spontaneous abortion. Am J Obstet Gynecol 104:973

Bräunig G, Lohe K (1968) Carcinosarkom des Uterus mit besonderer histologischer Differenzierung. Arch Gynäkol 206:51

Braitenberg H v (1941) Zur pathologischen Anatomie und Klinik des proliferierenden Adenoms der Matrone. Zentralbl Gynäkol 65:2050

Brandau H, Brandau L, Luh W (1969) Histochemische Lokalisierung von Hydroxysteroid-Dehydrogenasen im menschlichen Endometrium. Arch Gynäkol 208:138

Breinl H, Warnecke W (1967) Langzeitbehandlung mit Ovulationshemmern. Med Klin 62:1835

Breipohl W (1935) Schleimhautbilder in der Menopause. Zentralbl Gynäkol 59:1998

Breiter R (1938) Über gleichzeitiges getrenntes Vorkommen von Karzinom und Sarkom im Uterus. Zentralbl Gynäkol 62:2218

Bremer E, Ober KG, Zander J (1951) Histochemische Untersuchungen über das Verhalten der Nucleinsäuren im Endometrium. Arch Gynäkol 181:96

Breuker KH, Winkhaus-Schindl I, Citoler P (1978) Chromosomenanomalien bei Ehepaaren mit wiederholten Aborten. Geburtshilfe Frauenheilkd 38:11
Brewer JJ, Foley TJ (1953) Endometrial carcinoma and hepatic cirrhosis. Obstet Gynecol 1:67
Brewer JJ, Mazur MT (1981) Gestational chorio-carcinoma. Its origin in the placenta during seemingly normal pregnancy. Am J Surg Pathol 5:267
Briggs MH, Brotherton J (1970) Steroid biochemistry and pharmacology. Academic Press, London
Brinkley D, Haybittle JL, Murrell DS (1963) The X-ray menopause in 267 cases. J Obstet Gynaecol Br Cwlth 70:1010
Bromberg YM, Liban E, Laufer H (1959) Early endometrial carcinoma following prolonged estrogen administration in an ovariectomized woman. Obstet Gynecol 14:221
Brosens IA, Pijnenborg R (1976) Comparative study of the estrogenic effect of ethinylestradiol and mestranol on the endometrium. Contraception 14:679
Bruce DF, Dick A (1956) Uterine sarcoma simulating placenta praevia. J Obstet Gynaecol Br Emp 63:884
Bruntsch KH (1950) Beitrag zur Erscheinung der sogenannten Plattenepithelknötchen in der hyperplastischen Korpusschleimhaut. Geburtshilfe Frauenheilkd 10:944
Bruntsch KH (1954) Über das Verhalten des Endometriums bei Extrauteringravidität und seine Verwertbarkeit in der klinischen Differentialdiagnostik. Ärztl Wochenschr 9:852
Brux J de, Ancla M (1964) Arias-Stella endometrial atypias. Case study with the electron microscope. Am J Obstet Gynecol 89:661
Brux J de, Dupré-Froment J (1965) Étude anatomo-pathologique de la tuberculose génitale féminine cliniquement «latente». Déductions pathogéniques et therapeutiques. Rev Fr Gynécol 60:57
Brux J de, Palmer R, Ayoub-Despois H (1956) Les ossifications de l'endomètre. Gynecol Obstét 55:494
Buchholz R, Nocke W (1965) Wirkungsmechanismen der Ovulationshemmung. Fortschr Geburtshilfe Gynäkol 21:148
Buchholz R, Nocke L, Nocke W (1962) Untersuchungen über den Wirkungsmechanismus von Äthinyl-Nortestosteron bei der Unterdrückung der Ovulation. Geburtshilfe Frauenheilkd 22:923
Büchner F (1961) Die experimentelle Kanzerisierung der Parenchymzellen in der Synopsis klassischer und moderner morphologischer Methoden. Verh Dtsch Ges Pathol 45:37
Büchner F, Oehlert W, Noltenius H (1963) Desoxyribonukleinsäure, Ribonukleinsäure und Protein bei der Regeneration and Kanzerisierung im Experiment. Dtsch Med Wochenschr 88:2277
Buehl IA, Vellios F, Carter JE, Huber CP (1964) Carcinoma in situ of the endometrium. Am J Clin Pathol 42:594
Büngeler W (1935) Akute Miliartuberkulose nach Ausschabung bei tuberkulöser Endometritis. Frankfurt Z Pathol 47:313
Büngeler W, Dontenwill W (1959) Hormonell ausgelöste geschwulstartige Hyperplasien, hyperplasiogene Geschwülste und ihre Verhaltensweisen. Dtsch Med Wochenschr 84:1885
Bullough WS (1955) Hormones and mitotic activity. Vitam Horm 13:261
Bulmer D (1965) Esterase and acid phosphatase activities in the placenta. J Anat 99:513
Burger H (1958) Zur Steuerung des Menstruationszyklus. Alte und neue Anschauungen über die Steuerung und Auslösung der Menstruationsblutung. Dtsch Med Wochenschr 83:1991
Burke L, Rubin HW, Kim I (1973) Uterine abscess formation secondary to endometrial cryosurgery. Obstet Gynecol 41:224
Burkman RT, Tonascia JA, Atienza MF, King TM (1976) Untreated endocervical gonorrhea and endometritis following elective abortion. Am J Obstet Gynecol 126:648
Burrows S, Hosten EB, Pomerantz J (1964) Lymphosarcoma of the uterus. Obstet Gynecol 24:468
Busanni-Caspari W, Undeutsch D (1956) Zum Vorkommen von Glykogen bei der glandulär-zystischen Hyperplasie des Endometriums. Arch Gynäkol 188:1

Buscema J, Klein V, Rotmensch J, et al. (1987) Uterine hemangiopericytoma. Obstet Gynecol 69:104
Butenandt A (1949) Biochemische Untersuchungen zum Problem der Krebsentstehung. Verh Dtsch Ges Inn Med 55:342
Butenandt A (1952) Karzinogene Stoffe und Tumorgenese. Verh Dtsch Ges Pathol 35:70
Büttner O (1911) Die Gestationsveränderungen der Uterusgefäße. Arch Gynäkol 94:1
Buttram VC, Vanderheyden JD, Besch PK, Acosta AA (1974) Post "pill" amenorrhoea. Int J Fertil 19:37
Buxton CL (1950) The atypical secretory phase. In: Engle (ed) Menstruation and its disorders. Thomas, Springfield, p 270
Buxton CL, Herrmann W (1961) Induction of ovulation in the human with human gonadotropins. Am J Obstet Gynecol 81:584
Bychkov V, Toto PD (1987) Histochemical study of lectin binding to gestational endometrium. Int J Gynecol Pathol 6:66
Cadena D, Cavanzo FJ, Leone CL, Taylor HB (1973) Chronic endometritis. A comparative clinicopathologic study. Obstet Gynecol 41:733
Campbell PE, Barter RA (1961) The significance of atypical endometrial hyperplasia. J Obstet Gynaecol Br Cwlth 68:668
Cardell RR, Hisaw FL, Dawson AB (1969) The fine structure of granular cells in the uterine endometrium of the rhesus monkey (macaca mulatta) with a discussion of the possible function of these cells in relaxin secretion. Am J Anat 124:307
Carlström K, Furuhjelm M (1969) Mechanisms of action of clomiphene. Acta Obstet Gynecol Scand [Suppl 3] 48:35
Carr DH (1969) Cytogenetics and the pathology of hydatidiform degeneration. Obstet Gynecol 33:333
Carr DH (1970) Chromosome studies in selected spontaneous abortions. 1. Conception after oral contraceptives. Can Med Assoc J 103:343
Carter ER, McDonald JR (1960) Uterine mesodermal mixed tumors. Am J Obstet Gynecol 80:368
Carter WF, Faucher GL, Greenblatt RB (1964) Evaluation of a new progestational agent, 6,17α-dimethyl-6-dehydro-progesterone. Am J Obstet Gynecol 89:635
Cartier R, Moricard R (1959) Variations topographiques des ultrastructures de l'épithelium cylindrique du corps utérin humain en fonction du cycle ovarien. Gynécol Obstét 58:477
Cassmer O (1959) Hormone production of the isolated human placenta. Acta Endocrinol (Kbh) [Suppl 45] 32:1
Cederqvist LL, Fuchs F (1974) Cervical perforation by the copper-T intrauterine contraceptive device. Am J Obstet Gynecol 119:854
Centaro A, Serra G (1949) Le modificazioni del reticolo dell'endometrio nelle varie fasi del ciclo ovarico e nelle vetropatie ghiandolari iperplastische. Arch Vecchi Anat Nat 12:1031
Chalvardjian A (1978) Sarcoidosis of the female genital tract. Am J Obstet Gynecol 132:78
Chalvardjian A, Picard L, Shaw R, et al. (1980) Malakoplakia of the female genital tract. Am J Obstet Gynecol 138:391
Chambers JT, Merino M, Kohorn EI, et al. (1987) Uterine papillary serous carcinoma. Obstet Gynecol 69:109
Chamlian DL, Taylor HB (1970) Endometrial hyperplasia in young women. Obstet Gynecol 36:659
Chan L, O'Malley BW (1978) Steroid hormone action: recent advances. Ann Intern Med 89:694
Chang YC, Craig JM (1963) Vaginal-smear assessment of estrogen activity in endometrial carcinoma. Obstet Gynecol 21:170
Charles D (1964) Iatrogenic endometrial patterns. J Clin Pathol 17:205
Charles D (1965) Endometrial adenoacanthoma. Cancer (Philad) 18:737
Charles D, Barr W, Bell EJ et al. (1963) Clomiphene in the treatment of oligomenorrhea and amenorrhea. Am J Obstet Gynecol 86:913

Charles D, Loraine JA, Bell ET, Harkness RA (1964) The use of chlormadinone in gynecological practice. Am J Obstet Gynecol 90:364

Charles D, Bell ET, Loraine JA, Harkness RA (1965) Endometrial carcinoma-endocrinological and clinical studies. Am J Obstet Gynecol 91:1050

Charles D, Loraine JA, Bell ET, Harkness RA (1967) The mechanism of action of clomiphen. Proc 5th World Congr Fertil Steril Stockholm 1966. Excerpta Medica, Amsterdam, p 92

Charles D, Turner JH, Redmond C (1973) The endometrial karyotypic profils of women after clomiphene citrate therapy. J Obstet Gynaecol Br Cwlth 80:264

Charpin C, Martin PA, Lavaut MN et al. (1986) Estrogen receptor immunocytochemical assay (ER-ICA) in human endometrium Int J Gynecol Pathol 5:119

Check JH, Wu C-H, Adelson HG (1985) Decreased abortions in HMG-induced pregnancies with prophylactic progesterone therapy. Int J Fertil 30:45

Chen JL, Trost DC, Wilkinson EJ (1985) Endometrial papillary adenocarcinomas: 2 clinicopathological types. Int J Gynecol Pathol 4:279

Chiari H (1955) Pathologische Anatomie des Gebärmutterkarzinoms. In: Seitz-Amreich (ed) Biologie und Pathologie des Weibes, vol IV. Urban & Schwarzenberg, München, p 534

Choo YC, Mak KC, Hsu C, Wong TS (1985) Postmenopausal uterine bleeding of nonorganic cause. Obstet Gynecol 66:225

Chorlton I, Karnei RF, King FM, Norris HJ (1974) Primary malignant reticuloendothelial diseases involving the vagina, cervix, and corpus uteri. Obstet Gynecol 44:735

Christiaens GCML, Sixma JJ, Haspels AA (1980) Morphology of haemostasis in menstrual endometrium. Br J Obstet Gynaecol 87:425

Christopherson WM, Alberhasky RC, Connelly PJ (1982a) Carcinoma of the endometrium. I. A clinicopathologic study of clear-cell carcinoma and secretory carcinoma. Cancer (Philad) 49:1511

Christopherson WM, Alberhasky RC, Connelly PJ (1982b) Carcinoma of the endometrium. II. Papillary adenocarcinoma. A clinical pathologic study of 46 cases. Am J Clin Pathol 77:534

Christopherson WM, Alberhasky RC, Connelly PJ (1982c) Glassy cell carcinoma of the endometrium. Hum Pathol 13:418

Chu F, Leprow H, Goolsick W (1958) Primary squamous-cell carcinoma of the corpus uteri. Arch Pathol 65:13

Chuang JT, van Velden DJJ, Graham JB (1970) Carcinosarcoma and mixed mesodermal tumor of the uterine corpus. Obstet Gynecol 35:769

Cianfrani R (1955) Endometrial carcinoma after bilateral oophorectomy. Am J Obstet Gynecol 69:64

Clement RB, Scully RE (1974) Müllerian adenosarcoma of the uterus. Cancer (Philad) 34:1138

Clement PB, Scully RE (1976) Uterine tumors resembling ovarian sex-cord tumors. A clinicopathologic analysis of fourteen cases. Am J Clin Pathol 66:512

Climie ARW, Rachmaninoff N (1965) A ten year experience with endometrial carcinoma. Surg Gynecol Obstet 120:73

Clyman MJ (1963) Electron-microscopic changes produced in the human endometrium by norethindrone acetate with ethinyl estradiol. Fertil Steril 14:352

Clyman MJ (1963) A new structure observed in the nucleolus of the human endometrial epithelial cell. Am J Obstet Gynecol 86:430

Clyman MJ, Spiegelman I, Ross T (1982) Appearance of tonofilaments and absence of microtubules in human endometrial glandular epithelium. Diagn Gynecol Obstet 4:173

Cohen CJ, Deppe G (1977) Endometrial carcinoma and oral contraceptive agents. Obstet Gynecol 49:390

Cohen CJ, Gusberg SB, Koffler D (1974) Histologic screening for endometrial cancer. Gynecol Oncol 2:279

Cohen C, Shulman G, Budgeon CR (1982) Endocervical and endometrial adenocarcinoma. Am J Surg Pathol 6:151

Cohen JS, Ingley H, Gayl L (1949) Hemangioendothelioma of the uterus. Am J Obstet Gynecol 57:592
Cohen S, Bitensky L, Chayen J et al. (1964) Histochemical studies on the human endometrium. Lancet II:56
Collins J (1972) Combined hormone therapy for recurrent adenocarcinoma of the endometrium. Am J Obstet Gynecol 113:842
Connell EB, Sedlis A, Stone ML (1967) Endometrial enzyme histochemistry in oral contraceptive therapy. Fertil Steril 18:35
Connelly PJ, Alberhasky RC, Christopherson WM (1982) Carcinoma of the endometrium. III. Analysis of 865 cases of adenocarcinoma and adenoacanthoma. Obstet Gynecol 59:569
Cook CL, Schroeder JA, Yussman MA, Sanfilippo JS (1984) Induction of luteal phase defect with clomiphene citrate. Am J Obstet Gynecol 149:613
Cooke ID, Morgan CA, Parry TE (1972) Correlation of endometrial biopsy and plasma progesterone levels in infertile women. J Obstet Gynaecol Br Cwlth 79:647
Copeland WE, Nelson PK, Payne FL (1957) Intrauterine radium for dysfunctional bleeding. Am J Obstet Gynecol 73:615
Corscaden JA (1956) Gynecologic cancer, 2nd edn. Williams & Wilkins, Baltimore
Corscaden JA, Gusberg SB (1947) The background of cancer of the corpus. Am J Obstet Gynecol 53:419
Corscaden JA, Fertig JW, Gusberg SB (1946) Carcinoma subsequent to the radiotherapeutic menopause. Am J Obstet Gynecol 51:1
Cosbie WG, Anderson W, Millor OB, Bunker MC (1954) Carcinoma of the body of the uterus. Am J Obstet Gynecol 67:1014
Costolow WE (1941) Treatment of uterine fibromyomas. JAMA 116:464
Courey NG, Graham JB (1964) Characteristics of women with uterine body cancer. NY State J Med 64:1724
Coutinho EM, de Souza JC, Scapo AI (1966) Reversible sterility induced by medroxyprogesterone injections. Fertil Steril 17:261
Couzinet B, Le Strat N, Ulmann A et al. (1986) Termination of early pregnancy by the progesterone antagonist RU 486 (Mifepristone). N Engl J Med 315:1565
Cove H (1979) The Arias-Stella reaction occurring in the endocervix in pregnancy. Am J Surg Pathol 3:567
Cox LW, Cox RI, Black TL (1968) Induction of ovulation. Am J Obstet Gynecol 102:177
Craig JM, Danzinger S (1965) Histological distribution and nature of stainable lipids of the human endometrium. Am J Obstet Gynecol 93:1018
Cramer H (1952) Über die Pathogenese des Schleimhautödems im Corpus uteri. Zugleich ein Beitrag zum Entstehungsmechanismus pathologischer Blutungen. Arch Gynäkol 181:549
Cramer H (1957) Die Bedeutung der Perjod-Schiff-Reaktion am Endometrium für die Diagnose des uterinen Frühaborts und der gestörten Extrauteringravidität. Geburtshilfe Frauenheilkd 17:820
Cramer H, Klöss O (1955) Verbesserung der Funktionsdiagnostik am Endometrium durch routinemäßige Darstellung der Polysaccharide. Arch Gynäkol 185:739
Cramer H, Wadulla H (1950) Abortus bei Leptospirosis canicola. Arch Gynäkol 177:167
Cramer H, Wildner GP (1953) Die Ausscheidung der östrogenen und gonadotropen Hormone im Urin bei gutartigen und bösartigen Geschwülsten. Arch Geschwulstforsch 6:36
Crepet CC, Nuova VM (1967) Resultats cytologiques des adénocarcinoms du fond et des hyperplasies chez les femmes ménopausées. Arch Anat Pathol 15:29
Crisp TM, Dessouky DA, Denys FR (1970) The fine structure of the human corpus luteum of early pregnancy and during the progestational phase of the menstrual cycle. Am J Anat 127:37
Crossen RJ, Hobbs JE (1935) Relationship of late menstruation to carcinoma of the corpus uteri. J Miss Med Assoc 32:361
Crowson LB, Winer BA, Noyes RW (1965) Evaluation of a new progestin. Obstet Gynecol 26:349

Crum CP, Richart RM, Fenoglio CM (1981) Adenoacanthosis of the endometrium. Am J Surg Pathol 5:15

Cruz-Aquino M, Shenker L, Blaustein A (1967) Pseudosarcomas of the endometrium. Obstet Gynecol 29:93

Csermely T, Demers LM, Hughes EC (1969) Organ culture of human endometrium. Obstet Gynecol 34:252

Csermely T, Hughes EC, Demers LM (1971) Effect of oral contraceptives on human endometrium in culture. Am J Obstet Gynecol 109:1066

Cullen TS (1900) Cancer of the uterus. Appleton, New York

Cutler BS, Forbes AP, Ingersoll FM, Scully RE (1972) Endometrial carcinoma after stilbestrol therapy in gonadal dysgenesis. N Engl J Med 287:628

Czernobilsky B, Garcia C-R, Wallach EE (1969) Endometrial histology and parenteral estrogen-progestogen administration. Fertil Steril 20:75

Czernobilsky B, Katz Z, Lancet M, Gaton E (1980) Endocervical-type epithelium in endometrial carcinoma. Am J Surg Pathol 4:481

Czernobilsky B, Borash A, Lancet M (1982) Partial moles: a clinicopathologic study of 25 cases. Obstet Gynecol 59:75

Czernobilsky B, Hohlweg-Majert P, Dallenbach-Hellweg G (1983) Uterine adenosarcoma: a clinicopathologic study of 11 cases with a reevaluation of histologic criteria. Arch Gynecol 233:281

Czernobilsky B, Moll R, Franke WW et al. (1984) Intermediate filaments of hormonal and neoplastic tissues of the female genital tract with emphasis on problems of differential tumor diagnosis. Pathol Res Pract 179:31

Czernobilsky B, Gaedcke G, Dallenbach-Hellweg G (1985) Endometrioid differentiation in ovarian sex cord tumor with annular tubules accompanied by gestagenic effect. Cancer (Philad) 55:738

Dabbs DJ, Geisinger KR, Norris HT (1986) Intermediate filaments in endocervical carcinomas: the diagnostic utility of vimentin patterns. Am J Surg Pathol 10:568

Daichman I, Mackles A (1966) Diagnostic curettage. A 13 year study of 585 patients. Am J Obstet Gynecol 95:212

Dalemans P, Buytaert P, Meulyzer P (1979) The gonadotropin-resistant ovary syndrome in association with secondary amenorrhea. Eur J Obstet Gynecol Reprod Biol 9:327

Dallenbach CH, Sterzik K, Dallenbach-Hellweg G (1987) Histologische Endometriumbefunde bei Patientinnen am Tage eines geplanten Embryo-Transfers. Geburtshilfe Frauenheilkd 47:623

Dallenbach FD (1966) Experimentelle Untersuchungen zur Genese des Arias-Stella-Phänomens. Verh Dtsch Ges Pathol 50:413

Dallenbach FD (1971) Beziehungen zwischen Oestrogen und Karzinogenese. Fortschr Med 89:626

Dallenbach FD (1977) Fluoreszenzoptische Befunde am Endometrium bei Kuper-T-Pessar nach Acridinorangefluorochromierung. Verh Dtsch Ges Pathol 61:419

Dallenbach FD, Dallenbach-Hellweg G (1964) Immunohistologische Untersuchungen zur Lokalisation des Relaxins in menschlicher Plazenta and Dezidua. Virchows Arch Pathol Anat 337:301

Dallenbach FD, Dallenbach-Hellweg G (1968) Fluoreszenzmikroskopische Tagesdiagnostik des menstruellen Zyklus und erste Anzeichen der senilen Involution. Verh Dtsch Ges Pathol 52:342

Dallenbach FD, Rudolph E (1974) Foam cells and estrogen activity of the human endometrium. Arch Gynäkol 217:335

Dallenbach FD, Vonderlin D (1973) The innervation of the human endometrium. Arch Gynäkol 215:365

Dallenbach-Hellweg G (1961) "Kollageneinschlüsse" in Deziduazellen und ihre praktische Bedeutung für die Diagnose einer vorausgegangenen Schwangerschaft. Geburtshilfe Frauenheilkd 21:759

Dallenbach-Hellweg G (1961) Über die Rückbildung von Decidualzellen unter Auftreten von „Kollageneinschlüssen". Virchows Arch Pathol Anat 334:195

Dallenbach-Hellweg G (1964) Über die Schaumzellen im Stroma des Endometriums: Vorkommen und histochemische Befunde. Virchows Arch Pathol Anat 338:51

Dallenbach-Hellweg G (1964) Das Karzinom des Endometrium und sein Vorstufen. Verh Dtsch Ges Pathol 48:81
Dallenbach-Hellweg G (1967) Endometrial granulocytes and implantation. Proc 5th World Congr Fertil Steril Stockholm 1966. Excerpta Medica, Amsterdam, p 411
Dallenbach-Hellweg G (1972) Therapieschäden in der Gynäkologie. Morphologische Beobachtungen über die Auswirkungen weiblicher Sexualhormone und von Stoffen mit ähnlicher Wirkung. Verh Dtsch Ges Pathol 56:252
Dallenbach-Hellweg G (1978) Häufigkeit von Spontanaborten mit und ohne vorherige Einnahme von Ovulationshemmern anhand morphologischer Untersuchungen. Gynäkol Rundsch 18:213
Dallenbach-Hellweg G (1979) Krebsvorstadien und -frühstadien im Endometrium. Verh Dtsch Ges Pathol 63:613
Dallenbach-Hellweg G (1980) Zur Ursache entzündlicher Reaktionen des Endometrium auf Intrauterinpessare. Verh Dtsch Ges Pathol 536
Dallenbach-Hellweg G (1980) The stromal and myogenic sarcomas of the uterus. Pathol Res Pract 169:127
Dallenbach-Hellweg G (1982) Vorkommen und histologische Struktur des Adenokarzinoms der Zervixschleimhaut nach langjähriger Einnahme von Ovulationshemmern. Geburtshilfe Frauenheilkd 42:249
Dallenbach-Hellweg G (1984) The endometrium of infertility. A review. Pathol Res Pract 178:527
Dallenbach-Hellweg G, Bornebusch CG (1970) Histologische Untersuchungen über die Reaktion des Endometrium bei der verzögerten Abstoßung. Arch Gynäkol 208:235
Dallenbach-Hellweg G, Brähler HJ (1960) Über Histologie und Lokalisation der Uteruscarcinoma mit besonderer Berücksichtigung der drüsig-soliden Mischformen. Z Krebsforsch 64:64
Dallenbach-Hellweg G, Dallenbach FD (1966) Experimentelle Erzeugung von Endothelproliferationen in Kapillaren und Arteriolen des Endometriums durch Relaxin und ihre Bedeutung für die Implantation und Regeneration. Verh Dtsch Ges Pathol 50:422
Dallenbach-Hellweg G, Jäger M (1969) Der Vergleich cytologischer und histologischer Befunde am normalen und carcinomatösen Endometrium. 5. Tgg. Schweiz Ges Klin Zyt, Sils-Maria
Dallenbach-Hellweg G, Sievers S (1975) Die histologische Reaktion des Endometrium auf lokal applizierte Gestagene. Virchows Arch Pathol Anat [A] 368:289
Dallenbach-Hellweg G, Wittlinger H (1976) Über ein gutartiges solides Teratom des Uterus. Beitr Pathol 158:307
Dallenbach-Hellweg G, Dawson AB, Hisaw FL (1966) The effect of relaxin on the endometrium of monkeys. Histological and histochemical studies. Am J Anat 119:61
Dallenbach-Hellweg G, Weber J, Stoll P, Velten CH (1971) Zur Differentialdiagnose adenomatöser Endometriumhyperplasien junger Frauen. Arch Gynäkol 210:303
Dallenbach-Hellweg G, Dallenbach FD, Sievers S (1979) Histologische, histochemische und fluoreszenzoptische Befunde am Endometrium nach Einlage eines Kupfer-T-Pessars. Geburtshilfe Frauenheilkd 39:575
Dallenbach-Hellweg G, Czernobilsky B, Alleman J (1986) Medroxyprogesteron-acetat bei der adenomatösen Hyperplasie des Korpusendometriums. Klinische und morphologische Untersuchungen zur Frage der Dauer und Dosierung der Gestagentherapie. Geburtshilfe Frauenheilkd 46:601
Daly DC, Walters CA, Soto-Albors CE, Riddick P (1983) Endometrial biopsy during treatment of luteal phase defects is predictive of therapeutic outcome. Fertil Steril 40:305
Daly JJ, Balogh K (1968) Hemorrhagic necrosis of the senile endometrium ("apoplexia uteri"). N Engl J Med 278:709
Damewood MD, Rosenhein NB, Grumbine FC, Parmley TH (1980) Cutaneous metastasis of endometrial carcinoma. Cancer (Philad) 46:1471
Damewood MD, Zacur HA, Hoffman GJ, Rock JA (1986) Circulating antiovarian antibodies in premature ovarian failure. Obstet Gynecol 68:850
Danforth DN, Chapman JCF (1949) The isthmic mucous membrane of the human uterus. Science 109:383

Dardi LE, Ariano L, Ariano M, Gould VE (1982) Arias-Stella reaction with prominent nuclear pseudoinclusions simulating herpetic endometritis. Diagn Gynecol Obstet 4:127

Daron GH (1936) The arterial pattern of the tunica mucosa of the uterus in macacus rhesus. Am J Anat 58:349

Daron GH (1937) The veins of the endometrium (*Macacus rhesus*) as a source of the menstrual blood. Anat Rec [Suppl 3] 67:13

Davidson EH (1965) Hormones and genes. Sci Am 212:36

Davie R, Hopwood D, Levinson DA (1977) Intercellular spaces and cell junctions in endometrial glands: their possible role in menstruation. Br J Obstet Gynaecol 84:467

Davis EW (1964) Carcinoma of the corpus uteri. Am J Obstet Gynecol 88:163

Davis HJ (1972) Intrauterine contraceptive devices: present status and future prospects. Am J Obstet Gynecol 114:134

Davis HJ, Lesinski J (1970) Mechanism of action of intrauterine contraceptives in women. Obstet Gynecol 36:350

Davis ME, Wied GL (1957) Long-acting progestational agents. 17-Ethinyl-19-nortestosterone enanthate, 17 alpha-hydroxyprogesterone carproate, and 17-alpha-hydroxyprogesteron acetate. Geburtshilfe Frauenheilkd 17:916

Dawood MY, Birnbaum SJ (1975) Unilateral tubo-ovarian abscess and intrauterine contraceptive device. Obstet Gynecol 46:429

Dazo EP, Whitehead N, Solomon C (1970) Histogenesis of microvilli and cilia in the endometrial cells: morphologic and cytochemical study. Acta Cytol 14:586

Debiasi E (1962) Les vascularisations de la muqueùse utérine. Rev Fr Gynécol 57:1

Dede JA, Plentl AA, Moore JG (1968) Recurrent endometrial carcinoma. Surg Gynecol Obstet 126:533

Deelman HT (1933) Die Histopathologie der Uterusmucosa. Thieme, Leipzig

Dehner LP, Askin FB (1975) Cytomegalovirus endometritis. Obstet Gynecol 45:211

Delforge JP, Ferin J (1970) A histometric study of two estrogens: ethinyl-estradiol and its 3-methylether derivative (mestranol): their comparative effect upon the growth of human endometrium. Contraception 1:57

Deligdisch L, Cohen GJ (1985) Histologic correlates and virulence implications of endometrial carcinoma associated with adenomatous hyperplasia. Cancer (Philad) 56:1452

Deligdisch L, Holinka CF (1986) Progesterone receptors in 2 groups of endometrial carcinoma. Cancer (Philad) 57:1385

Deligdish L, Loewenthal M (1970) Endometrial changes associated with myomata of the uterus. J Clin Pathol 23:676

Del Pozo E, Wyss H, Tolis G et al. (1979) Prolactin and deficient luteal function. Obstet Gynecol 53:282

Delprado WJ, Stevens SMB, Baird PJ (1985) Atypical polypoid adenomyoma: a case report with ultrastructural examination. Pathology 17:522

Demers LM, Csermely T, Hughes EC (1970) Culture of human endometrium. Effects of estradiol. Obstet Gynecol 36:275

Demol R, Ferin J (1964) The uterine gonadotropin content during treatment with lynestrenol. Int J Fertil 9:197

Demopoulos RI, Greco MP (1983) Mucinous metaplasia of the endometrium: ultrastructural and histochemical characteristics. Int J Gynecol Pathol 1:383

Demopoulos RI, Dubin N, Noumoff J et al. (1986) Prognostic significance of squamous differentiation in stage I endometrial adenocarcinoma. Obstet Gynecol 68:245

Denis R, Barnett JM, Forbes SE (1973) Diagnostic suction curettage. Obstet Gynecol 42:301

Derichsweiler H (1934) Über das Ödem des Endometriums. Arch Gynäkol 155:408

Dhom G (1952) Histologische Kurettagebefunde bei Frauen über 50 Jahren. Dtsch Med Wochenschr 77:77

Dhom G (1952) Über die senile Hyperplasie des Endometriums und ihre Genese. Beitr Pathol Anat 112:216

Dibbelt L, Müller HG, Ehlers F (1962) Die Häufigkeit konstitutioneller und exogener Faktoren bei Kranken mit einem Karzinom des Corpus uteri. Z Geburtshilfe Gynäkol 160:1

Dickey RP, Stone SC (1976) Progestational potency of oral contraceptives. Obstet Gynecol 47:106
Diczfalusy E (1968) Mode of action of contraceptive drugs. Am J Obstet Gynecol 100:136
Diczfalusy E, Goebelsmann U, Johannisson E et al. (1969) Pituitary and ovarian function in women on continuous low dose progestogens; effect of chlormadinone acetate and norethisterone. Acta Endocrinol (Kbh) 62:679
Dietz W (1958) Über den röntgenologischen Nachweis von Lungenmetastasen bei Genitalcarcinomen der Frau. Z Krebsforsch 62:316
Dmowski WP, Cohen MR (1975) Treatment and endometriosis with an antigonadotropin, Danazol. Obstet Gynecol 46:147
Dmowski WP, Greenblatt RB (1969) Asherman's syndrome and risk of placenta accreta. Obstet Gynecol 34:288
Dobbie BMW, Taylor CW, Waterhouse JAH (1965) A study of carcinoma of the endometrium. J Obstet Gynaecol Br Cwlth 72:659
Dockerty MB, Lovelady SB, Foust GT (1951) Carcinoma of the uterus in young women. Am J Obstet Gynecol 61:966
Dockerty MB, Smith RA, Symmonds RE (1959) Pseudomalignant endometrial changes induced by administration of new synthetic progestins. Proc Mayo Clin 34:321
Dodek OI, Kotz HL (1967) Syndrome of anovulation following the oral contraceptives. Am J Obstet Gynecol 98:1065
Döring GK (1963) Über die relative Häufigkeit des anovulatorischen Zyklus im Leben der Frau. Arch Gynäkol 199:115
Döring GK (1965) Unsere Erfahrungen mit der Ovulationsauslösung durch Clomiphen. Arch Gynäkol 202:185
Döring GK (1968) Über den anovulatorischen Zyklus als Sterilitätsursache und seine Behandlung mit Clomiphen. Fortschr Med 86:395
Dominguez H, Simowitz F, Greenblatt RB (1962) Clinical evaluation of a new oral progestin-chlormadinone. Am J Obstet Gynecol 84:1478
Donkers B, Kazzaz BA, Meijering JH (1972) Rhabdomyosarcoma of the corpus uteri. Am J Obstet Gynecol 114:1025
Dontenwill W (1961) Die endokrinen Regulationen hyperplastischer und maligner Gewebsproliferationen. Verh Dtsch Ges Pathol 45:74
Dontenwill W (1965) Krebs und Hormone. Hippokrates 36:89
Dontenwill W (1966) Erzeugung von Tumoren durch endogenhormonelle Faktoren. In: Handbuch der experimentellen Pharmakologie, vol 16, part 13: Tumoren II. Springer, Berlin Heidelberg New York, p 74
Dorfman RI (1957) Comments of the metabolism of steroid hormones. Cancer Res 17:535
Doss LL, Llorens AS, Henriquez EM (1984) Carcinosarcoma of the uterus: a 40-year experience from the state of Missouri. Gynecol Oncol 18:43
Douglas CF, Weed JC (1959) Endometriosis treated with prolonged administration of Diethylstilbestrol. Obstet Gynecol 13:744
Dowling EA, Gravlee LC, Hutchins KE (1969) A new technique for the detection of adenocarcinoma of the endometrium. Acta Cytol 13:496
Downs KA, Gibson M (1983) Clomiphene citrate therapy for luteal phase defect. Fertil Steril 39:34
Doyle LL, Clewe T (1968) Preliminary studies on the effect of hormone-releasing intrauterine devices. Am J Obstet Gynecol 101:564
Driessen LF (1914) Endometritis, Folge abnormaler Menstruation. Ursache profuser Blutungen. Zentralbl Gynäkol 38:618
Dubrauzsky V (1950) Histologische Untersuchungen der Gebärmutterschleimhaut im Wochenbett und während der Lactation. Arch Gynäkol 178:174
Dubrauszky V, Pohlmann G (1960) Strukturveränderungen am Nukleolus von Korpusendometriumzellen während der Sekretionsphase. Naturwissenschaften 47:523
Dubrauszky V, Schmitt H (1958) Mikroskopische und elektronenmikroskopische Untersuchungen am Gitterfasersystem der Corpusmucosa während des Zyklus und der Gestation. Arch Gynäkol 191:212

Dubrauszky V, Schmitt H (1961) Die Ultrastruktur des Korpusendometriums während des Cyclus. Arch Gynäkol 196:180
Dubs I (1923) Xanthomazellenbildung in der Uterusschleimhaut bei Funduskarzinom. Zentralbl Allg Pathol Anat 34:145
Dunn LJ, Merchant JA, Bradbury JT, Stone DB (1968) Glucose tolerance and endometrial carcinoma. Arch Intern Med 121:246
Dunn TB, Green AW (1963) Cysts of the epididymis, cancer of the cervix, granular cell myoblastoma, and other lesions after estrogen injection in newborn mice. JNCI 31:425
Duperroy G (1951) Morphological study of the endocervical mucosa in relation to the menstrual cycle and to leucorrhea. Gynaecologia (Basel) 131:73
Dutra F (1959) Intraglandular morules of the endometrium. Am J Clin Pathol 31:60
Dykova H, Vacek Z, Havranek F (1963) Pseudodeciduální transformace stromatu endometria u sterilnich żen. Čs Gynekol 28:439
Eastwood J (1978) Mesonephroid (clear cell) carcinoma of the ovary and endometrium. A comparative prospective clinico-pathological study and review of literature. Cancer (Philad) 41:1911
Eberl M, Pfleiderer A, Teufel G et al. (1980) Sarcomas of the uterus. Morphologic criteria and clinical course. Pathol Res Pract 189:165
Eckert J (1955) Über das Verhalten des Schleimhautstromas bei der glandulär-cystischen Hyperplasie. Arch Gynäkol 185:452
Eckman TR, Carrow LA (1962) Placental lesions in spontaneous abortion. Am J Obstet Gynecol 84:222
Eckstein RP, Russell P, Friedlander ML et al. (1985) Metastasizing placental site trophoblastic tumor: a case study. Hum Pathol 16:632
Edgar DG (1952) Progesterones in body fluids. Nature (Lond) 543
Edwards R, Brush MG, Taylor RW (1969) The uptake and intracellular distribution of (1,2-^{3}H) progesterone by human endometrium. J Endocrinol 45/1: III–IV
Edwards RG, Surani MAH (1978) The primate blastocyst and its environment. Upsala J Med Sci [Suppl] 22:39
Egger H, Kindermann G (1974) Effect of estrogens at high dosage on the human endometrium. Arch Gynäkol 216:399
Ehrlich CE, Young PCM, Cleary RE (1981) Cytoplasmic progesterone and estradiol receptors in normal, hyperplastic, and carcinomatous endometria: therapeutic implications. Am J Obstet Gynecol 141:539
Eichner E, Abellera M (1971) Endometrial hyperplasia treated by progestins. Obstet Gynecol 38:739
Eifel P, Hendrickson M, Ross J et al. (1982) Simultaneous presentation of carcinoma involving the ovary and the uterine corpus. Cancer (Philad) 50:163
El-Fiky SM, Taha YM (1976) Cytoenzymology of benign and malignant tumours of the corpus uteri. I. Respiratory enzymes. Acta Histochem 56:1
Elias EA, Elias RA, Kooistra AM et al. (1983) Fluctuations in the enzymatic activity of the human endometrium. Histochemistry 77:159
Elster K, Spanknebel G (1959) Histologische Strukturanalysen regressiv veränderten Gewebes im Abrasionsmaterial. Arch Gynäkol 192:27
Elston CW, Bagshawe KD (1972) The value of histological grading in the management of hydatidiform mole. J Obstet Gynaecol Br Cwlth 79:717
Elton XW (1942) Morphologic variations in adenocarcinoma of the fundus of the uterus, with reference to secretory activity and clinical interpretations. Am J Clin Pathol 12:32
Emmelot P, Benedetti EL (1960) Changes in the fine structure of rat liver brought about by dimethyl-nitrosamine. J Biophys Biochem Cytol 7:393
Emmrich P (1967) Zur Diagnostik von Abortiveiern an retinierten Aborten. Frankfurt Z Pathol 77:1
Engeler V, Wyss R, Koehler R (1972) Die Aspirationscurettage als diagnostischer und therapeutischer Eingriff. Schweiz Rundsch Med 61:1384
Epifanova OI (1966) Mitotic cycles in estrogen treated mice: a radioautographic study. Exp Cell Res 42:562

Epstein JA, Kupperman HS, Cutler A (1958) Comparative pharmacological and clinical activity of 19-nortestosterone and 17-hydroxyprogesterone derivatives in man. Ann NY Acad Sci 71:560

Epstein NA (1976) Prostatic biopsy. A morphologic correlation of aspiration cytology with needle biopsy histology. Cancer (Philad) 38:2078

Erb H, Ludwig KS (1965) Corpus-Luteumbildung während Einnahme eines hormonalen Antikonzeptivums. Gynaecologia (Basel) 159:309

Eriksen B (1947) Endometritis tuberculosa. Acta Obstet Gynecol Scand 27:249

Erkkola R, Liukko P (1977) Intrauterine device and ectopic pregnancy. Contraception 16:569

Esch (1929) Ein Fall von Mammakarzinom mit Metastase in die Portio und Vagina und ein Fall von Korpuskarzinom mit Pagetkrebs der Mamma. Monatsschr Geburtshilfe Gynäkol 81:451

Eufinger H (1952) Zur Frage des Menstruationsmechanismus. Geburtshilfe Frauenheilkd 12:1014

Evans HL (1982) Endometrial stromal sarcoma and poorly differentiated endometrial sarcoma. Cancer (Philad) 50:2170

Evans LH, Hähnel R (1972) Oestrogen receptors in human uterine tissue. J Endocrinol 50:209

Factor SM (1974) Papillary adenocarcinoma of the endometrium with psammoma bodies. Arch Pathol 98:201

Falconer B (1948) Investigations into the uterine mucosa. V. Normal cyclic changes of the endometrium; a critical study of phase determination. Acta Obstet Gynecol Scand 27:339

Fanger H, Barker BE (1961) Capillaries and arterioles in normal endometrium. Obstet Gynecol 17:543

Farber ER, Leahy MS, Meadows TR (1968) Endometrial blastomycosis acquired by sexual contact. Obstet Gynecol 32:195

Farrer-Brown G, Beilby JOW, Tarbit MH (1970) The blood supply of the uterus. J Obstet Gynaecol Br Cwlth 77:673, 682

Farrer-Brown G, Beilby JOW, Tarbit MH (1971) Venous changes in the endometrium of myomatous uteri. Obstet Gynecol 38:743

Farrow GM, Conventry MB, Dockerty MB (1968) Endometrial sarcoma, "stromal endometriosis". Am J Obstet Gynecol 100:301

Fasske E, Morgenroth K, Themann H, Verhagen A (1965) Vergleichende elektronenmikroskopische Untersuchungen von Proliferationsphase, glandulär-cystischer Hyperplasie und Adenocarcinom der Schleimhaut des Corpus uteri. Arch Gynäkol 200:473

Fathalla MF (1967) The occurrence of granulosa and theca tumours in clinically normal ovaries. A study of 25 cases. J Obstet Gynecol Br Cwlth 74:279

Fechner RE, Kaufman RH (1974) Endometrial adenocarcinoma in Stein-Leventhal Syndrome. Cancer (Philad) 34:444

Fechner RE, Bossart MI, Spjut HJ (1979) Ultrastructure of endometrial stromal foam cells. Am J Clin Pathol 72:628

Feichter GE, Höffken H, Heep J et al. (1982) DNA-flow cytometric measurements on the normal, atrophic, hyperplastic and neoplastic human endometrium. Virchows Arch Pathol Anat [A] 398:53

Fekete PS, Vellios F (1984) The clinical and histologic spectrum of endometrial stromal neoplasias. Int J Gynecol Pathol 3:198

Fekete PS, Vellios F, Patterson BD (1985) Uterine tumor resembling an ovarian sex-cord tumor: report of a case of an endometrial stromal tumor with foam cells and ultrastructural evidence of epithelial differentiation. Int J Gynecol Pathol 4:378

Feldhaus FJ, Themann H, Wagner H, Verhagen A (1977) Feinstrukturelle Untersuchungen über das Nuclear-Channel-System im menschlichen Endometrium. Arch Gynäkol 223:195

Fenoglio CM, Crum CP, Ferenczy A (1982) Endometrial hyperplasia and carcinoma. Are ultrastructural, biochemical and immunocytochemical studies useful in distinguishing between them? Pathol Res Pract 174:257

Ferenczy A (1976) Studies on the cytodynamics of human endometrial regenerations.

I. Scanning electron microscopy. II. Transmission electron microscopy and histochemistry. Am J Obstet Gynecol 124:64, 582
Ferenczy A (1976) The ultrastructural morphology of gynecologic neoplasms. Cancer (Philad) 38:463
Ferenczy A (1980) Morphological effects of exogenous gestagens on abnormal human endometrium. In: Dallenbach-Hellweg G (ed) Functional morphologic changes in female sex organs induced by exogenous hormones. Springer, Berlin Heidelberg New York, p 101
Ferenczy A, Richart RM, Agathe FJ et al. (1972) Scanning electron microscopy of the human endometrial surface epithelium. Fertil Steril 23:515
Ferenczy A, Shore M, Guralnick M, Gelfand MM (1979) The Kevorkian curette. An appraisal of its effectiveness in endometrial evaluation. Obstet Gynecol 54:262
Ferenczy A, Bertardo G, Gelford MM (1979) Studies on the cytodynamics of human endometrial regeneration. III. In vitro short-term incubation historadioautography. Am J Obstet Gynecol 134:297
Feria-Velasco A, Aznar-Ramos R, Gonzales-Angulo A (1972) Ultrastructural changes found in the endometrium of women using megestrol for contraception. Contraception 5:187
Ferin J (1954) In: Colloques sur la fonction lutéale. Biologie, exploration fonctionnelle et pathologie. Masson, Paris
Ferin J (1955) Les critères endometriaux de l'action progestinique. Bull Soc R Belge Gynecol Obstet 25:384
Ferin J (1963) Critères endométriaux de l'activité du corps jaune non gravidique. D'insuffisance lutéale. Masson, Paris, p 235
Ferin J (1964) Hypoestrogenic amenorrhea and/or sterility induced by lynestrenol. Int J Fertil 9:29
Fettig O (1965) ^{3}H-Index-Bestimmungen und Berechnungen der mittleren Generationszeit (Lebensdauer) der Einzelabschnitte des gesunden und krankhaften Endometriums nach autoradiographischen Untersuchungen mit ^{3}H-Thymidin. Arch Gynäkol 200:659
Fettig O (1965) Autoradiographische Untersuchungen der DNS-, RNS- und Protein-Synthese im menschlichen Endometrium in Abhängigkeit von der Ovulation. Arch Gynäkol 202:246
Fettig O, Kopecky P (1968) Klinische und morphologische Untersuchungen zur hormonellen Antikonzeption mit der Sequential-Methode. Geburtshilfe Frauenheilkd 28:540
Fettig O, Oehlert W (1964) Autoradiographische Untersuchungen der DNS- und Eiweiß-Neubildung im gynäkologischen Untersuchungsmaterial. Arch Gynäkol 199:649
Fettig O, Sievers R (1966) Die primäre karzinomatöse Entartung der Zervixpolypen. Zentralbl Gynäkol 88:808
Feyrter F (1952) Zur Frage der hellen Zellen der menschlichen Gebärmutterschleimhaut. Virchows Arch Pathol Anat 321:134
Feyrter F (1957) Über den zelligen Bestand des Stromas der menschlichen Corpusmucosa. Arch Gynäkol 190:47
Feyrter F, Froewis J (1949) Zur Frage der „hellen Zellen" in der Schleimhaut der menschlichen Gebärmutter. Gynaecologia (Basel) 127:33
Feyrter F, Klima R (1958) Zur Frage der sog. monozytären Rundzellen in der menschlichen Corpusmucosa. Virchows Arch Pathol Anat 331:456
Fields PA, Larkin LH (1981) Purification and immunohistochemical localization of relaxin in the human term placenta. J Clin Endocrinol Metab 52:79
Fienberg R (1958) Ovarian estrogenic tumors and diffuse estrogenic thecomatosis in postmenopausal colporrhagia. The importance of the benign endometrial mitosis. Am J Obstet Gynecol 76:851
Fienberg R (1963) Thecosis: a study of diffuse stromal thecosis of the ovary and superficial collagenization with follicular cysts (Stein-Leventhal ovary). Obstet Gynecol 21:687
Fienberg R (1969) The stromal theca cell and postmenopausal endometrial adenocarcinoma. Cancer (Philad) 24:32

Fienberg R, Lloyd HED (1974) The Arias-Stella reaction in early normal pregnancy – an involutional phenomenon. Hum Pathol 5:183
Filipe MI, Dawson IMP (1968) Qualitative and quantitative enzyme histochemistry of the human endometrium and cervix in normal and pathological conditions. J Pathol Bacteriol 95:243
Finke L (1950) Ergebnisse fluorescenzmikroskopischer Untersuchungen zum Nachweis von Tuberkelbacillen bei der weiblichen Genitaltuberkulose. Arch Gynäkol 177:440
Fischer H (1957) Obduktionsbefunde beim Corpus-Carcinom des Uterus. Arch Gynäkol 188:329
Fleming S, Tweeddale DN, Roddick JW (1968) Ciliated endometrial cells. Am J Obstet Gynecol 102:186
Flowers CE, Wilborn WH (1978) New observations on the physiology of menstruation. Obstet Gynecol 51:16
Flowers CE, Wilborn WN, Enger J (1974) Effects of quingestanol acetate on the histology, histochemistry, and ultrastructure of the human endometrium. Am J Obstet Gynecol 120:589
Fluhmann CF (1928) Squamous epithelium in the endometrium in benign and malignant conditions. Surg Gynecol Obstet 46:309
Fluhmann CF (1953) The histogenesis of squamous cell metaplasia of the cervix and endometrium. Surg Gynecol Obstet 97:45
Fluhmann CF (1954) Comparative studies of squamous metaplasia of the cervix uteri and endometrium. Am J Obstet Gynecol 68:1447
Foix A, Bruno RO, Davison T, Lema B (1966) The pathology of postcurettage intrauterine adhesions. Am J Obstet Gynecol 96:1027
Foraker AG, Celi PA, Denham SW (1954) Dehydrogenase activity in normal and hyperplastic endometrium. Cancer (Philad) 7:100
Forbes JA, Heinz JC (1953) Glycogen synthesis in human endometrium. A histochemical study using frozen dried material. Aust NZ J Surg 22:297
Forbes TR (1953) Pre-ovulatory progesterons in the peripheral blood of the rabbit. Endocrinology 53:79
Foss BA, Horne HW, Hertig AT (1958) The endometrium and sterility. Fertil Steril 9:193
Foster LN, Montgomery R (1965) Endometrial carcinoma. A review of prior biopsies. Am J Clin Pathol 43:26
Fox H (1984) Endometrial carcinogenesis and its relation to oestrogens. Pathol Res Pract 179:13
Fox H, More JRS (1965) Primary malignant lymphoma of the uterus. J Clin Pathol 18:723
Fox H, Harilal KR, Youell A (1979) Müllerian adenosarcoma of the uterine body: a report of nine cases. Histopathology 3:167
Frampton J (1963) Fluorescence microscopy applied to frozen tissue sections of the uterine cervix and endometrium. J Obstet Gynaecol Br Cwlth 70:976
Franz G (1965) Beurteilung von Behandlungsergebnissen beim Endometriumkarzinom unter Berücksichtigung des Malignitätsindex. Krebsarzt 20:193
Fraser IS, Baird DT (1972) Endometrial cystic glandular hyperplasia in adolescent girls. J Obstet Gynaecol Br Cwlth 79:1009
Frederiksen T (1958) The Arias-Stella reaction as an aid in the diagnosis of ectopic pregnancy. Acta Obstet Gynecol Scand 37:86
Freischütz G, Jopp H (1964) Ein neuentwickeltes Gerät für die Endometrium-Saugbiopsie. Geburtshilfe Frauenheilkd 24:1060
Frick HC (1965) Progestational drugs in the management of endometrial cancer. Metabolism 14:348
Frick HC, Munnell EW, Richart RM et al. (1973) Carcinoma of the endometrium. Am J Obstet Gynecol 115:663
Fridhandler L (1968) Gametogenesis to implantation. In: Assali NS (ed) Biology of gestation, vol I: The material organism. Academic Press, New York, p 67
Friedley NJ, Rosen S (1975) Carbonic anhydrase activity in the mammalian ovary, fallopian tube, and uterus: histochemical and biochemical studies. Biol Reprod 12:293

Friedman S, Goldfien A (1969) Amenorrhea and galactorrhea following oral contraceptive therapy. JAMA 210:1888

Friedrich ER (1967) Effects of contraceptive hormone preparations on the fine structure of the endometrium. Obstet Gynecol 30:201

Friedrich ER, Meyer JS (1982) Estrogen-progestin pharmacodynamics of the postmenopausal endometrium studied by thymidine labeling. Am J Obstet Gynecol 143:352

Froboese C (1924) Die Verfehlung des Endometriums. Beitrag zur normalen und pathologischen Anatomie der Uterusschleimhaut. Virchows Arch Pathol Anat 250:296

Froewis J, Ulm R (1957) Weitere tierexperimentelle Untersuchungen zur Frage der inneren Sekretion des Uterus. Acta Neuroveg (Wien) 15:101

Fruin DH, Tighe JR (1967) Tubal metaplasia of the endometrium. J Obstet Gynaecol Br Cwlth 74:93

Fuchs M (1959) Über die "hellen Zellen" im Epithel der menschlichen Uterusschleimhaut. Acta Anat (Basel) 39:244

Fuhrmann K (1959) Kolorimetrische Bestimmung und histochemischer Nachweis der Aminopeptidase an Geweben weiblicher Genitalorgane. Zentralbl Gynäkol 81:1105

Fuhrmann K (1961) Hormone und Fermente des Endometriums. Gynaecologia (Basel) 152:1

Fujikura T, Ezaki K, Nishimura H (1971) Chorionic villi and syncytial sprouts in spontaneous and induced abortions. Am J Obstet Gynecol 110:547

Fukuma K, Fukushima T, Matsuo I et al. (1983a) A graduated regimen of clomiphene citrate, its correlation to glycogen content of the endometrium and serum levels of estradiol and progesterone in infertile patients at the midluteal phase. Fertil Steril 39:780

Fukuma K, Mimori H, Matsuo I et al. (1983b) Hormone dependency of carcinoma of the human endometrium. Effect of progesterone on glycogen metabolism in the carcinoma tissue. Cancer (Philad) 51:288

Funder JW, Mercer J, Hood J (1976) SC 23992: radioreceptor assays for therapeutic and side effects. Clin Sci Mol Med [Suppl 3] 51:333

Furth J, Butterworth J (1936) Neoplastic diseases occurring among mice subjected to general irradiation with X-ray. Am J Cancer 28:66

Gambrell RD (1977) Estrogens, progestogens and endometrial cancer. J Reprod Med 18:301

Gambrell RD (1978) The role of hormones in endometrial cancer. South Med J 71:1280

Gambrell RD, Massey FM, Castaneda TA et al. (1980) Use of the progestogen challenge test to reduce the risk of endometrial cancer. Obstet Gynecol 55:732

Ganem KJ, Parsons L, Friedell GH (1962) Endometrial ossification. Am J Obstet Gynecol 83:1592

Garcia CR (1967) The oral contraceptive, an appraisal and review. Am J Med Sci 253:718

Garcia J, Jones GS, Wentz AC (1977) The use of clomiphene citrate. Fertil Steril 28:707

Garcia-Bunuel R, Brandes D (1966) Lysosomal enzymes in human endometrium. A histochemical study of acid phosphatase, nonspecific esterase, and E-600 resistant esterase. Am J Obstet Gynecol 94:1045

Gardner JM, Mishell DR (1970) Analysis of bleeding patterns and resumption of fertility following discontinuation of a long acting injectable contraceptive. Fertil Steril 21:286

Gardner WU (1939) Estrogens in carcinogenesis. Arch Pathol 27:138

Gardner WU, Pfeiffer CA, Trentin JJ, Wolstenholme JT (1959) Hormonal factors in experimental carcinogenesis. In: Homburger, Fishman (eds) The physiology of cancer, 2nd edn. Hoeber-Harper, New York

Garnet JD (1958) Constitutional stigmas associated with endometrial carcinoma. Am J Obstet Gynecol 76:11

Gauribazaz-Malik Maheshwari B, Neera L (1983) Tuberculous endometritis: a clinicopathological study of 1000 cases. Br J Obstet Gynaecol 90:84

Gebhard C (1903) Eine Mischgeschwulst des Uterus (Endothelium mit Fett- und Knorpelgewebe). Z Geburtshilfe Gynäkol 48:111

Gehring U, Tomkins GM, Ohne S (1971) Effect of the androgen-insensitivity mutation on a cytoplasmic receptor for dihydrotestosterone. Nature (Lond) 232:106

Geiger W (1980) Diagnostik und Pathophysiologie endokriner Störungen bei der Frau. In: Kaiser R, Schumacher GFB (eds) Die menschliche Fortpflanzung und ihre Störungen. Thieme, Stuttgart
Geisinger KK, Marshall RB, Kute TE, Homesley HD (1986) Correlation of female sex steroid hormone receptors with histologic and ultrastructural differentiation to adenocarcinoma of the endometrium. Cancer (Philad) 58:1506
Geisler HE, Gibbs CP (1968) Invasive carcinoma of the endometrium. Am J Obstet Gynecol 102:516
Geist SH, Walter RI, Salmon VJ (1941) Are estrogens carcinogenic in the human female? Am J Obstet Gynecol 42:242
Geller HF, Lohmeyer H (1959) Über die Endokrinie der menschlichen Gebärmutterschleimhaut. Arch Gynäkol 192:44
Gemzell C (1966) Human pituitary gonadotropins in the treatment of sterility. Fertil Steril 17:149
Gerdes H, Schulte H (1966) Über das Vorkommen von kernhaltigen Erythrozyten in den Chorionzotten bei Aborten. Frankfurt Z Pathol 75:141
Gerschenson LE, Fennell R (1982) A developmental view of endometrial hyperplasia and carcinoma based on experimental research. Pathol Res Pract 174:285
Gigon U, Herzer H, Stamm O, Zarro D (1970) Endometriumveränderungen und luteotrope Sekretionsanomalien bei Gelbkörperinsuffizienz. Z Geburtshilfe Gynäkol 173:304
Gillam JS (1955) Study of the inadequate secretion phase endometrium. Fertil Steril 6:18
Glass SJ, Miller W, Rosenblum G (1955) Secretory hypoplasia of the endometrium. Fertil Steril 6:344
Gloor E (1979) Müllerian adenosarcoma of the uterus. Am J Surg Pathol 3:203
Gloor E, Dialdes J, Hurlimann J et al. (1983) Placental site trophoblastic tumor (trophoblastic pseudotumor) of the uterus with metastases and fatal outcome: clinical and autopsy observations of a case. Am J Surg Pathol 7:483
Goecke H (1932) Thrombopenie als Ursache juveniler Blutungen und ihre Behandlung. Arch Gynäkol 151:330
Goecke H, Schwanitz G, Muradow I, Zerres K (1985) Pathomorphologie und Genetik in der Frühschwangerschaft. Pathologe 6:249
Gold JJ, Borushek S, Smith L, Scommegna A (1965) Synthetic progestins: a review. Int J Fertil 10:99
Goldberg B, Jones HW (1956) Acid phosphatase of the endometrium. Histochemical demonstration in various normal and pathologic conditions. Obstet Gynecol 7:542
Goldfarb AF (1964) Advances in the treatment of menstrual dysfunction. Lea & Febiger, Philadelphia
Golditch IM (1972) Postcontraceptive amenorrhea. Obstet Gynecol 39:903
Goldman JA, Gans B (1967) Stromal endometriosis or endometrial sarcoma. Obstet Gynecol 29:12
Goldman RL (1970) Herpetic inclusions in the endometrium. Obstet Gynecol 36:603
Goldzieher JW, Rice-Wray E (1966) Oral contraception; mechanism and management. Thomas, Springfield
Goldzieher JW, Rice-Wray E, Schulz-Contreras M, Aranda-Rosell A (1962) Fertility following termination of contraception with norethindrone-endometrial morphology and conception rate. Am J Obstet Gynecol 84:1474
Goldzieher JW, Becerra C, Gual S et al. (1964) New oral contraceptiva. Sequential estrogen and progestin. Am J Obstet Gynecol 90:404
Gompel C (1962) The ultrastructure of the human endometrial cell studied by electron microscopy. Am J Obstet Gynecol 84:1000
Gompel C (1964) Structure fine des mitochondries de la cellule glandulaire endométriale humaine au cours du cycle menstrual. J Microsc 3:427
Gonzalez-Angulo A, Aznar-Ramos R (1976) Ultrastructural studies on the endometrium of women wearing TCu-200 intrauterine devices by means of transmission and scanning electron microscopy and x-ray dispersive analysis. Am J Obstet Gynecol 125:170

Good RG, Moyer DL (1968) Estrogen-progesterone relationships in the development of secretory endometrium. Fertil Steril 19:37

Gordon M, Kohorn EI, Gore BZ, Rice SI (1973) Effect of postovulatory oestrogens on the fine structure of the epithelial cell in human endometrium. J Reprod Fertil 34:375

Gore BZ, Gordon M (1974) Fine structure of epithelial cell of secretory endometrium in unexplained primary infertility. Fertil Steril 25:103

Gore H, Hertig AT (1962) Premalignant lesions of the endometrium. Clin Obstet Gynecol 5:1148

Gore H, Hertig AT (1962) The pathologic anatomy of uterine carcinoma. Acad Med NJ Bull 8:218

Gore H, Hertig AT (1966) Carcinoma in situ of endometrium. Am J Obstet Gynecol 94:134

Gorlitzsky GA, Kase NG, Speroff L (1978) Ovulation and pregnancy rates with clomiphene citrate. Obstet Gynecol 51:265

Gorski J, Gannon F (1976) Current models of steroid hormone action: a critique. Annu Rev Physiol 38:425

Gosch J (1949) Bilder des klimakterischen und senilen Korpusendometrium bei starken hormonellen und entzündlichen Reizen. Geburtshilfe Frauenheilkd 9:201

Gräfenberg E (1931) Einfluß der intrauterinen Konzeptionsverhütung auf die Uterusschleimhaut. Arch Gynäkol 114:345

Graham CE, McClure HM, Collins DC (1980) Uterine tumors in nonhuman primates after estrogen exposure. In: Dallenbach-Hellweg G (ed) Functional morphologic changes in female sex organs induced by exogenous hormones. Springer, Berlin Heidelberg New York, p 29

Grattarola R (1969) Misdiagnosis of endometrial adenocarcinoma in young women with polycystic ovarian disease. Am J Obstet Gynecol 105:498

Grattarola R (1973) Misdiagnosis of endometrial adenoacanthoma in a 27-year-old woman with adrenocortical tumor. Oncology 28:246

Gray JD (1956) The problem of spontaneous abortion. II. Changes in the placental villi. Am J Obstet Gynecol 72:615

Gray JD, Barnes ML (1964) Histogenesis of endometrial carcinoma. Ann Surg 159:976

Gray JD, Christopherson WM, Hoover RN (1977) Estrogens and endometrial carcinoma. Obstet Gynecol 49:385

Greenblatt RB, Zarate A (1967) Endometrial studies following Quinestrol administration. Int J Fertil 12:187

Greenblatt RB, Hammond DO, Clark SL (1954) Membrane dysmenorrhea: studies in etiology and treatment. Am J Obstet Gynecol 68:835

Greenblatt RB, Barfield WE, Jungck EC, Ray AW (1961) Induction of ovulation with M.R.L.41. JAMA 178:101

Greenblatt RB, Gambrell RD, Stoddard LD (1982) The protective role of progesterone in the prevention of endometrial cancer. Pathol Res Pract 174:297

Greene GL, Nolan C, Engler JP, Jensen EV (1980) Monoclonal antibodies to human estrogen receptor. Proc Natl Acad Sci USA 77:5115

Greene GL, Sobel NB, King WJ, Jensen EV (1984) Immunochemical studies of estrogen receptors. J Steroid Biochem 2:51

Greene HSN (1941) Uterine adenomata in the rabbit. III. Susceptibility as a function of constitutional factors. J Exp Med 73:273

Greene RR, Gerbie AB (1954) Hemangiopericytoma of the uterus. Obstet Gynecol 3:150

Greene RR, Peckham BM (1951) Carcinogenic cells in the ovary? Am J Obstet Gynecol 61:657

Greenwald P, Caputo TA, Wolfgang PE (1977) Endometrial cancer after menopausal use of estrogens. Obstet Gynecol 50:239

Greenwood SM, Moran JJ (1981) Chronic endometritis: morphologic and clinical observations. Obstet Gynecol 58:176

Greenwood SM, Wright DJ (1979) Evaluation of the office endometrial biopsy in the detection of endometrial carcinoma and atypical hyperplasia. Cancer (Philad) 43:1474

Gremme A (1932) Über die Ursache und Ursprung von Genitalblutungen der Frau bei der essentiellen Thrombopenie. Arch Gynäkol 149:515

Grimalt M, Arguelles M, Ferenczy A (1975) Papillary cystadenofibroma of endometrium: A histochemical and ultrastructural study. Cancer (Philad) 36:137

Gropp A (1967) Chromosomenuntersuchungen bei Spontanabortus. Verh Dtsch Ges Pathol 51:278

Gross SJ (1964) Ribonucleoprotein, glucuronidase, and phosphamidase in normal and abnormal endometrium. Am J Obstet Gynecol 90:166

Gross SJ (1964) Histochemistry of normal and abnormal endometrium. Nonspecific esterase, acid phosphatase, and alkaline phosphatase. Am J Obstet Gynecol 88:647

Gross SJ, Lee OK, Maeck JS van, Sims EAH (1957) The immediate puerperium. II. Endometrium and urinary lactose. Obstet Gynecol 10:504

Grosser O (1948) Über die Ursachen des Abortus. Arch Gynäkol 176:1

Gruenwald P (1965) Decidual sloughing in abortion, premature birth and abruptio placentae. Bull Johns Hopkins Hosp 116:363

Grund G, Siegel P (1954) Gemeinsames Auftreten von Hämangiomen der Haut und des Endometrium. Zentralbl Gynäkol 76:1232

Gruner W (1942) Anatomische Bilder zur sekretorischen Umwandlung der glandulären Hyperplasie. Arch Gynäkol 172:465

Gruner W (1942) Ein Beitrag zum anatomischen, klinischen und hormonalen Bilde der glandulären Hyperplasie des Endometriums und deren sekretorischer Umwandlung. Virchows Arch Pathol Anat 308:265

Gumbrecht P (1936) Schleimhautveränderungen (Metaplasie) des Uterus bei Dauerzufuhr von Follikelhormonen. Arch Gynäkol 160:525

Gunning JE, Moyer D (1967) The effect of medoxyprogesterone acetate on endometriosis in the human female. Fertil Steril 18:759

Günther J (1967) Histologische Formen und Malignitätsgrade der Uterussarkome. Zentralbl Gynäkol 89:1185

Gupta RK, Schueller ES (1967) Acid mucopolysaccharide and mast cell variations in endometrium and some uterine tumors. Obstet Gynecol 30:510

Gusberg SB (1947) Precursors of corpus carcinoma: I. Estrogens and adenomatous hyperplasia. Am J Obstet Gynecol 54:905

Gusberg SB (1967) Views and reviews. Hormone-dependence of endometrial cancer. Obstet Gynecol 30:287

Gusberg SB (1976) The individual at high risk for endometrial carcinoma. Am J Obstet Gynecol 126:535

Gusberg SB, Hall RE (1961) Precursors of corpus cancer. III. The appearance of cancer of the endometrium in estrogenically conditioned patients. Obstet Gynecol 17:397

Gusberg SB, Kaplan AL (1963) Precursors of corpus cancer. IV. Adenomatous hyperplasia as stage 0 carcinoma of the endometrium. Am J Obstet Gynecol 87:662

Gusberg SB, Kardon P (1971) Proliferative endometrial response to theca-granulosa cell tumors. Am J Obstet Gynecol 111:633

Gusberg SB, Moore DB, Martin F (1954) Precursors of corpus cancer. II. A clinical and pathologic study of adenomatous hyperplasia. Am J Obstet Gynecol 68:1472

Haake KW, Ruckhäberle KE, Bilek K (1982) Histochemische Untersuchungen am Endometrium nach laparoskopischer Follikelpunktion zur Eizellgewinnung. Zentralbl Gynäkol 104:1072

Haberlandt L (1921) Über hormonale Sterilisierung des weiblichen Tierkörpers. Münch Med Wochenschr 68:1577

Hachisuga T (1986) Endometrial carcinoma. A histopathologic analysis of 155 cases with special reference to prognostic factors and background lesions. Fukuoka Igaku Zasshi 77:314

Hackl H (1968) Der Effekt peroraler Antikonzeptionsmittel auf den in vitro-Glucosestoffwechsel des Endometrium. Arch Gynäkol 205:398

Hackl H (1968) Hormonbehandeltes Corpuscarcinom und dessen in vitro-Glucosemetabolismus. Arch Gynäkol 206:252

Hafez ESE, Ludwig H, Metzger H (1975) Human endometrial fluid kinetics as observed by scanning electron microscopy. Am J Obstet Gynecol 122:929

Hagenfeldt K (1972) Intrauterine contraception with the copper-T-device. Contraception 6:37, 191, 207, 219
Haines M, Taylor CW (1962) Gynaecological pathology. Churchill, London
Halban J (1922) Keimdrüse und Geschlechtsentwicklung. Arch Gynäkol 117:289
Halbert DR, Chistian CD (1969) Amenorrhea following oral contraceptives. Obstet Gynecol 34:161
Halbrecht I (1965) Endometrial and tubal sequelae of latent nonspecific infections. Int J Fertil 10:121
Hale RW, Reich LA, Joiner JM et al. (1976) Histopathologic evaluation of uteri curetted by flexible suction cannula. Am J Obstet Gynecol 125:805
Hall EV van, Mastboom JL (1969) Luteal phase insufficiency in patients treated with clomiphene. Am J Obstet Gynecol 103:165
Hall HH, Sedlis A, Chabon I, Stone ML (1965) Effect of intrauterine stainless steel rings on endometrial structure and function. Am J Obstet Gynecol 93:1031
Hall JE (1950) Alkaline phosphatase in human endometrium. Am J Obstet Gynecol 60:212
Hall JE, Nelms WF (1953) Carcinosarcoma of the endometrium. Am J Obstet Gynecol 65:433
Hall KU (1957) Irregular hyperplasias of the endometrium. Acta Obstet Gynecol Scand 36:306
Haller J (1966) Wahrscheinlicher Wirkungsmechanismus der oralen Kontrazeptiva. Dtsch Med Wochenschr 91:7
Haller U, Kubli F, Bräunig G et al. (1973) Die diagnostische Aspirationskürettage. Geburtshilfe Frauenheilkd 33:1
Hameed K, Morgan DA (1972) Papillary adenocarcinoma of endometrium with psammoma bodies. Cancer (Philad) 29:1326
Hamilton TH (1964) Sequences of RNA und protein synthesis during early estrogen action. Proc Natl Acad Sci (USA) 51:83
Hamilton TH, Teng CS, Means AR (1968) Early estrogen action: nuclear synthesis and accumulation of protein correlated with enhancement of two DNA-dependent RNA polymerase activities. Biochemistry 59:1265
Hammerstein J (1965) Die Ausscheidung von Steroiden und Gonadotropinen im anovulatorischen Cyklus der Frau. Arch Gynäkol 200:638
Hammond CB, Jelovsek FR, Lee KL et al. (1979) Effects of long-term estrogen replacement therapy. II. Neoplasia. Am J Obstet Gynecol 133:537
Hamperl H (1950) Über die "hellen" Flimmerepithelzellen der menschlichen Uterusschleimhaut. Virchows Arch Pathol Anat 319:265
Hamperl H (1952) Über Gutartigkeit und Bösartigkeit von Geschwülsten. Verh Dtsch Ges Pathol 35:29
Hamperl H (1954) Über die endometrialen Granulozyten (endometriale Körnchenzellen). Klin Wochenschr 32:665
Hamperl H (1956) Die Morphologie der Tumoren. In: Büchner F, Letterer E, Roulet F (eds) Handbuch der Allgemeinen Pathologie, vol VI/3. Springer, Berlin Göttingen Heidelberg
Hamperl H (1957) Über die Entwicklung (Progression) von Tumoren. Wien Klin Wochenschr 69:201
Hamperl H (1958) Über „Kollageneinschlüsse" in Dezidualzellen. Klin Wochenschr 36:939
Hamperl H, Kaufmann C, Ober KG (1959) Wuchernde Glia im Endometrium. Geburtshilfe Frauenheilkd 19:978
Hando T, Okada DM, Zamboni L (1968) Atypical cilia in human endometrium. J Cell Biol 39:475
Hanski W (1971) Gliomatosis uteri. Pol Med J 10:273
Hanson DJ (1959) Studies of the endometrial stroma in cystic glandular hyperplasia. Am J Clin Pathol 32:152
Harkin HC (1956) Deoxyribonucleic acid (DNA) content of human endometrium. A microspectrophotometric study of the endometrial glandular nuclei in the physiologic cycle and in atrophy. Arch Pathol 61:24

Harnett LW (1949) A statistical report on 955 cases of cancer of the cervix uteri and 321 cases of cancer of the corpus uteri. Br J Cancer 3:433
Harris HR (1958) Foam cells in the stroma of carcinoma of the body of the uterus and uterine cervical polyps. J Clin Pathol 11:19
Hartmann CG, Geschikter GF, Speert H (1941) Effects of continuous estrogen administration in very large doses. Anat Rec [Suppl 2] 79:31
Harvey WF, Hamilton TD (1935) Carcino-sarcoma: a study of the microscopic anatomy and meaning of a peculiar cancer. Edinb Med J 42:337
Haskins AL, Moszkowski EF, Whitelock VP (1968) The estrogenic potential of estriol. Am J Obstet Gynecol 102:665
Haspels AA (1970) Depot-gestagen voor contraceptic. Ned Tijdschr Geneeskd 114:61
Haspels AA (1973) Anwendung der Intrauterinpessare. Arch Gynäkol 214:464
Haspels AA, Andriesse R (1973) The effect of large dosis of estrogens post coitum in 2000 women. Eur J Obstet Gynecol Reprod Biol 3/4:113
Haspels AA, Linthorst GA, Kicovic PM (1977) Effect of postovulatory administration of a "morning-after" injection on corpus luteum function and endometrium. Contraception 15:105
Hasselgren PO, Bolin T (1977) Postmenopausal tuberculous pyometra. Acta Obstet Gynecol Scand 56:23
Hata Y, Isaihama A, Kudo N et al. (1969) The effect of long-term use of intrauterine devices. Int J Fertil 14:246
Hathcock EW, Williams GA, Engelhardt III SM, Murphy AL (1974) Office aspiration curettage of the endometrium. Am J Obstet Gynecol 120:205
Haude H (1956) Betrachtungen über Fremdkörperschäden im Peritoneum und Endometrium. Ärztl Forsch 10:110
Hausknecht RU, Gusberg SB (1973) Estrogen metabolism in patients at high risk for endometrial carcinoma. Am J Obstet Gynecol 116:981
Heckeroth V, Ziegler HK (1986) Zur Kenntnis der Ichthyosis uteri. Geburtshilfe Frauenheilkd 46:248
Heinen G (1971) The discriminating use of combination and sequential preparations in the hormonal inhibition of ovulation. Contraception 4:393
Heinicke G (1959) Schleimhautbefunde bei Uterus myomatosus. Zentralbl Allg Pathol Anat 99:263
Held E (1969) Kritische Bemerkungen zur neuen Einteilung des Korpuskarzinoms. Ein Beitrag zur Pathologie, Prognose und Therapie. Geburtshilfe Frauenheilkd 29:301
Hellweg G (1954) Über endometriale Körnchenzellen (endometriale Granulozyten). Arch Gynäkol 185:150
Hellweg G (1956) Untersuchungen zur Charakterisierung der Granula in endometrialen Körnchenzellen. Virchows Arch Pathol Anat 329:111
Hellweg G (1957) Über Auftreten und Verhalten der endometrialen Körnchenzellen im Verlauf der Schwangerschaft, im krankhaft veränderten Endometrium und außerhalb des Corpus uteri. Virchows Arch Pathol Anat 330:658
Hellweg G (1959) Über körnchenhaltige Zellen im menschlichen und tierischen Endometrium (endometriale Körnchenzellen, metachromasierende Zellen). Z Zellforsch 49:555
Hellweg G, Sandritter W (1956) Ultraviolettmikrospektrophotometrische Untersuchungen an den Körnchen der endometrialen Körnchenzellen. Klin Wochenschr 34:1040
Hellweg G, Shaka JA (1959) Über den Nachweis der endometrialen Körnchenzellen in der Gewebekultur. Virchows Arch Pathol Anat 332:375
Hempel E, Böhm W (1976) Elektronenmikroskopische Untersuchung der Proliferation und Regression des menschlichen Endometriums nach Applikation des neuen Depotöstrogens Äthinylöstradiolsulfonat. Zentralbl Gynäkol 98:1508
Hempel E, Böhm W, Carol W, Klinger G (1977) Zur Problematik von Bestimmung und Beurteilung der Östrogen-Aufbaudosis am menschlichen Endometrium. Zentralbl Gynäkol 99:1060
Henderson SR, Roxburgh DR, Bobrow LG et al. (1975) Endometrial washings. Histological and cytological assessment of material obtained with an intrauterine jet washing device. Br J Obstet Gynaecol 82:976

Hendrickson MR, Kempson RL (1980) The differential diagnosis of endometrial adenocarcinoma. Some viewpoints concerning a common diagnostic problem. Pathology 12:35

Hendrickson MR, Kempson RL (1980) Endometrial epithelial metaplasias: proliferations frequently misdiagnosed as adenocarcinoma. Report of 89 cases and proposed classification. Am J Surg Pathol 4:525

Hendrickson MR, Kempson RL (1983) Ciliated carcinoma – a variant of endometrial adenocarcinoma: a report of 10 cases. Int J Gynecol Pathol 2:1

Hendrickson MR, Scheithauer BW (1986) Primitive neuroectodermal tumor of the endometrium: report of two cases, one with electron-microscopic observations. Int J Gynecol Pathol 5:249

Hendrickson M, Ross J, Eifel P et al. (1982) Uterine papillary serous carcinoma. Am J Surg Pathol 6:93

Henriksen E (1960) Estrogen and endometrial carcinoma. Obstet Gynecol 15:663

Henriksen E, Murrieta T (1950) Adenocarcinoma of the corpus uteri: a clinico-pathological study. West J Surg 58:331

Henzl M, Jirasek J, Horsky J, Presl J (1964) Die Proliferationswirkung des 17-α-Äthinyl-19-Nor-Testosterons. Arch Gynäkol 199:335

Henzl M, Smith RE, Magoun RE, Hill R (1968) The influence of estrogens on rabbit endometrium. Fertil Steril 19:914

Henzl M, Smith RE, Boost G, Tyler ET (1972) Lysosomal concept of menstrual bleeding in humans, J Clin Endocrinol Metab 34:860

Hernández O, Aznar R, Hicks JJ et al. (1975) Subcellular distribution of trace metals in the normal and in the copper treated human secretory endometrium. Contraception 11:451

Herrell WE (1939) Studies on the endometrium in association with the normal menstrual cycle, with ovarian dysfunctions and cancer of the uterus. Am J Obstet Gynecol 37:559

Herrell WE, Broders AC (1935) Histological studies of endometrium during various phases of menstrual cycle. Surg Gynecol Obstet 61:751

Hertig AT (1944) The aging ovary-A preliminary note. J Clin Endocrinol 4:581

Hertig AT (1957) Endocrine ovarian-cancer relationships. Cancer (Philad) 10:838

Hertig AT (1967) Human trophoblast: normal and abnormal. A plea for the study of the normal so as to understand the abnormal. Am J Clin Pathol 47:249

Hertig AT (1968) Human trophoblast. The Carl Vernon Weller Lecture Series. Thomas, Springfield

Hertig AT, Edmonds HW (1940) Genesis of hydatidiform mole. Arch Pathol 30:260

Hertig AT, Gore H (1960) Tumors of the female sex organs, part 2. In: Atlas of tumor pathology, sect. IX, fasc. 33. Armed Forces Institute of Pathology, Washington DC

Hertig AT, Gore H (1963) Precancerous lesions of endometrium. Z Krebsforsch 65:201

Hertig AT, Livingstone RG (1944) Spontaneous, threatened and habitual abortion: their pathogenesis and treatment. N Engl J Med 230:797

Hertig AT, Mansell H (1956) Hydatidiform mole and choriocarcinoma. In: Atlas of tumor pathology, sect. IX, fasc. 33. Armed Forces Institute of Pathology, Washington DC

Hertig AT, Sheldon WH (1943) Minimal criteria required to prove prima facie case of traumatic abortion or miscarriage. Ann Surg 117:596

Hertig AT, Sommers SC (1949) Genesis of endometrial carcinoma. I. Study of prior biopsies. Cancer (Philad) 2:946

Hertig AT, Sommers SC, Bengloff A (1949) Genesis of endometrial carcinoma. III. Carcinoma in situ. Cancer (Philad) 2:964

Hertz R (1968) Experimental and clinical aspects of the carcinogenic potential of steroid contraceptives. Int J Fertil 13:273

Herxheimer G (1907) Über heterologe Cancroide. Beitr Pathol Anat 41:348

Herzer H, Cavegn B, Stamm O, Siebenmann R (1969) Endometriumveränderungen durch das Retrosteroid RO-4-8347. Gynaecologia (Basel) 168:1

Hester LL, Kellett WW, Spicer SS et al. (1968) Effects of a sequential oral contraceptive

on endometrial enzyme and carbohydrate histochemistry. Am J Obstet Gynecol 102:771
Hester LL, Kellett WW, Spicer SS (1970) Effects of the intrauterine contraceptive device on endometrial enzyme and carbohydrate histochemistry. Am J Obstet Gynecol 106:1144
Hibbard LT, Schwinn CE (1971) Diagnosis by endometrial jet washings. Am J Obstet Gynecol 111:1039
Hicks JJ, Rosado A (1976) Molecular distribution of trace metals in the normal and in the Copper treated human secretory endometrium. Int J Fertil 21:55
Hienz HA, Stoll P (1962) Sex determinations in intra-uterine death by means of sex chromatin. Acta Cytol 6:108
Hiersche H-D, Meinen K (1971) Funktionelle Morphologie des fetalen und infantilen endometrialen Stroma. Arch Gynäkol 210:164
Hill RP, Miller NF (1951) Combined mesenchymal sarcoma and carcinoma (carcinosarcoma) of the uterus. Cancer (Philad) 4:803
Hilliard GD, Norris HJ (1979) Pathologic effects of oral contraceptives. Cancer Res 66:49
Hinselmann H (1930) Die Ätiologie, Symptomatologie und Diagnostik des Uteruscarcinoms. In: Stoeckel W (ed) Handbuch der Gynaekologie, vol 6/1. Springer, Berlin, p 864
Hintze O (1928) Plattenepithelknötchen in hyperplastischen Drüsen der Korpusschleimhaut. Zentralbl Gynäkol 52:2209
Hinz W (1952) Ein Beitrag zum Carcinosarkom der Gebärmutterschleimhaut. Arch Gynäkol 182:301
Hinz W (1953) Die zeitgerechte Ausschabung bei funktionellen Blutungsstörungen, vom Standpunkt der Zusammenarbeit zwischen Kliniker und Histologen. Geburtshilfe Frauenheilkd 13:43
Hinz W (1954) Die Bedeutung der Blutungsanamnese für die funktionelle Schleimhautdiagnostik. Geburtshilfe Frauenheilkd 14:518
Hinz W (1957) Zur Abstoßung der Gebärmutterschleimhaut bei anovulatorischen Blutungen. Geburtshilfe Frauenheilkd 17:835
Hinz W, Solth K (1959) Zum Hämosiderinvorkommen im Endometrium. Zentralbl Gynäkol 81:617
Hinz W, Terbrüggen H (1952) Extrauteringravidität und Mucosa uteri. Arch Gynäkol 182:230
Hirschfield L, Kahn LB, Chen S et al. (1986) Müllerian adenosarcoma with ovarian sex cord-like differentiation. Cancer (Philad) 57:1197
Hisaw FL (1926) Experimental relaxation of the pubic ligament of the guinea pig. Proc Soc Exp Biol (NY) 23:661
Hisaw FL (1935) The physiology of menstruation of monkeys. Am J Obstet Gynecol 29:638
Hisaw FL (1944) The placental gonadotropin and luteal function in monkeys (*Macaca mulatta*). Yale J Biol Med 17:119
Hisaw FL, Hisaw FL (1961) Action of estrogen and progesterone on the reproductive tract of lower primates. In: Young WC (ed) Sex and internal secretions. Williams & Wilkins, Baltimore, p 556
Hisaw FL, Hisaw FL (1964) Effect of relaxin on the uterus of monkeys (*Macaca mulatta*) with observations on the cervix and symphysis pubis. Am J Obstet Gynecol 89:141
Hitschmann F (1903) Ein Beitrag zur Kenntnis des Corpuscarcinoms. Arch Gynäkol 69:629
Hitschmann F (1904) Zur mikroskopischen Diagnose des Abortus. Zentralbl Gynäkol 28:961
Hitschmann F, Adler L (1907) Die Lehre von der Endometritis. Z Geburtshilfe Gynäkol 60:63
Hitschmann F, Adler L (1908) Der Bau der Uterusschleimhaut des geschlechtsreifen Weibes mit besonderer Berücksichtigung der Menstruation. Monatsschr Geburtshilfe Gynäkol 27:1

Hoffbauer J (1931) The etiology of hyperplasia of the endometrium. Surg Gynecol Obstet 52:223
Hoffmann F (1947) Untersuchungen über die Entstehung der Hypomenorrhoe. Zentralbl Gynäkol 69:1052
Hoffmann F (1948) Über die Progesteronbildung im Zyklus und der Schwangerschaft. Zentralbl Gynäkol 70:1177
Hoffmann F (1951) Primäre Amenorrhoe mit zyklischer Ovarialfunktion. Geburtshilfe Frauenheilkd 11:163
Hoffmann I, Ober KG, Schmitt A (1953) Beobachtungen an einer Scheidenendometriose. Geburtshilfe Frauenheilkd 13:881
Hoffmeister H, Hanschke HJ (1960) Maligner Mischtumor des Uterus. Geburtshilfe Frauenheilkd 20:1265
Hoffmeister H, Schulz H (1961) Lichtoptische und elektronenoptische Befunde am Endometrium der geschlechtsreifen Frau während der Proliferations- und Sekretionsphase unter besonderer Berücksichtigung der Faserstrukturen. Beitr Pathol Anat 124:415
Hofmann D (1960) Zur Frage der Geschwulstentstehung nach früherer Anwendung ionisierender Strahlen in der Gynäkologie. Geburtshilfe Frauenheilkd 20:749
Hofmann D, Legerlotz C (1968) Untersuchungen zur Differentialdiagnose der ektopischen Schwangerschaft und über die diagnostische Bedeutung der Arias-Stella-Reaktion. Geburtshilfe Frauenheilkd 28:50
Hofmeister FJ, Vondrak BF (1970) Endometrial carcinoma in patients with bilateral oophorectomy or irradiation castration. Am J Obstet Gynecol 107:1099
Hohman WR, Shaw ST, Macaulay L, Moyer DL (1977) Vascular defects in human endometrium caused by intrauterine contraceptive devices. Contraception 16:507
Holmstrom EG, McLennan CE (1947) Menorrhagia associated with irregular shedding of the endometrium. Am J Obstet Gynecol 53:727
Holzner JH, Lassmann G (1967) Neurofibromatosis uteri (Neurofibrom encapsulée-Masson). Arch Gynäkol 204:43
Homma H (1955) Chronische Endometritis und Zykluspathologie. Wien Klin Wochenschr 67:361
Homma H (1958) Über die Diagnostik der extrauterinen Gravidität am Abrasionsmaterial. Gynaecologia (Basel) 146:193
Honoré LH (1976) Midtrimester prostaglandin-induced abortion: gross and light microscopic findings in the placenta. Prostaglandins 11:1019
Honoré LH (1979) Benign obstructive myxometra: report of a case. Am J Obstet Gynecol 133:227
Hoogerland DL, Buchler DA, Crowley JJ, Carr WF (1978) Estrogen use – risk of endometrial carcinoma. Gynecol Oncol 6:451
Hooker CW, Forbes TR (1947) A bio-assay for minute amounts of progesterone. Endocrinology 41:158
Hopkin ID, Harlow RA, Stevens PJ (1970) Squamous carcinoma of the body of the uterus. Br J Cancer 24:71
Hopkins M, Nunez C, Murphy JR, Wentz B (1985) Malignant placental site trophoblastic tumor. Obstet Gynecol 66:95S
Horie A, Yasumoto K, Ueda H et al. (1977) Clear cell adenocarcinoma of the uterus- ultrastructural and hormonal study. Acta Pathol Jpn 27/6:907
Hörmann C (1908) Die Bindegewebsfasern in der Schleimhaut des Uterus. Arch Gynäkol 86:404
Hörmann G, Lemtis H (1965) Die menschliche Placenta. In: Schwalm H, Döderlein G (eds) Klinik der Frauenheilkunde und Geburtshilfe. Urban & Schwarzenberg, München
Horne HW, Hertig AT, Kundsin RB, Kosasa TS (1973) Sub-clinical endometrial inflammation and T-mycoplasma. Int J Fertil 18:226
Hsu C (1975) Endometrial ossification. Br J Obstet Gynaecol 82:836
Hsueh AJW, Peck EJ, Clark JH (1975) Progesterone antagonism of the oestrogen receptor and oestrogen-induced uterine growth. Nature (Lond) 254:337
Huang K, Muechler EK, Bonfiglio TA (1984) Follicular phase treatment of luteal phase defect with follicle-stimulating hormone in infertile women. Obstet Gynecol 64:32

Huber A, Michael S, Feik K (1971) Funktionelle Veränderungen am fetalen und kindlichen Endometrium. Arch Gynäkol 211:583
Huber CP, Melin JR, Vellios H (1957) Changes in chorionic tissue of aborted pregnancy. Am J Obstet Gynecol 73:569
Huber H (1951) Zur Klinik des Schleimhautpolypen des Uterus. Geburtshilfe Frauenheilkd 11:675
Huber H (1960) Tumorbildung am Genitale nach Röntgenkastration. Geburtshilfe Frauenheilkd 20:745
Hüffer E (1922) Über Aktinomykose des weiblichen Genitales, speziell des Uterus. Monatsschr Geburtshilfe 58:197
Hughes EC (1976) The effect of enzymes upon metabolism, storage, and release of carbohydrates in normal and abnormal endometria. Cancer (Philad) 38:487
Hughes EC, Csermely TV (1965) Chromosome constitution of human endometrium. Am J Obstet Gynecol 93:777
Hughes EC, Jacobs RD, Rubulis A (1964) Effect of treatment for sterility and abortion upon the carbohydrate pathways of the endometrium. Am J Obstet Gynecol 89:69
Hughes EC, Demers LM, Csermely T, Jones DB (1969) Organ culture of human endometrium. Effect of ovarian steroids. Am J Obstet Gynecol 105:707
Hughesdon PE, Cocks DP (1955) Endometrial sarcoma complicating cystic hyperplasia. With remarks on "carcino-sarcoma". J Obstet Gynaecol Br Emp 62:567
Humason GL (1962) Animal tissue techniques. Freeman, San Francisco
Hung LHY, Kurtz DM (1985) Hodgkin's disease of the endometrium. Arch Pathol Lab Med 109:952
Hunter DT, Coggins FW (1965) Endometrial hemangiomata. Report of a case. Obstet Gynecol 25:538
Hunter WC, Nohlgren JE, Lancefield SM (1956) Stromal endometriosis or endometrial sarcoma. Am J Obstet Gynecol 72:1072
Hunziker H (1911) Über Plattenepithel in der Schleimhaut des Cavum uteri. Frankfurt Z Pathol 8:1
Husslein H (1948) Hyperplasia endometrii im Senium. Wien Klin Wochenschr 60:45, 63
Husslein H (1950) Die Bedeutung des Follikelhormons für die Entstehung des Corpuscarcinoms. Wien Klin Wochenschr 62:740
Husslein H, Schüller E (1952) Corpuscarcinom in der Geschlechtsreife. Arch Gynäkol 182:125
Hussy P, Wallart J (1915) Interstitielle Drüse und Röntgenkastration. Z Geburtshilfe Gynäkol 77:177
Hustin J (1970) Endometrial carcinoma and synthetic progestogens: results of intrauterine treatment. J Obstet Gynaecol Br Cwlth 77:915
Hustin J (1975) Effect of protein hormones and steroids on tissue cultures of endometrial carcinoma. Br J Obstet Gynaecol 82:493
Hustin J (1976) Morphology and DNA content of endometrial cancer nuclei under progestogen treatment. Acta Cytol 20:556
Iglesias R (1965) Hormones and tumors. In: Taylor S (ed) Proc 2nd Int Congr Endocr London 1964. Excerpta Medica, Amsterdam, p 1072
Ingerslev M, Jeppesen T, Ramsing E-M (1976) Secondary amenorrhoea and oral contraceptives. Acta Obstet Gynecol Scand 55:233
Ingersoll FM (1965) Carcinoma of the corpus uteri. Postgrad Med 37:539
Inglis RM, Weir JH (1976) Endometrial suction biopsy: appraisal of a new instrument. Am J Obstet Gynecol 125:1070
Ingram JM, Novak E (1951) Endometrial carcinoma associated with feminizing ovarian tumors. Am J Obstet Gynecol 61:774
Inhoffen HH (1940) Übergang von Sterinen in aromatische Verbindungen. Angew Chem 53:471
Inoue M, Ueda G, Yamasaki M et al. (1982) Endometrial argyrophil cell adenocarcinoma with indole-or catecholamine precursor uptake and decarboxylation. Int J Gynecol Pathol 1:47

Irey NS, Manion WC, Taylor HB (1970) Vascular lesions in women taking oral contraceptives. Arch Pathol 89:1
Irwin JB (1956) The lymphoid apparatus of the endometrium with report of a case of primary lymphoma of the endometrium. Am J Obstet Gynecol 72:915
Isaacson PG, Pilot LMJR, Gooselaw JG (1964) Foam cells in the stroma in carcinoma of the endometrium. Obstet Gynecol 23:9
Ishihara M, Hasegawa G, Mori M (1964) Histochemical observations of oxydative enzymes in malignant tumors of female genital organs. Am J Obstet Gynecol 90:183
Ishikawa S, Kaneko H, Sumida T, Sekiya M (1979) Ultrastructure of mesodermal mixed tumor of the uterus. Acta Pathol Jpn 29:801
Israel SL (1942) The clinical similarity of corpus luteum cyst and ectopic pregnancy. Am J Obstet Gynecol 44:22
Israel SL (1959) Menstrual disorders and sterility. Hoeber, New York
Israel SL, Roitman HB, Clancy C (1963) Infrequency of unsuspected endometrial tuberculosis. JAMA 183:63
Jackson MCN (1963) Oral contraception in practice. J Reprod Fertil 6:153
Jackson RL, Dockerty MB (1957) The Stein-Leventhal syndrome: analysis of 43 cases with special reference to association with endometrial carcinoma. Am J Obstet Gynecol 73:161
Jacobson CB, Barter RH (1967) Some cytogenetic aspects of habitual abortion. Am J Obstet Gynecol 97:666
Jaeger J, Dallenbach-Hellweg G (1969) Elektronenmikroskopische Befunde an den endometrialen Körnchenzellen des Menschen. Gynaecologia (Basel) 168:117
Jafari K, Javaheri G, Ruiz G (1978) Endometrial adenocarcinoma and the Stein-Leventhal-Syndrome. Obstet Gynecol 51:97
Jahoda E, Tatra G (1972) Die Tumormultiplizität beim Endometriumcarcinom. Arch Gynäkol 213:1
Jain AK (1975) Safety and effectiveness of intrauterine devices. Contraception 11:243
Jakobovits A (1956) Todesursachen und anatomische Verteilung der Metastasen beim Uteruskrebs. Zentralbl Allg Pathol Anat 95:346
Jakobovits A (1963) Endometrial manifestations of ovarian feminizing mesenchymomas. Acta Morphol Acad Sci Hung 12:141
James VHT, Folkerd EJ, Bonney RC et al. (1982) Factors influencing estrogen production and metabolism in postmenopausal women with endocrine cancer. J Endocrinol Invest 5:335
Janovski NA, Weir JA (1962) Comparative histologic and histochemical studies of mesonephric derivates and tumors. Obstet Gynecol 19:57
Janssen P, Piekarski G, Korte W (1970) Zum Problem des Abortes bei latenter Toxoplasmainfektion der Frau. Klin Wochenschr 48:25
Javert CT, Hofammann K (1952) Observations on the surgical pathology, selective lymphadenectomy, and classification of endometrial adenocarcinoma. Cancer (Philad) 5:485
Javert CT, Renning EL (1963) Endometrial cancer. Survey of 610 cases treated at woman's hospital (1919–1960). Cancer (Philad) 16:1057
Jeffrey JF, Krepart GV, Lotocki RJ (1986) Papillary serous adenocarcinoma of the endometrium. Obstet Gynecol 67:670
Jensen EV (1963) Über die Wirkungsweise von Oestrogenen. Dtsch Med Wochenschr 88:1229
Jensen EV (1979) Interaction of steroid hormones with the nucleus. Pharmacol Rev 30:477
Jensen EV, Østergaard E (1954) Clinical studies concerning the relationship of estrogens to the development of cancer of the corpus uteri. Am J Obstet Gynecol 67:1094
Jensen EV, Suzuki T, Numata M et al. (1969) Estrogen-binding substances of target tissues. Steroids 13:417
Jensen PA, Dockerty MB, Symmonds ER, Wilson RB (1966) Endometrioid sarcoma ("stromal endometriosis"). Report of 15 cases including 5 with metastases. Am J Obstet Gynecol 95:79

Jessen DA, Lane RE, Greene RR (1963) Intra-uterine foreign body: a clinical and histopathologic study on the use of the Grafenberg ring. Am J Obstet Gynecol 85:1023

Jewelewicz R, Khalaf S, Neuwirth RS, Wiele RLV (1976) Obstetric complications after treatment of intrauterine synechiae (Asherman's syndrome). Obstet Gynecol 47:701

Jick H, Watkins RN, Hunter JR et al. (1979) Replacement estrogens and endometrial cancer. N Engl J Med 300:218

Jirasek JE, Dykova H (1964) Esterasepositive endometriale Stromazellen. Gynaecologia (Basel) 157:3

Johannisson E (1973) Recent developments with intrauterine devices. Contraception 8:99

Johannisson E, Hagenfeldt K (1971) Isolation and cytochemical properties of human endometrial cells. Acta Endocrinol 153:81

Johannisson E, Nilsson L (1972) Scanning electron microscopy study of the human endometrium. Fertil Steril 23:613

Johannisson E, Landgren B-M, Hagenfeldt MD (1977) The effect of intrauterine progesterone on the DNA-content in isolated human endometrial cells. Acta Cytol 21:441

John HA, Cornes JS, Jackson WD, Bye P (1974) Effect of a systemically administered progestogen on histopathology of endometrical carcinoma. J Obstet Gynaecol Br Cwlth 81:786

Jones GS (1973) Luteal phase insufficiency. Clin Obstet Gynecol 16:255

Jones GS, Askel S, Wentz AC (1974) Serum progesterone values in the luteal phase defects. Obstet Gynecol 44:26

Jones HO, Brewer JI (1941) A study of the ovaries and endometriums of patients with fundal carcinomas. Am J Obstet Gynecol 42:207

Jopp H (1965) Karzinom und Sarkom des Endometrium als Koinzidenztumoren. Zentralbl Gynäkol 87:1663

Jopp H, Krone HA (1962) Zum Problem der Histogenese carcinomhaltiger heterologer mesodermaler Mischtumoren des Uterus. Arch Gynäkol 197:387

Jörgensen SEB, Starup J, Roos J, Micic S (1976) Studies of the mode of action of clomiphene citrate. Acta Obstet Gynecol Scand 55:337

Jørgensen V, Enevoldsen B (1963) The occurrence of the first menstruation after curettage. Acta Obstet Gynecol Scand [Suppl 6] 42

Junkmann K (1963) Experimentelle Gesichtspunkte bei der Prüfung synthetischer Gestagene. Dtsch Med Wochenschr 13:629

Jurkovic I, Muzelak R (1970) Frequency of pathologic changes in the young human chorion in therapeutic abortions of normal pregnancies. Am J Obstet Gynecol 108:382

Kadar NR, Kohorn EI, Li Volsi VA, Kapp DS (1982) Histologic variants of cervical involvement by endometrial carcinoma. Obstet Gynecol 59:85

Kaeser O (1949) Studien an menschlichen Aborteiern mit besonderer Berücksichtigung der frühen Fehlbildungen und ihrer Ursachen. 11. Mitt.: Die Fehleier oder Molen und ihre hormonale Aktivität. Schweiz Med Wochenschr 79:780, 803

Kahanpää KV, Wahlström T, Gröhn P et al. (1986) Sarcomas of the uterus: a clinicopathologic study of 119 patients. Obstet Gynecol 67:417

Kahler VL, Creasy RK, Morris JA (1969) Value of the endometrial biopsy. Obstet Gynecol 34:91

Kahner S, Ferenczy A, Richart RM (1975) Homologous mixed müllerian tumors (carcinosarcoma) confined to endometrial polyps. Am J Obstet Gynecol 121:278

Kaiser J, Wide L, Gemzell C (1966) Sequential and combined therapy in oral contraception. Acta Obstet Gynecol Scand 45:53

Kaiser R (1959) Die Wirkung von Gestagenen beim Corpuscarcinom. Arch Gynäkol 193:195

Kaiser R (1963) Hormonale Ovulationshemmung. Dtsch Med Wochenschr 88:2325

Kaiser R (1963) Die Reaktion des fetalen und mütterlichen Endometriums und die Hormone der Plazenta. Arch Gynäkol 198:128

Kaiser R (1969) Ätiologie und Prophylaxe des Endometriumkarzinoms. Geburtshilfe Frauenheilkd 29:431

Kaiser R, Schneider E (1968) Funktionszustände und mitotische Aktivität des Endometrium bei Frauen mit und ohne Endometrium-Carcinom. Arch Gynäkol 205:151

Kaiserling H (1950) Ist die Cytometrie eine Ergänzung der histologischen Cyclusdiagnostik? Med Klin 45:367
Kaltenbach FJ, Fettig O, Welter J (1973) Histologische und autoradiographische Untersuchungen am menschlichen Endometrium unter der 2-Phasen-Therapie mit Mestranol-Lynestrenol. Arch Gynäkol 215:325
Kanbour A, Stock J (1978) Squamous cell carcinoma in situ of the endometrium and fallopian tube as superficial extension of invasive cervical carcinoma. Cancer (Philad) 42:570
Kanbour A, Klionsky B, Cooper R (1974) Cytohistologic diagnosis of uterine jet wash preparations. Acta Cytol 18:51
Kantor HI, Harrel DG (1953) Treatment of the underdeveloped secretory phase of the endometrium. Am J Obstet Gynecol 65:602
Kapadia SB, Krause JR, Kanbour AI, Hartsock RJ (1978) Granulocytic sarcoma of the uterus. Cancer (Philad) 41:687
Kaplan M, Grumbach R, Strauss P et al. (1960) Tuberculose congénitale due a une endométrite tuberculeuse de la mère. Guérison bactériologique. Mort par insuffisance respiratoire. Ann Pédiatr 36:133
Karlen JR, Sternberg LB, Abbott JN (1972) Carcinoma of the endometrium co-existing with pregnancy. Obstet Gynecol 40:334
Karlson P (1965) Mechanismus of hormone action. Thieme, Stuttgart
Karlson P (1967) Colloquien der Ges. für biologische Chemie. 18. Colloquium: Wirkungsmechanismen der Hormone. Springer, Berlin Heidelberg New York
Karow WG, Gentry WC, Skeels RF, Payne SA (1971) Endometrial biopsy in the luteal phase of the cycle of conception. Fertil Steril 22:482
Karpas CM, Speer FD (1957) Carcinosarcoma of the endometrium. An unusual case receiving estrogen therapy for eleven years. Arch Pathol 63:17
Kase N, Cohn GL (1967) Clinical implications of extragonadal estrogen production. J Med 276:29
Katzenstein AAL, Askin FB, Feldman PS (1977) Müllerian adenosarcoma of the uterus: an ultrastructural study of four cases. Cancer (Philad) 40:2233
Kaufman DW, Shapiro S, Rosenberg L et al. (1980) Intrauterine contraceptive device use and pelvic inflammatory disease. Am J Obstet Gynecol 136:159
Kaufmann C (1933) Echte menstruelle Blutung bei kastrierten Frauen nach Zufuhr von Follikel- and Corpus luteum-Hormon. Klin Wochenschr 12:217
Kaufmann C (1939) Die praktische Verwendung der Hormone in der Frauenheilkunde. Geburtshilfe Frauenheilkd 1:313
Kauppila A, Jänne O, Stenbäck F, Vihko R (1982a) Cytosolic estrogen and progestin receptors in human endometrium from different regions of the uterus. Gynecol Oncol 14:225
Kauppila A, Kujansuu E, Vihko R (1982b) Cytosol estrogen and progestin receptors in endometrial carcinoma of patients treated with surgery, radiotherapy, and progestin. Cancer (Philad) 50:2157
Kay S (1957) Clear cell carcinoma of the endometrium. Cancer (Philad) 10:124
Kay S (1974) Squamous-cell carcinoma of the endometrium. Am J Clin Pathol 61:264
Kayser HW (1959) Besondere Verlaufsformen des weiblichen Genitalkarzinoms. Zugleich ein Beitrag zum Systemkarzinomproblem. Z Geburtshilfe Gynäkol 152:52
Kazzaz BA (1975) Granular cell sarcoma of endometrium. Eur J Obstet Gynecol Reprod 5/4:233
Keller DW, Wiest WG, Askin FB et al. (1979) Pseudocorpus luteum insufficiency: a local defect of progesterone action on endometrial stroma. J Clin Endocrinol Metab 48:127
Keller R (1911) Gefäßveränderungen in der Uterusschleimhaut zur Zeit der Menstruation. Z Geburtshilfe Gynäkol 69:333
Keller R, Andrian J (1939) L'atrophie sénile de la muqueuse utérine. Gynécol Obstét 40:400
Kelley HW, Miles PA, Buster JE, Scragg WH (1976) Adenocarcinoma of the endometrium in women taking oral contraceptives. Obstet Gynecol 47:200

Kelley RM, Baker WH (1961) Progestational agents in the treatment of carcinoma of the endometrium. N Engl J Med 264:216
Kelley RM, Baker WH (1965) Role of progesterone in human endometrial cancer. Cancer Res 25:1190
Kempson RL, Pokorny GE (1968) Adenocarcinoma of the endometrium in women aged forty and younger. Cancer (Philad) 21:650
Kendall JZ, Plopper CG, Bryant-Greenwood GD (1978) Ultrastructural immunoperoxidase demonstration of relaxin in corpora lutea from a pregnant sow. Biol Reprod 18:94
Kennedy BJ (1969) Progestogens in the treatment of carcinoma of the endometrium. Surg Gynecol Obstet 127:103
Kepp R (1961) Das Problem des Zusammenhangs der Strahlentherapie gutartiger Erkrankungen mit der Entstehung von bösartigen Tumoren in der Gynäkologie. Zentralbl Gynäkol 83:1
Kerger H (1949) Primäres Plattenepithelcarcinom des Corpus uteri und Plattenepithelinseln im Myometrium. Zentralbl Gynäkol 71:1185
Kern-Bontke E, Wächter M (1962) Morphologie des Gewebes im Frischgefrier- und Paraffinschnitt an gynäkologischem Material. Virchows Arch Pathol Anat 336:1
Kerr M, Rashad MN (1966) Chromosome studies on spontaneous abortions. Am J Obstet Gynecol 94:322
Khoo SK, Mackay EV, Adam RR (1971) Contraception with a six-monthly injection of progestogen. Part 3. Effects on the endometrium. Aust NZ J Obstet Gynaecol 11:226
Kief H, Muth H (1951) Extrauteringravidität – Glanduläre Hyperplasie. Geburtshilfe Frauenheilkd 11:990
Kindler KF (1956) Vergleichende Untersuchungen am Endometrium bei Hyperfollikulinie in Beziehung zur Karzinomentstehung. Geburtshilfe Frauenheilkd 16:716
King ME, Kramer EE (1980) Malignant mullerian mixed tumors of the uterus. Cancer (Philad) 45:188
King RJB (1967) Fixation of steroids to receptors. Arch Anat Microsc Morphol Exp 56:570
King RJB, Gordon J (1967) The association of (6,7-^{3}H) oestradiol with a nuclear protein. J Endocrinol 39:533
King WJ, Desombre ER, Jensen EV, Greene GL (1985) Comparison of immunocytochemical and steroid binding assays for estrogen receptor in human tumors. Cancer (Philad) 45:293
Kirchhoff H (1955) Die Genitaltuberkulose der Frau. Arch Gynäkol 186:279
Kirchhoff H, Haller J (1964) Klinische Erfahrungen mit einer ovulationsunterdrückenden Oestrogen-Kombination (Anovlar). Med Klin 59:681
Kirkpatrick AF, Milholland RJ, Rosen F (1971) Stereospecific glucocorticoid binding to subcellular fractions of the sensitive and resistant lymphosarcoma. Nature (Lond) 232:216
Kistner RW (1959) Histological effects of progestins on hyperplasia and carcinoma in situ of the endometrium. Cancer (Philad) 12:1106
Kistner RW (1965) Induction of ovulation with clomiphene citrate. Obstet Gynecol Surv 20:873
Kistner RW (1965) Further observations of the effects of clomiphene citrate in anovulatory females. Am J Obstet Gynecol 92:380
Kistner RW (1969) The pill: facts and fallacies about today's oral contraceptives. Delacorte, New York
Kistner RW (1982) Treatment of hyperplasia and carcinoma in situ of the endometrium. Clin Obstet Gynecol 25:63
Kistner RW, Smith OW (1960) Observations on the use of a nonsteroidal estrogen antagonist: MER-25. Surg Forum 10:725
Kistner RW, Duncan CJ, Mansell H (1956) Suppression of ovulation by tri-p-anisyl chlorethylene (TCE). Obstet Gynecol 8:399
Kistner RW, Griffiths CT, Craig JM (1965) Use of progestational agents in the management of endometrial cancer. Cancer (Philad) 18:1563

Kistner RW, Leais JL, Steiner GJ (1966) Effects of clomiphene citrate on endometrial hyperplasia in the premenopausal female. Cancer (Philad) 19:115

Klaer W, Holm-Jensen S (1972) Metastases to the uterus. Acta Pathol Microbiol Scand [A] 80:835

Klinger HP, Glasser M, Kawa HW (1976) Contraceptives and the conceptus. I. Chromosome abnormalities of the fetus and neonate related to maternal contraceptive history. Obstet Gynecol 48:40

Knorr G (1960) Talkumgranulome des Endometrium. Dtsch Med Wochenschr 85:1804

Knörr K, Knörr-Gärtner H (1977) Das Abortgeschehen unter genetischen Aspekten. Gynäkologe 10:3

Koch F (1949) Über die Karzinom- und Sarkombildung am Genitale nach Kastrationsbestrahlung. Z Geburtshilfe Gynäkol 131:195

Kofinas AD, Suarez J, Calame RJ, Chipeco Z (1984) Chondrosarcoma of the uterus. Gynecol Oncol 19:231

Kofler E (1954) Glandulär-zystische Hyperplasie und Korpuskarzinom. Zentralbl Gynäkol 76:2242

Kohorn EI (1976) Gestagens and endometrial carcinoma. Gynecol Oncol 4:398

Kohorn EI, Rice SI, Gordon M (1970) In vitro production of nucleolar channel system by progesterone in human endometrium. Nature (Lond) 228:671

Kohrman AF, Greenberg RE (1968) Permanent effects of estradiol on cellular metabolism of the developing mouse vagina. Dev Biol 18:632

Komorowski RA, Garancis JC, Clowry LJ (1970) Fine structure of endometrial stromal sarcoma. Cancer (Philad) 26:1042

Koninckx PR, Brosens IA (1977) The "gonadotropin-resistant ovary" syndrome as a cause of secondary amenorrhea and infertility. Fertil Steril 28:926

Koninckx PR, Brosens IA (1982) Clinical significance of the luteinized unruptured follicle syndrome as a cause of infertility. Eur J Obstet Gynecol Reprod Biol 13:355

Koninckx PR, Goddeeris PG, Lauweryns JM et al. (1977) Accuracy of endometrial biopsy dating in the relation of the midcycle luteinizing hormone peak. Fertil Steril 28:443

Koppen K (1950) Histologische Untersuchungsergebnisse von der Nervenversorgung des Uterus. Arch Gynäkol 177:354

Koss LG, Spiro RH, Brunschwig A (1965) Endometrial stromal sarcoma. Surg Gynecol Obstet 121:531

Kottmeier HL (1947) Über Blutungen in der Menopause. Acta Obstet Gynecol Scand [Suppl 6] 27

Kottmeier HL (1953) Carcinoma of the female genital tract. The Abraham Flexner lecture series, no 11. Williams & Wilkins, Baltimore

Kottmeier HL (1959) Carcinoma of the corpus uteri. Diagnosis and therapy. Am J Obstet Gynecol 78:1127

Kottmeier HL (1962) Erfahrungen mit Progesteron in Fällen von Corpuskarzinom. Geburtshilfe Frauenheilkd 22:1070

Krantz KE (1959) Innervation of the human uterus. Ann NY Acad Sci 75:770

Kräubig H (1972) Die Toxoplasmose der Schwangeren. Gynäkologe 5:203

Krause W, Böhm W, Müller W (1968) Vergleichende zytologische und histologische Studien nach Behandlung mit einer ovulationsunterdrückenden Östrogen-Gestagen-Kombination (Ovosiston). Gynaecologia (Basel) 166:432

Kremer H, Narik G (1953) Über das gleichzeitige Vorkommen von Uterusschleimhautpolypen und Karzinomen der weiblichen Genitalorgane. Krebsarzt 8:7

Kreutner A, Johnson D, Williamson HO (1976) Histology of the endometrium in longterm use of a sequential oral contraceptive. Fertil Steril 27:905

Krone HA (1961) Die Bedeutung der Eibettstörungen für die Entstehung menschlicher Mißbildungen. Veröff Morphol Pathol 62

Krone HA, Littig G (1959) Über das Vorkommen von Schaumzellen im Stroma von Adeno-Karzinomen des Corpus uteri. Arch Gynäkol 191:432

Krupp PJ, Sternberg WH, Clark WH et al. (1961) Malignant mixed Müllerian neoplasms (mixed mesodermal tumors). Am J Obstet Gynecol 81:959

Kruschwitz S (1967) Glandulär-zystische Hyperplasie und Korpuskarzinom. Zentralbl Gynäkol 89:1199

Kucera F (1964) Alkalische Phosphatasen im Endometrium. Zentralbl Gynäkol 86:1332
Kühne D, Seidl St, Göretzlehner G (1972) Contraceptive treatment with chlormadinone and its effect on the endometrium. A histological investigation. Endokrinologie 59:295
Kullander S (1956) Studies in spayed rats with ovarian tissue autotransplanted to the spleen. Acta Endocrinol (Kbh) [Suppl 27] 22
Kumar NB, Hart WR (1982) Metastases to the uterine corpus from extragenital cancers. A clinicopathologic study of 63 cases. Cancer (Philad) 50:2163
Kumar NB, Schneider V (1983) Metastases to the uterus from extrapelvic primary tumors. Int J Gynecol Pathol 2:134
Kupryjanczyk J, Dallenbach FD, Dallenbach-Hellweg G (1986) Immunohistochemischer Nachweis von Oestrogenrezeptoren im Endometrium. Verh Dtsch Ges Pathol 70:494
Kurman RJ, Norris HJ (1982) Evaluation of criteria for distinguishing atypical endometrial hyperplasia from well-differentiated carcinoma. Cancer (Philad) 49:2547
Kurman J, Scully RE (1976) Clear cell carcinoma of the endometrium. An analysis of 21 cases. Cancer (Philad) 37:872
Kurman RJ, Scully RE, Norris HJ (1976) Trophoblastic pseudotumor of the uterus. An exaggerated form of "syncytial endometritis" simulating a malignant tumor. Cancer (Philad) 38:1214
Kurman RJ, Kaminski PF, Norris HJ (1985) The behavior of endometrial hyperplasia. Cancer (Philad) 56:403
Küstermann H (1930) Systematische histologische Untersuchungen über die Venen des Uterus. Z Mikrosk Anat Forsch 20:417
Kutlik JE (1962) Pseudoichthyosis endometrii. Zentralbl Allg Pathol 104:10
Kwak HM (1965) Studies on the effects of intra-uterine contraceptive device: with particular reference on the endometrial changes. Kor J Obstet Gynecol 8:253
Laatikainen T, Anderson B, Kärkkäinen J, Wahlström T (1983) Progestin receptor levels in endometria with delayed or incomplete secretory changes. Obstet Gynecol 62:592
Laffargue P, Cabanne F, Nosny Y (1966) Sarcomes du corps utérin. Memoires Originaux. Gynécol Obstét 65:423
Lahm W (1928) Das Karzinom des Uterus. In: Halban-Seitz (ed) Biologie und Pathologie des Weibes, vol IV. Urban & Schwarzenberg, Wien, p 864
Lajos L, Illi G, Kecskés L et al. (1963) Hyperoestrogenism after the menopause. J Obstet Gynaecol Br Cwlth 70:1016
Lancet M, Liban E (1970) Carcinosarcoma of the uterus in a young girl with survival. Int J Gynaecol Obstet 8:316
Lang FJ, Schneider H (1960) Die Organstruktur des Genitaltraktes als Grundlage der Organleistung und Organerkrankung. In: Büchner F, Letterer E, Roulet F (eds) Handbuch der allgemeinen Pathologie, vol III/2. Springer, Berlin Göttingen Heidelberg, p 489
Langer H (1963) Intrauterine Toxoplasma-Infektion. Thieme, Stuttgart
Langer H (1966) Die Bedeutung der latenten mütterlichen Toxoplasma-Infektion für die Gestation. In: Kirchhoff, Kräubig (eds) Toxoplasmose, praktische Fragen und Ergebnisse. Thieme, Stuttgart
Langhans T (1901) Syncytium und Zellschicht. Placentarreste nach Aborten. Chorionepitheliome. Hydatidenmole. Hegars Beitr Z Geburtshilfe Gynäkol 5:1
Larranaga A, Winterhaltel M, Sartoretto JN (1975) Evaluation of d-Norgestrel 1.0 mg as a post-coital contraceptive. Int J Fertil 20:165
Larsen JF (1973) Ultrastructure of the abnormal human trophoblast. Acta Anat [Suppl 1] (Basel) 86:47
Larson JA (1954) Estrogens and endometrial carcinoma. Obstet Gynecol 3:551
Larson SL, Titus JL (1970) Chromosomes and abortions. Mayo Clin Proc 45:60
Larsson B, Liedholm P, Sjöberg N-O, Åstedt B (1974) Increased fibronolytic activity in the endometrium of patients using copper-IUD. Contraception 9:531
Lassmann G (1965) Die Nervenversorgung der Uterusschleimhaut. Arch Gynäkol 200:500
Last PA (1974) Pregnancy and the intrauterine contraceptive device. Contraception 9:439
Lau H, Stoll P (1962) Das Adenom des Corpus uteri. Dtsch Med Wochenschr 87:1005

Lau H, Stoll P (1963) Leistungsfähigkeit und Grenzen der Endometriumdiagnostik. Landarzt 39:719

Lauchlan SC (1968) Conceptual unity of the müllerian tumor group. Cancer (Philad) 22:601

Laufer A (1968) The influence of steroids on the endometrium. Int J Fertil 13:373

Lauritsen JG (1975) The significance of oral contraceptives in causing chromosome anomalies in spontaneous abortions. Acta Obstet Gynecol Scand 54:261

Lauterwein G (1941) Die Bedeutung der Strichcurettage bei der Behandlung von Zyklusanomalien. Zentralbl Gynäkol 65:822

Lawn AM, Wilson EW, Finn CA (1971) The ultrastructure of human decidual and predecidual cells. J Reprod Fertil 26:85

Leavitt WW, Chen TJ, Allen TC (1977) Regulation of progesterone receptor formation by estrogen action. Ann NY Acad Sci 286:210

Leduc M, Delcroix M, Gautier PJ (1981) Biopsie d'endomètre et stérilité. Gynécologie 32:21

Lee CH, Chow LP, Cheng TY, Wei PY (1967) Histologic study of the endometrium of intrauterine contraceptive device users. Am J Obstet Gynecol 98:808

Lee MC, Damjanov I (1985) Pregnancy-related changes in the human endometrium revealed by lectin-histochemistry. Histochemistry 82:275

Lee RA (1969) Contraceptive and endometrial effects of medroxyprogesterone acetate. Am J Obstet Gynecol 104:130

Lehfeldt H, Kulka EW, Liebmann HC (1965) Comparative study of intrauterine contraceptive devices. Obstet Gynecol 26:679

Lehfeldt H, Tietze C, Gorstein F (1970) Ovarian pregnancy and the intrauterine device. Am J Obstet Gynecol 108:1005

Lemon HM (1956) quoted from Sommers SC, Meissner WA. Cancer (Philad) 10:516 (1957)

Lendrum AC (1947) The phloxine-tartrazin method as general histological stain and for the demonstration of inclusion bodies. J Pathol Bacteriol 59:399

Leroy F (ed) (1980) Blastocyst-endometrium relationships. 7. Sem on Reprod Physiol and Sex. Endocr. Springer, Berlin Heidelberg New York

Leroy F, Manavian D, Hubinont PO (1967) Nuclear DNA estimations in the Hooker and Forbes test with sex hormones. J Endocrinol 39:277

Lester WM, Bartholomew RA, Colvin ED et al. (1956) The role of retained placental fragments in immediate and delayed postpartum hemorrhage. Am J Obstet Gynecol 72:1214

Letterer E (1948) Die Morphologie der hormonal bedingten Veränderungen des Endometriums und der weiblichen Brustdrüse. Ärztl Wochenschr 3:230

Letterer E, Masshoff W (1941) Funktionelle Diagnostik der Uterusschleimhaut. Dtsch Med Wochenschr 67:859

Leventhal ML (1958) The Stein-Leventhal syndromes. Am J Obstet Gynecol 76:825

Levine AJ (1969) Endometrial adenocarcinoma evaluated by histologic and functional criteria. Cancer (Philad) 24:229

Levine B (1963) Sex steroids, alkaline phosphatase, and endometrial carcinoma. Obstet Gynecol 22:563

Lewin E (1960) Histochemische Untersuchungen an Schleimhäuten von Extrauteringraviditäten. II. Mitt. Gynaecologia (Basel) 149:216

Lewin E (1961) Histochemische Untersuchungen an Uterusschleimhäuten. Z Geburtshilfe Gynäkol 157:196

Liebig W, Stegner H-E (1977) Die Dezidualisation der endometrialen Stromazelle. Elektronenmikroskopische Untersuchungen. Arch Gynäkol 223:19

Liedholm P, Sjöberg N (1974) Two year experience with copper-T 200 in a Swedish population. Contraception 10:55

Lifschitz-Mercer B, Czernobilsky B, Dgani R, Dallenbach-Hellweg G et al. (1987) Immunocytochemical study of an endometrial diffuse clear cell stromal sarcoma and other endometrial stromal sarcomas. Cancer (Philad) 59:1494

Limburg H (1947) Zur Frage der Thecazelltumoren des Ovariums und ihrer hormonalen Funktion. Z Geburtshilfe Gynäkol 128:186

Limburg H (1951) Die Bedeutung spontaner Oestrogenbildung in der Menopause. Arch Gynäkol 180:260
Limpaphayom K, Lee C, Jacobson HI, King TM (1971) Estrogen receptor in human endometrium during the menstrual cycle and early pregnancy. Am J Obstet Gynecol 111:1064
Linde Te RW, Henriksen E (1940) Decidua-like changes in the endometrium without pregnancy. Am J Obstet Gynecol 39:733
Lipin T, Davison C (1947) Metastases of uterine carcinoma to the central nervous system. A clinico-pathologic study. Arch Neurol Psychiatry 57:186
Lippes L, Zielezny M (1975) The loop after 10 years. In: Hefnawi, Segal (eds) Analysis of intrauterine contraception. North-Holland, Amsterdam, p 225
Lipschütz A (1950) Steroid hormones and tumors. Williams & Wilkins, Baltimore
Liu CT (1972) A study of endometrial adenocarcinoma with emphasis on morphologically variant types. Am J Clin Pathol 57:562
Liu DTY, Melville HAH, Measday B, Melcher D (1975) Assessment of diagnostic aspiration curettage as an outpatient procedure. Am J Obstet Gynecol 122:106
Liu W (1955) Vaginal cornification in women with uterine cancer. Cancer (Philad) 8:779
Liukko P, Erkkola R, Laakso L (1977) Ectopic pregnancies during use of low-dose progestogens for oral contraception. Contraception 16:575
Livolsi VA (1977) Adenocarcinoma of the endometrium with psammoma bodies. Obstet Gynecol 50:725
Lohmeyer H, Velten CH (1957) Die Beziehungen zwischen Uterus myomatosus und Endometriumstroma. Arch Gynäkol 189:467
Lomax CW, Harbert GM, Thornton WN (1976) Actinomycosis of the female genital tract. Obstet Gynecol 48:341
Long ME, Doko F (1959) Cytochemical studies on non-malignant and malignant human endometria. Ann NY Acad Sci 75:504
Loraine JA, Bell ET (1968) Fertility and contraception in the human female. Williams & Wilkins, Baltimore
Lucas M, Wallace I, Hirschhorn K (1972) Recurrent abortions and chromosome abnormalities. J Obstet Gynaecol Br Cwlth 79:1119
Lüdinghausen M von, Anastasiadis P (1984) Anatomic basis of endometrial cytology. Acta Cytol 28:555
Ludwig H (1980) Intrauterine devices: reactions of the endometrium and alterations of the devices after varying time of exposure in situ. Verh Dtsch Ges Pathol 64:523
Ludwig H (1982) The morphologic response of the human endometrium to long-term treatment with progestational agents. Am J Obstet Gynecol 142:796
Ludwig H, Metzger H (1976) The re-epithelization of endometrium after menstrual desquamation. Arch Gynäkol 221:51
Luh W, Brandau H (1967) Enzymologische Studien am normalen menschlichen Endometrium. Z Geburtshilfe Gynäkol 168:14
Lukeman JM (1974) An evaluation of the negative pressure "jet washing" of the endometrium in menopausal and post-menopausal patients. Acta Cytol 18:462
Lunan CB, Green B (1975) Oestradiol-17β uptake in vitro into the nuclei of endometrium from different regions of the human uterus. Acta Endocrinol 78:353
Lunenfeld B (1964) The ovarian response to exogenous human gonadotropins alone and during simultaneous administration of progestagens. Int J Fertil 9:167
Lunenfeld B (1965) Urinary gonadotropins. In: Taylor S (ed) Proc Second Int Congr Endocrinology, London 1964. Excerpta Medica, Amsterdam, p 814
Lynch HT, Krush AJ, Larsen AL, Magnuson CW (1966) Endometrial carcinoma: multiple primary malignancies, constitutional factors and heredity. Am J Med Sci 252:381
Lynch HT, Krush AJ, Larsen AL (1967) Heredity and endometrial carcinoma. South Med J 60:231
Lyon FA (1975) The development of adenocarcinoma of the endometrium in young women receiving long-term sequential oral contraception. Report of 4 cases. Am J Obstet Gynecol 123:299
Lyon FA, Frisch MJ (1976) Endometrial abnormalities occurring in young women on long-term sequential oral contraception. Obstet Gynecol 47:639

MacCarthy J (1955) Actinomycosis of the female pelvic organs with involvement of the endometrium. J Pathol 69:175

MacDonald PC, Grodin JM, Edman CD et al. (1976) Origin of estrogen in a postmenopausal woman with a nonendocrine tumor of the ovary and endometrial hyperplasia. Obstet Gynecol 47:644

MacMahon B, Hertig A, Ingalls T (1954) Association between maternal age and pathologic diagnosis in abortion. Obstet Gynecol 4:477

Maddi FV, Papanicolaou GN (1961) Diagnostic significance of ciliated cells in human endometrial tissue cultures. Am J Obstet Gynecol 82:99

Mainwaring WIP (1975) Steroid hormone receptors: a survey. Vitamins and Hormones 33:223

Mainwaring WIP (1977) The mechanism of action of androgens. Springer, Berlin Heidelberg New York

Mall-Haefeli M, Ludwig KS, Spornitz UM, Uettwiller A (1976) Die Low-Dosis-Gestagen-Therapie. Geburtshilfe Frauenheilkd 36:645

Mandl L (1911) Flimmerndes und sezernierendes Uterusepithel. Monatsschr Geburtshilfe Gynäkol 34:150

Mandruzzato GP (1964) Die Endometritis tuberculosa bei sterilen Frauen. In: Fikentscher R (ed) Beiträge zur Fertilität und Sterilität. Beilageh zu Z Geburtshilfe Gynäkol 162:125

Manning JP, Hisaw FL, Steinetz BG, Kroc RL (1967) The effects of ovarian hormones on uterine phosphatases of the rhesus monkey (*Macaca mulatta*). Anat Rec 157:465

Mansour FS, Baradi AF (1967) Enzyme histochemical study on postmenopausal endometrium in symptom-free patients. Am J Obstet Gynecol 97:109

Maqueo M, Becerra C, Mungiua W, Goldzieher JW (1964) Endometrial histology and vaginal cytology during oral contraception with sequential estrogen and progestin. Am J Obstet Gynecol 90:395

Maqueo M, Perez-Vega E, Goldzieher JW et al. (1963) Comparison of the endometrial activity of three synthetic progestins used in fertility control. Am J Obstet Gynecol 85:427

Maqueo M, Gorodovsky J, Rice-Wray E, Goldzieher W (1970) Endometrial changes in women using hormonal contraceptives for periods up to ten years. Contraception 1:115

Maqueo M, Rice-Wray E, Gorodovsky J, Goldzieher JW (1970) Endometrial regeneration in patients discontinuing oral contraceptives. Fertil Steril 21:224

Marchand D (1895) Über die sogenannten dezidualen Geschwülste im Anschluß an normale Geburt, Blasenmole und Extrauterinschwangerschaft. Monatsschr Geburtshilfe Gynäkol 1:419, 513

Marcus CC (1961) Relationship of adenomyosis uteri to endometrial hyperplasia and endometrial carcinoma. Am J Obstet Gynecol 82:408

Marcus CC (1963) Relationship of ovarian hilus cells to benign and malignant endometrium. Obstet Gynecol 22:73

Marcus SL (1961) Adenoacanthoma of the endometrium. Am J Obstet Gynecol 81:259

Marcuse PM (1957) Dehydrogenase activity of endometrium. Application of tetrazolium staining methods to smears and sections from surgical specimens. Am J Clin Pathol 28:539

Mariani LP, Chardier MP, Fabiano A (1957) Tumeurs à double souche de l'endomètre. Bull Assoc Fr Cancer 44:311

Mark J, Hulka J (1978) Luteinized unruptured follicle syndrome: a subtle cause of infertility. Fertil Steril 29:270

Markee JE (1940) Menstruation in intraocular endometrial transplants in the rhesus monkey. Contrib Embryol Carnegie Inst 518, 28:219

Markee JE (1950) The morphological and endocrine basis for menstrual bleeding. In: Meigs, Sturgis (eds) Progress in gynecology, vol II. Grune & Stratton, New York

Marks F (1979) Molekulare Biologie der Hormone. Fischer, Stuttgart

Marsh R (1950) Angioma of the uterus. Arch Pathol 49:490

Marshall RJ, Braye SG (1985) α-1-Antitrypsin, α-1-antichymotrypsin, actin, and myosin in uterine sarcomas. Int J Gynecol Pathol 4:346

Martin E (1951) Untersuchung zur Frage des Gewebsschadens nach intrauteriner Sulfonamidanwendung. Geburtshilfe Frauenheilkd 11:800
Martin E, Scholes J, Richart RM, Fenoglio CM (1979) Benign cystic teratoma of the uterus. Am J Obstet Gynecol 135:429
Martin JF, Cabanne F, Fournie G (1956) A propos des "tumeurs mixtes" du corps utérin. (Tumeurs malignes du blastème Müllérien: Mülleroblastomes.) Ann Anat Pathol 1:428
Martins AG (1960) Adenocarcinoma of the uterus in infancy. Br J Cancer 14:165
Martz G (1968) Die hormonale Therapie maligner Tumoren. Springer, Berlin Heidelberg New York
Maruffo CA, Casavilla F, van Nynatten B, Perez V (1974) Modifications of the human endometrial fine structure induced by low-dose progestogen therapy. Fertil Steril 25:778
Massei M (1947) I follicoli linfatica nella mucosa uterine in fase premestruale e nella decidua. Ann Obstet Ginecol 69:250
Masshoff W (1941) Die Uterusschleimhaut bei Sterilität. Zentralbl Gynäkol 65:1519
Masshoff W (1941) Morphologische Beiträge zur Kenntnis der zystisch-glandulären Hyperplasie des Endometriums und ihre funktionelle Bedeutung. Z Geburtshilfe Gynäkol 122:15
Masshoff W, Kraus L (1955) Über das quantitative Verhalten der Gefäße bei verschiedenen Zuständen der Uterusmucosa, Virchows Arch Pathol Anat 327:259
Mathews DD, Kakani A, Bhattacharya A (1973) A comparison of vacuum aspiration of the uterus and conventional curettage in the management of abnormal uterine bleeding. J Obstet Gynaecol Br Cwlth 80:176
Mathieu P, Rahier J, Thomas K (1981) Localization of relaxin in human gestational corpus luteum. Cell Tissue Res 219:213
Mauthner E (1921) Das Verhalten des Kapillarsystems bei der zyklischen Wandlung der Uterusmukosa. Monatsschr Geburtshilfe Gynäkol 54:81
Mazer C, Ziserman AJ (1932) Pseudomenstruation in the human female. Am J Surg 18:332
Mazur MT (1981) Atypical polypoid adenomyomas of the endometrium. Am J Surg Pathol 5:473
Mazur MT, Hendrickson MR, Kempson RC (1983) Optically clear nuclei. An alteration of endometrial epithelium in the presence of trophoblast. Am J Surg Pathol 7:415
Mazur MT, Hsueh S, Gersell DJ (1984) Metastases to the female genital tract. Analysis of 325 cases. Cancer (Philad) 53:1978
McBride JM (1954) The normal postmenopausal endometrium. J Obstet Gynaecol Br Emp 61:691
McCarty KS, Barton TK, Peete CH, Creasman WT (1978) Gonadal dysgenesis with adenocarcinoma of the endometrium. An electron microscopic and steroid receptor analysis with a review of the literature. Cancer (Philad) 42:512
McCarty KS, Barton TK, Fetter BF et al. (1979) Correlation of estrogen and progesterone receptors with histologic differentiation in endometrial adenocarcinoma. Am J Pathol 96:171
McCarthy VP, Cho CT (1979) Endometritis and neonatal sepsis due to streptococcus pneumoniae. Obstet Gynecol 53:47S
McCracken AW, D'Agostino AN, Brucks AB, Kingsley WB (1974) Acquired cytomegalovirus infection presenting as viral endometritis. Am J Clin Pathol 61:556
McDonald JR, Waugh JM (1939) Chronic lymphatic leukemia with infiltration into endometrium. Proc Mayo Clin 14:465
McDonald JR, Broders AC, Counseller VS (1940) Sarcoma of the endometrial stroma. Surg Gynecol Obstet 70:223
McGarvey RN, Gibson WE (1952) Adenocarcinoma of the endometrium. Am J Obstet Gynecol 63:836
McKay DG (1950) Metachromasia in the endometrium. Am J Obstet Gynecol 59:875
McKay DG (1962) The interrelation of the ovary and endometrium in carcinoma of the endometrium. Acad Med NJ Bull 8:258

McKay DG, Robinson D (1947) Observations on the fluorescence, birefrigence and histochemistry of the human ovary during the menstrual cycle. Endocrinology 41:378

McKay DG, Hertig AT, Hickey WF (1953) The histogenesis of granulosa and theca cell tumors of the human ovary. Obstet Gynecol 1:125

McKay DG, Hertig AT, Bardawil W, Velardo JT (1956) Histochemical observations on the endometrium: I. Normal endometrium. II. Abnormal endometrium. Obstet Gynecol 8:22, 140

McKelvey JL (1942) Irregular shedding of the endometrium. Lancet II:434

McKelvey JL, Samuels LT (1947) Irregular shedding of the endometrium. Am J Obstet Gynecol 53:627

McLennan C (1969) Endometrial regeneration after curettage. Am J Obstet Gynecol 104:185

McLennan C, Rydell AH (1965) Extent of endometrial shedding during normal menstruation. Obstet Gynecol 26:605

Mead PB, Beecham JB, Maeck JVS (1976) Incidence of infections associated with the intrauterine contraceptive device in an isolated community. Am J Obstet Gynecol 125:79

Mears E (1965) Handbook on oral contraception. Churchill, London

Meinrenken H (1949) Genitaltuberkulose und Schwangerschaft. Zentralbl Gynäkol 71:418

Meinrenken H (1952) Zur Frage der Rückbildung der Uterusschleimhaut bei lebender und abgestorbener Extrauteringravidität. Geburtshilfe Frauenheilkd 12:602

Meinrenken H (1956) Die Cervixveränderungen in der Schwangerschaft. Beitrag zur Frage der Epidermisation. Arch Gynäkol 187:501

Meissner WA, Sommers SC (1950) Postpartum endometrial hyperplasia in diabetics treated with stilbestrol and progesterone. J Clin Endocrinol 10:603

Meissner WA, Sommers SC, Sherman G (1957) Endometrial hyperplasia, endometrial carcinoma, and endometriosis produced experimentally by estrogen. Cancer (Philad) 10:500

Melin JR, Wanner L, Schulz DM, Cassel EE (1979) Primary squamous cell carcinoma of the endometrium. Obstet Gynecol 53:115

Menge C (1922) Das Korpusadenom der Matrone. Zentralbl Gynäkol 46:1

Mercado E, Aznar R, Gallegos AJ et al. (1977) Subcellular distribution of lysosomal enzymes in the human endometrium. II. Effect of the inert, and copper and progesterone-releasing T intrauterine devices. Contraception 16:299

Merker HJ, Diaz-Encinas J (1969) Das elektronenmikroskopische Bild des Ovars juveniler Ratten und Kaninchen nach Stimulierung mit PMS und HCG. I. Theka und Stroma (interstitielle Drüse). Z Zellforsch 94:605

Merker HJ, Herbst R, Kloss K (1968) Elektronenmikroskopische Untersuchungen an den Mitochondrien des menschlichen Uterusepithels während der Sekretionsphase. Z Zellforsch 86:139

Mester J, Martel D, Psychoyos A, Baulieu EE (1974) Hormonal control of oestrogen receptor in the uterus and receptivity for ovoimplantation in the rat. Nature (Lond) 250:776–778

Mestwerdt W, Brandau H, Müller O (1972) Struktur und Funktion steroidaktiver Zellen im Postmenopausenovar. Arch Gynäkol 212:268

Mey R (1961) Ätiologie und Pathogenese der Abortiveier. Veröff Morphol Pathol 63

Meyer R (1922) Plattenepithelknötchen in hyperplastischen Drüsen der Corpusschleimhaut des Uterus und bei Karzinomen. Arch Gynäkol 115:394

Meyer R (1923) Über seltenere gutartige und zweifelhafte Epithelveränderungen der Uterusschleimhaut im Vergleich mit den ihnen ähnlichen Karzinomformen. 1. Endometritis, 2. Schleimhauthyperplasie, 3. Plattenepithelknötchen, 4. Polypen, 5. Papillome. Z Geburtshilfe Gynäkol 85:440

Meyer R (1925) Über Blut- und Lymphgefäßwucherungen in der Uterusmuskulatur (Teleangiektasie und Hämangiome, Hyperplasie und Lymphangiocystofibrom des Uterus). Arch Gynäkol 126:609

Meyer R (1930) Pathologie der Bindegewebsgeschwülste und Mischgeschwülste des Uterus. In: Veit-Stoeckel (ed) Handbuch der Gynäkologie, vol VI/I. Bergmann, München

Meyer R (1930) Die pathologische Anatomie der Gebärmutter. In: Henke-Lubarsch (ed) Handbuch der speziellen pathologischen Anatomie und Histologie, vol VII/I. Springer, Berlin

Meyer WC, Malkasian GD, Dockerty MB, Decker DG (1971) Postmenopausal bleeding from atrophic endometrium. Obstet Gynecol 38:731

Meyer-Fürst P (1961) Zwei Fälle von Endometropathia osteoplastica. Gynaecologia (Basel) 151:185

Mikamo K (1970) Anatomic and chromosomal anomalies in spontaneous abortion. Am J Obstet Gynecol 106:243

Miles PA, Greenberg H, Herrera GA, Trujillo I (1982) Müllerian adenofibroma of the endometrium. Diagn Gynecol Obstet 4:215

Milgrom E, Luu Thi M, Atger M, Baulieu EE (1973) Mechanisms regulating the concentration and the conformation of progesterone receptors in the uterus. J Biol Chem 248:6366

Milton PJD, Metters JS (1972) Endometrial carcinoma: an analysis of 355 cases treated at St. Thomas' Hospital, 1945-69. J Obstet Gynaecol Br Cwlth 79:455

Mishell DR, El Habashy MA, Good RG, Moyer DL (1968) Contraception with an injectable progestin. Am J Obstet Gynecol 101:1046

Mitani Y, Yukimari S, Jimi S, Jwasaki H (1964) Carcinomatous infiltration into the uterine body in carcinoma of the uterine cervix. Am J Obstet Gynecol 89:984

Moe N (1972) Short-term progestogen treatment of endometrial carcinoma. Acta Obstet Gynecol Scand 51:55

Moegen P (1951) Über komplizierte carcinomhaltige Mischgeschwülste des Uterus und ihre Histogenese. Frankfurt Z Pathol 62:562

Moghissi KS, Marks C (1971) Effects of microdose norgestrel on endogenous gonadotropic and steroid hormones, cervical mucus properties, vaginal cytology, and endometrium. Fertil Steril 22:424

Moghissi KS, Syner FN (1975) Studies on the mechanism of action of continuous microdose quingestanol acetate. Fertil Steril 26:818

Moghissi KS, Syner FN, McBride LC (1973) Contraceptive mechanism of microdose norethindrone. Obstet Gynecol 41:585

Mohamed NC, Cardenas A, Villasanta U et al. (1978) Hilus cell tumor of the ovary and endometrial carcinoma. Obstet Gynecol 52:486

Moll R, Levy R, Czernobilsky B et al. (1983) Cytokeratins of normal epithelia and some neoplasms of the female genital tract. Lab Invest 49:599

Molnar JJ, Poliak A (1983) Recurrent endometrial malakoplakia. Am J Clin Pathol 80:762

Mönch G (1918) Über Rundzellenknötchen im Endometrium. Arch Gynäkol 108:483

Montgomery JB, Long JP, Hoffman J (1952) A clinical evaluation of the use of radiumtherapy in the uterine bleeding. Am J Obstet Gynecol 64:1011

Mookerjea G (1961) Cytochemical patterns of the normal and abnormal human endometrium. Nucleus 4:81

Moore RB, Reagan JW, Schoenberg MD (1959) The mucins of the normal and cancerous uterine mucosa. Cancer (Philad) 12:215

Mordi VPN, Nnatu SNN (1986) Endometrial carcinoma in Nigerians. Cancer (Philad) 57:1840

More IAR, Masterston RG (1975) The fine structure of the human endometrial ciliated cell. J Reprod Fertil 45:343

More IAR, Armstrong EM, Carty M, McSeveney D (1974) Cyclical changes in the ultrastructure of the normal human endometrial stroma cell. J Obstet Gynaecol Br Cwlth 81:337

More IAR, Armstrong EM, McSeveney D, Chatfield WR (1974) The morphogenesis and fate of the nucleolar channel system in the human endometrial glandular cell. J Ultrastruct Res 47:74

Morese KN, Peterson WF, Allen ST (1966) Endometrial effects of an intrauterine contraceptive device. Obstet Gynecol 28:323

Morf E, Müller JH (1966) Endometriumsveränderungen unter Ovulationshemmung mit „Planovin-Novo". Geburtshilfe Frauenheilkd 26:1569

Moricard R (1954) Critères morphologiques utérins et vaginaux de l'exploration cytohormonale dans la phase lutéale. In: Colloques sur "La fonction lutéale". Masson, Paris, p 185

Moricard R (1966) Modifications cytologiques ultrastructurales provoquées par certains équilibres hormonaux dans la muqueuse utérine corporéale humaine. Arch Gynäkol 203:85

Moricard R, Moricard F (1964) Modifications cytoplasmiques et nucléaires ultrastructuralés utérines au cours de l'état follicolutéinique aglycogène massif. Gynécol Obstét 63:203

Morris JM (1973) Mechanisms involved in progesterone contraception and estrogen interception. Am J Obstet Gynecol 117:167

Morris JM, Wagenen G van (1966) Compounds interfering with ovum implantation and development. III. The role of estrogens. Am J Obstet Gynecol 96:804

Mortel R, Nedwich A, Lewis GC, Brady LW (1970) Malignant mixed Müllerian tumors of the uterine corpus. Obstet Gynecol 35:468

Mortel R, Koss LG, Lewis JL, d'Urso JR (1974) Mesodermal mixed tumors of the uterine corpus. Obstet Gynecol 43:248

Moss WT (1947) Common preculiarities of patients with adenocarcinoma of the endometrium. With special reference to obesity, body build, diabetes and hypertension. Am J Roentgenol 58:203

Mostoufi-Zadeh M, Berkowitz RS, Driscoll SG (1987) Persistence of partial mole. Am J Clin Pathol 87:377

Moszkowski E, Woodruff JD, Jones GES (1962) The inadequate luteal phase. Am J Obstet Gynecol 83:363

Moukhtar M (1966) Functional disorders due to bilharzial infection of the female genital tract. J Obstet Gynaecol Br Cwlth 73:307

Moukhtar M, Aleem FA, Hung HC et al. (1977) The reversible behavior of locally invasive endometrial carcinoma in a chromosomally mosaic. (45, X/46, Xr (X)) young woman treated with Clomid. Cancer (Philad) 40:2957

Moukhtar M, Higgins G (1965) The early diagnosis of carcinoma of the female genital tract. I. 6-Phosphogluconate dehydrogenase activity and carcinoma of the female genital tract. J Obstet Gynaecol Br Cwlth 72:677

Moyer DL, Mishell DR (1971) Reactions of human endometrium to the intrauterine foreign body. Am J Obstet Gynecol 111:66

Muenzer RW, Girgis ZA, Rigal RD, Bennett AD (1974) An acceptable yearly screening device for endometrial carcinoma. Am J Obstet Gynecol 119:31

Mühlbock O (1959) Hormones in the genesis of cancer. Acta Un Int Cancer 15:62

Mühlbock O (1963) Hormones in the genesis of cancer. Neoplasma (Bratisl) 10:337

Müller HG (1951) Das Vorkommen heller epithelialer Zellen in der Mucosa uteri der Frau. Zentralbl Gynäkol 73:1187

Müller JH, Keller M (1957) Atypische Proliferationserscheinungen des Endometriums und ihre Beziehung zum manifesten und latenten Corpus-Carcinom. Gynaecologia (Basel) 144:31

Müntefering H, Becker K, Schleiermacher E, Kessel E (1982) Korrelation zwischen morphologischen und zytogenetischen Befunden bei Spontanaborten. Verh Dtsch Ges Pathol 66:373

Mussey E, Malkasian GD (1966) Progesterone treatment of recurrent carcinoma of the endometrium. Am J Obstet Gynecol 94:78

Myhre E (1966) Endometrial biopsy and ovarian hormonal failure. Acta Obstet Gynecol Scand [Suppl 9] 45:143

Nachlas MM, Seligman AM (1949) The comparative distribution of esterase in the tissues of live mammals by a histochemical technique. Anat Rec 105:677

Nakao K, Meyer DJ, Noda Y (1971) Progesterone-specific protein crystals in the endometrium: an electron-microscopic study. Am J Obstet Gynecol 111:1034

Nathan E, Knoth M, Nilsson BO (1978) Scanning electron microscopy of the effect of short-term hormonal therapy on postmenopausal endometrium. Upsala J Med Sci 83:175

Naujoks H, Pallaske HJ (1968) Chromosomenanalysen bei primärer und sekundärer Amenorrhoe unter Anwendung der Lymhocytenkultur. Arch Gynäkol 205:162
Nayak SK (1968) Pathology of abortion: Essential abortion. Obstet Gynecol 32:316
Neumann HO (1927) Zur Metastasierung primärer Ovarialkarzinome in den Uterus. Z Geburtshilfe Gynäkol 92:350
Neumann HO (1929) Über Blut- und Lymphgefäßwucherungen in der Uterusmuskulatur und in Uterusmyomen. Teleangiektasien in der Uteruswand, Hämangioma uteri, teleangiektatische und lymphoangiektatische Myome. Ihre pathologische und klinische Bedeutung. Arch Gynäkol 139:161
Neumann HO (1930) Zur Frage des lymphatischen Apparates in der Gebärmutterschleimhaut. Arch Gynäkol 141:425
Nevinny-Stickel H (1952) Über die Schleimhautfunktion bei Endometriumtuberkulose. Zentralbl Gynäkol 74:2045
Nevinny-Stickel H (1964) Die gestagene Wirkung von zwei halogenierten Derivaten des 17α-Hydroxyprogesteronacetats bei der Frau. Z Geburtshilfe Gynäkol 161:168
Newton CW, Abell MR (1972) Iatrogenic fetal implants. Obstet Gynecol 40:686
Ng ABP, Reagan JW (1970) Incidence and prognosis of endometrial carcinoma by histologic grade and extent. Obstet Gynecol 35:437
Ng ABP, Reagan JW, Storaasli JP, Wentz WB (1973) Mixed adenosquamous carcinoma of the endometrium. Am J Clin Pathol 52:765
Nicolaisen HH, Pedersen H, Guttorm E, Rebbe H (1973) Postovulatory endometrial development in women with IUD. Acta Obstet Gynecol Scand 52:253
Nielsen JC (1960) Cancer of the corpus uteri after radiotherapy. Ugeskr Læger 122:1239
Nieminen U (1962) Studies on the vascular pattern of ectopic endometrium with special reference to cyclic changes. Acta Obstet Gynecol Scand [Suppl 3] 41
Nilsson O (1962) Electron microscopy of the glandular epithelium in human uterus. I. Follicular phase. II. Early and late luteal phase. J Ultrastruct Res 6:413, 422
Nilsson O, Hagenfeldt K, Johannisson E (1974) Ultrastructural signs of an interference in the carbohydrate metabolism of human endometrium produced by the intrauterine copper-T device. Acta Obstet Gynecol Scand 53:139
Nilsson O, Bergström S, Håkansson S et al. (1978) Ultrastructure of implantation. Upsala J Med Sci [Suppl] 22:27
Nishikawa Y, Kaseki S, Tomoda Y et al. (1985) Histopathologic classification of uterine choriocarcinoma. Cancer (Philad) 55:1044
Nissen-Meyer R, Sverdrup A (1961) The influence of oophorectomy, ovarian irradiation, corticoids and hypophysectomy on the urinary excretion of estrogens and pregnanediol. In: Progress in endocrinology, part II. Cambridge University Press, Cambridge
Niven PAR, Stansfeld AG (1973) "Glioma" of the uterus. a fetal homograft. Am J Obstet Gynecol 115:534
Noer T (1961) The histology of the senile endometrium. Acta Pathol Microbiol Scand 51:193
Nogales F, Beato M, Martinez H (1966) Funktionelle Veränderungen des tuberkulösen Endometriums. Arch Gynäkol 203:75
Nogales F, Martinez H, Beato M (1966) Erwägungen über die Pathogenese der Endometritis tuberculosa. Arch Gynäkol 203:45
Nogales F, Martinez H, Parache J (1969) Abstoßung und Wiederaufbau des menschlichen Endometriums. Gynäkol Rundsch 7:292
Nogales-Ortiz F, Puerta J, Nogales FF (1978) The normal menstrual cycle. Chronology and mechanism of endometrial desquamation. Obstet Gynecol 51:259
Nogales-Ortiz F, Tarancón I, Nogales FF (1979) The pathology of female genital tuberculosis. Obstet Gynecol 53:422
Nordqvist S (1964) Hormone effects on carcinoma of the human uterine body studied in organ culture. Acta Obstet Gynecol Scand 43:296
Nordqvist S (1969) Hormonal responsiveness of human endometrial carcinoma studied in vitro and in vivo. Studentlitteratur, Lund
Nordqvist S (1970) The synthesis of DNA and RNA in normal human endometrium in short-term incubation in vitro and its response to oestradiol and progesterone. J Endocrinol 48:17

Norris CC, Behney CA (1936) Radium irradiation for benign hemorrhage. Am J Obstet Gynecol 32:661
Norris HJ (1985) Editorial comments. Int J Gynecol Pathol 4:177
Norris HJ, Taylor HB (1965) Post irradiation sarcomas of the uterus. Obstet Gynecol 26:689
Norris HJ, Taylor HB (1966) Mesenchymal tumors of the uterus. I. A clinical and pathological study of 53 endometrial stromal tumors. Cancer (Philad) 19:755
Norris HJ, Roth E, Taylor HB (1966) Mesenchymal tumors of the uterus. II. A clinical and pathologic study of 31 mixed mesodermal tumors. Obstet Gynecol 28:57
Norris HJ, Tavassoli FA, Kurman RJ (1983) Endometrial hyperplasia and carcinoma. Am J Surg Pathol 7:839
Novak E (1929) The pathologic diagnosis of early cervical and corporeal cancer with special reference to the differentiation from pseudomalignant inflammatory lesions. Am J Obstet Gynecol 18:449
Novak E (1933) Recent advances in the physiology of menstruation. Can menstruation occur without ovulation? JAMA 94:833
Novak E (1935) A suction curet apparatus for endometrial biopsy. JAMA 104:1497
Novak E (1937) The diagnostic and therapeutic applications of the uterine suction curette. Surg Gynecol Obstet 1:610
Novak E (1940) Der anovulatorische Zyklus der Frau. Geburtshilfe Frauenheilkd 2:168
Novak E (1953) Gynecologic and obstetric pathology. Saunders, Philadelphia
Novak E, Richardson EH (1941) Proliferation changes in the senile endometrium. Am J Obstet Gynecol 42:564
Novak E, Rutledge F (1948) Atypical endometrial hyperplasia simulating adeno-carcinoma. Am J Obstet Gynecol 55:46
Novak E, Yui E (1936) Relations of endometrial hyperplasia to adenocarcinoma of the uterus. Am J Obstet Gynecol 32:674
Novak ER (1956) Postmenopausal endometrial hyperplasia. Am J Obstet Gynecol 71:1312
Novak ER (1970) Ovulation after fifty. Obstet Gynecol 36:903
Novak ER, Mohler DI (1953) Ovarian changes in endometrial cancer. Am J Obstet Gynecol 65:1099
Novak ER, Goldberg B, Jones GS, O'Toole RV (1965) Enzyme histochemistry of the menopausal ovary associated with normal and abnormal endometrium. Am J Obstet Gynecol 93:669
Noyes RW (1956) Uniformity of secretory endometrium. Obstet Gynecol 7:221
Noyes RW (1959) The underdeveloped secretory endometrium. Am J Obstet Gynecol 77:929
Noyes RW, Haman JO (1953) Accuracy of endometrial dating. Fertil Steril 4:504
Noyes RW, Hertig AT, Rock J (1950) Dating the endometrial biopsy. Fertil Steril 1:3
Nuckols HH, Hertig AT (1938) Pneumococcus infection of the genital tract in women. Am J Obstet Gynecol 35:782
Nugent FB (1963) Office suction biopsy of the endometrium. Obstet Gynecol 22:168
Numers CV (1942) Über die Zellformen des Stromagewebes der menschlichen Gebärmutterschleimhaut. Acta Obstet Gynecol Scand [Suppl 3)] 22
Numers CV, Nieminen U (1961) Beobachtungen über das Vorkommen von Schaumzellen im Endometriumstroma bei Hyperplasie. Acta Pathol Microbiol Scand 52:133
Nunes A (1945) Três tumores raros do utero: papiloma xantomatoso, adenocárcinocondrossarcoma, polipo mucoso do corpo invadido por endometriose. Anat Lusit 4:461
Nygren K-G, Johansson EDB (1974) Retrograde cervical perforation by the copper-T device. Acta Obstet Gynecol Scand 53:383
Ober KG (1949) Die zyklischen Veränderungen der Endometriumgefäße. Geburtshilfe Frauenheilkd 9:736
Ober KG (1950) Die wechselnde Aktivität der alkalischen Phosphatase im Endometrium und Ovar während des menstuellen Zyklus, sowie im Myometrium unter der Geburt. Klin Wochenschr 28:9

Ober KG, Schneppenheim P, Hamperl H, Kaufmann C (1958) Die Epithelgrenzen im Bereiche des Isthmus uteri. Arch Gynäkol 190:346
Ober WB (1959) Uterine sarcomas: histogenesis and taxonomy. Ann NY Acad Sci 75:568
Ober WB (1966) Synthetic progestagen-estrogen preparations and endometrial morphology. J Clin Pathol 19:138
Ober WB (1977) Effects of oral and intrauterine administration of contraceptives on the uterus. Hum Pathol 8:513
Ober WB, Bernstein J (1955) Observations on the endometrium and ovary in the newborn. Pediatrics 16:445
Ober WB, Bronstein SB (1967) Endometrial morphology following oral administration of quinestrol. Int J Fertil 12:210
Ober WB, Grady WG (1961) Subinvolution of the placental site. Bull NY Acad Med 37:713
Ober WB, Jason S (1953) Sarcoma of the endometrial stroma. Arch Pathol 56:301
Ober WB, Tovell HMM (1959) Mesenchymal sarcomas of the uterus. Am J Obstet Gynecol 77:246
Ober WB, Clyman MJ, Decker A, Roland M (1964) Endometrial effects of synthetic progestagens. Int J Fertil 9:597
Ober WB, Decker A, Clyman MJ, Roland M (1966) Endometrial morphology after sequential medication with mestranol and chlormadinone. Obstet Gynecol 28:247
Ober WB, Sobrero AJ, Kurman R, Gold S (1968) Endometrial morphology and polyethylene intrauterine devices. A study of 200 endometrial biopsies. Obstet Gynecol 32:782
Obiditsch-Mayer I (1951) Über sekundäre Karzinose des Uterus und ihre Diagnose aus dem Probeküretement und der Portioexcision. Zentralbl Gynäkol 73:1142
O'Brien PK, Lea PJ, Roth-Moyo LA (1985) Structure of a radiate pseudocolony associated with an intrauterine contraceptive device. Hum Pathol 16:1153
O'Connor KI (1964) Mixed mesodermal tumors of the body of the uterus following irradiation therapy for carcinoma of the cervix. J Obstet Gynaecol Br Cwlth 71:281
Oehlert GK, Neumann K, Hansmann H (1954) Histochemische Untersuchungen über die Lokalisation des Enzyms Phosphoamidase im menschlichen Endometrium und über seine Aktivitätsschwankungen während des Zyklus. Arch Gynäkol 184:414
Ohama K, Ueda K, Okamoto E et al. (1986) Cytogenetic and clinicopathologic studies of partial moles. Obstet Gynecol 68:250
Okagaki T, Brooker DC, Adcock LL, Prem KA (1979) Müllerian adenosarcoma of the uterus with rapid progression: an ultrastructural study. Gynecol Oncol 7:361
Okkels H (1950) The histophysiology of the human endometrium. In: Engel (ed) Menstruation and its disorders. Thomas, Springfield, p 139
O'Leary JL (1929) Form changes in the human uterine gland during the menstrual cycle and in early pregnancy. Am J Anat 43:289
Olesen H, Albeck V (1949) Primary tubal carcinoma with metastasis to the endometrium and the mesovarium. Acta Obstet Gynecol Scand 29:246
Olson N, Twiggs L, Sibley R (1982) Small-cell carcinoma of the endometrium: light microscopic and ultrastructural study of a case. Cancer (Philad) 50:760
O'Malley BW (1971) Mechanisms of action of steroid hormones. N Engl J Med 284:370
O'Malley BW, Schrader WT (1976) The receptors of steroid hormones. Sci Am 234:32
Ongkasuwan C, Taylor JE, Tang C-K, Prempree T (1982) Angiosarcomas of the uterus and ovary: clinicopathologic report. Cancer (Philad) 49:1469
Orlans FB (1974) Copper IUDs: a review of the literature. Contraception 10:543
Oster G, Salgo MP (1975) The copper intrauterine device and its mode of action. N Engl J Med 293:432
Ostergaard E (1974) Malignant and pseudomalignant hyperplasia adenomatosa of the endometrium in postmenopausal women treated with oestrogen. Acta Obstet Gynecol Scand 53:97
Ostergard DR (1974) Intrauterine contraception in multiparas with the Dalcon Shield. Am J Obstet Gynecol 119:1033
Östör AG, Fortune DW (1980) Benign and low grade variants of mixed Müllerian tumor of the uterus. Histopathology 4:369

Overbeck L (1953) Das Endometrium bei abgestorbener Tubargravidität. Virchows Arch Pathol Anat 324:409

Overbeck L (1959) Die Bedeutung der „hellen Drüsen" im Endometrium für die Diagnose des uterinen Abortes. Zugleich ein Beitrag zur verzögerten menstruellen Abstoßung. Geburtshilfe Frauenheilkd 19:1098

Overbeck L (1962) Die funktionelle Rückbildung der Uterusschleimhaut bei ektopischer Schwangerschaft. Enke, Stuttgart

Overstreet EW (1948) An evaluation of infertility factors. Calif Med 69:1

Palmer JP, Reinhard MC, Sadugor MG, Goltz HL (1949) A statistical study of cancer of the corpus uteri. Am J Obstet Gynecol 58:457

Pane A, Sabatalle R, Reyniak JV (1970) Ovarian pregnancy with in situ IUCD: report of 2 cases. Am J Obstet Gynecol 108:672

Panella J (1960) Sulla vera natura della dismenorrea membranosa. Rapporti con l'endometrio in fase preamenorroica e gravidica iniziali. Clin Ginecol 2:171

Pankow O (1924) Über Uterusblutungen, bedingt durch Regenerationsstörungen des Endometrium. Monatsschr Geburtshilfe Gynäkol 67:71

Papadia S (1959) Contributo allo studio delle cellule chiare di Feyrter nell'endometrio. Monit Ostet Ginecol 1:1

Pardo R, Larkin LH, Fields PA (1980) Immunocytochemical localization of relaxin in endometrial glands of the pregnant guinea pig. Endocrinology 107:2110

Parks RD, Scheerer PP, Greene RR (1958) The endometria of normal postmenopausal women. Surg Gynecol Obstet 106:409

Payan H, Daino J, Kish M (1964) Lymphoid follicles in endometrium. Obstet Gynecol 23:570

Pearse AGE (1968) Histochemistry, theoretical and applied. Churchill, London

Peck JG, Boyes DA (1969) Treatment of advanced endometrial carcinoma with a progestational agent. Am J Obstet Gynecol 103:90

Peel JH (1956) Observations upon the etiology and treatment of carcinoma of the corpus uteri. Am J Obstet Gynecol 71:718

Pellillo D (1968) Proliferative stromatosis of the uterus with pulmonary metastases. Remission following treatment with a long-acting synthetic progestin: a case report. Obstet Gynecol 31:33

Pentecost MP, Brack CB (1959) Carcinoma of the endometrium. South Med J 52:190

Pepler WJ, Fouche W (1968) Spontaneous polyovulation in the human and its effect on the endometrial patterns. S Afr J Obstet Gynaecol 6:50

Perez CA, Zivnuska F, Askin F et al. (1975) Prognostic significance of endometrial extension from primary carcinoma of the uterine cervix. Cancer (Philad) 35:1493

Peris LA, Jernstrom P, Bowers PA (1958) Primary squamous-cell carcinoma of the uterine corpus. Report of a case and review of the literature. Am J Obstet Gynecol 75:1019

Perkins MB (1960) Pneumopolycystic endometritis. Am J Obstet Gynecol 80:332

Perlmutter JF (1974) Experience with the Dalcon Shield as a contraceptive device. Obstet Gynecol 43:443

Pertschuk LP, Beddoe AM, Gorelic LS, Shain SA (1986) Immunocytochemical assay of estrogen receptors in endometrial carcinoma with monoclonal antibodies. Cancer (Philad) 57:1000

Peterson WF, Novak ER (1956) Endometrial polyps. Obstet Gynecol 8:40

Pfleiderer A (1968) Enzymhistochemische Untersuchungen am Carcinom des Corpus uteri. Fortschr Geburtshilfe Gynäkol 36:1

Pfleiderer A (1974) Enzyme-histochemical studies on the cycle in the endocervix and on the isthmus. Arch Gynäkol 216:317

Pharriss BB, Erickson R, Bashaw J et al. (1974) Progestasert: a uterine therapeutic system for long-term contraception. I. Philosophy and clinical efficacy. Fertil Steril 25:915

Philippe E (1973) Morphologie et morphométrie des placentas d'aberration chromosomique léthale. Rev Fr Gynécol 68:645

Philippe E, Boué JG (1969) Le placenta des aberrations chromosomiques léthales. Ann Anat Pathol 14:249

Philippe E, Ritter J, Renaud R, Gandar R (1965) Le cycle endométrial normal biphasique. Rev Fr Gynécol 60:405

Philippe E, Ritter J, Gandar R (1966) L'endomêtre biphasique normal en période menstruelle. Gynécol Obstét 65:515
Philippe E, Ritter J, Renaud R et al. (1968) Les métrorragies tardives du post-partum par anomalie d'involution des artères utéro-placentaires. Rev Fr Gynécol 63:255
Photopulos GJ, Carney CN, Edelman DA et al. (1979) Clear cell carcinoma of the endometrium. Cancer (Philad) 43:1448
Picard D (1949) Anomalies nucleaires et perturbations mitotiques dans l'épithélium utérin chez la femme; Rôle possible des oestrogènes. Bull Histol Appl 26:199
Picard D (1950) Sur les noyaux de l'épithélium utérin au cours de l'hyperfolliculinie. C R Assoc Anat 59:581
Piekarski G (personal communication)
Pildes RB (1965) Induction of ovulation with clomiphene. Am J Obstet Gynecol 91:466
Pileri S, Martinelli G, Serra L, Bazzocchi F (1980) Endodermal sinus tumor arising in the endometrium. Obstet Gynecol 56:391
Pilleron JP, Durand JC (1968) Les carcinosarcomes du corps utérin. A propos de 6 cas observés à la Fondation Curie de 1950 à 1966. Bull Cancer 55:215
Pincus G (1965) The control of fertility. Academic Press, New York
Pincus G, Graubard M (1940) Estrogen metabolism in cancerous and noncancerous women. Endocrinology 26:427
Piver MS (1966) Distant metastasis of adenoacanthoma of the endometrium. Am J Obstet Gynecol 96:1011
Piver MS, Barlow JJ, Lurain JR, Blumenson LE (1980) Medoxyprogesterone acetate (Depo-Provera) vs Hydroxyprogesterone caproate (Delalutin) in women with metastatic endometrial adenocarcinoma. Cancer (Philad) 45:268
Pizarro E, Gomez-Rogers C, Rowe PJ, Lucero S (1977) Comparative study of the progesterone T (65 mg daily) and copper 7 IUD. Contraception 16:313
Plate WP (1971) Post-pil-anovulatie. Ned Tijdschr Geneeskd 115:1694
Plaut H (1950) Human infection with cryptococcus glabratus. Report of case involving uterus and fallopian tube. Am J Clin Pathol 20:377
Plotz J (1950) Der Wert der Basaltemperatur für die Diagnose der Menstruationsstörungen. Arch Gynäkol 177:521
Plotz J, Wiener M, Stein AA, Hahn BD (1967) Enzymatic activities related to steroidogenesis in postmenopausal ovaries of patients with and without endometrial carcinoma. Am J Obstet Gynecol 99:182
Podvoll EM, Goodman StJ (1967) Cellular dynamics: hormones. Science 155:226
Poland BJ (1970) Conception control and embryonic development. Am J Obstet Gynecol 106:365
Pollow K, Boquoi E (1976) Oestradiol- and Progesteron-bindende Rezeptoren sowie 17β-Hydroxysteroiddehydrogenase in Endometriumkarzinomen der Frau vor und nach Gestagenbehandlung. Z Krebsforsch 86:231
Pollow K, Boquoi E, Lübbert H, Pollow B (1975) Effect of gestagen therapy upon 17β-Hydroxysteroid dehydrogenase in human endometrial adenocarcinoma. J Endocrinol 67:131
Pollow K, Lübbert H, Boquoi E, Pollow B (1975) Progesterone metabolism in normal human endometrium during the menstrual cycle and in endometrial carcinoma. J Clin Endocrinol Metab 41:729
Pollow K, Lübbert H, Boquoi E et al. (1975) Studies on 17β-hydroxysteroid dehydrogenase in human endometrium and endometrial carcinoma. Acta Endocrinol (Kbh) 79:134
Pollow K, Lübbert H, Boquoi E et al. (1975) Characterization and comparison of receptors for 17-β-estradiol and progesterone in human proliferative endometrium and endometrial carcinoma. Endocrinology 96:319
Pollow K, Schmidt-Gollwitzer M, Boquoi E (1977) Verhalten der Sexualsteroid-Rezeptoren des Endometriums während des menstruellen Zyklus und bei Endometriumkarzinomen. Arch Gynäkol 224:291
Post RC, Cohen T, Blaustein A, Shenker L (1966) Carcinoid tumor metastatic to the cervix and corpus uteri. Report of case. Obstet Gynecol 27:171

Potter VR (1965) Summary of 1965 biology research conference. J Cell Comp Physiol 66:175
Potts M, Pearson RM (1976) A light and electron microscope study of cells in contact with intrauterine contraceptive devices. J Obstet Gynaecol Br Cwlth 74:129
Poulsen HE, Taylor CW, Sobin L (1975) Histological typing of female genital tract tumors. WHO, Genf
Prade M, Gadenne C, Duvillard P et al. (1982) Endometrial carcinoma with argyrophil cells. Hum Pathol 13:870
Press MF, Scully RE (1985) Endometrial "sarcomas" complicating ovarian thecoma, polycystic ovarian disease and estrogen therapy. Gynecol Oncol 21:135
Press MF, Nousek-Goebl N, King WJ et al. (1984) Immunohistochemical assessment of estrogen receptor distribution in the human endometrium throughout the menstrual cycle. Lab Invest 51:495
Pribor HC (1951) Innervation of the uterus. Anat Rec 109:339
Printer KD (1963) Pituitary hyperactivity and adrenogenitalism associated with endometrial carcinoma. J Obstet Gynaecol Br Cwlth 70:303
Procope B-J (1968) Studies on the urinary excretion, biological effects and origin of oestrogens in post-menopausal women. Acta Endocrinol [Suppl 135] (Kbh) 60
Pryse-Davies J, Dewhurst CJ (1971) The development of the ovary and uterus in the foetus, new-born and infant: a morphological and enzyme histochemical study. J Pathol 103:5
Puck A, Korte W, Hübner KA (1957) Die Wirkung des Östriol auf Corpus uteri, Cervix uteri and Vagina der Frau. Dtsch Med Wochenschr 82:1864
Pugh WE, Vogt RF, Gibson RA (1973) Primary ovarian pregnancy and the intrauterine device. Obstet Gynecol 42:218
Puri S, Aleem F, Schulman H (1976) A histologic study of the placentas of patients with saline- and prostaglandin-induced abortion. Obstet Gynecol 48:216
Püschel W, Möbius G (1967) Histologischer Typ und Prognose des Korpuskarzinoms. Geburtshilfe Frauenheilkd 27:50
Pyörälä T, Allonen H, Nygren KG et al. (1982) Return of fertility after the removal of nova T or copper T 200. Contraception 26:113
Quagliarello J, Goldsmith L, Steinetz B et al. (1980) Induction of relaxin secretion in nonpregnant women by human chorionic gonadotropin. J Clin Endocrinol Metab 51:74
Rachmaninoff N, Climie ARW (1966) Mixed mesodermal tumors of the uterus. Cancer (Philad) 19:1705
Rahn J (1968) Zur nosologischen Bewertung der Infiltrate des menschlichen Endometriums. Gegenbaurs Morphol Jahrb 111:605
Rahn J, Uebel J (1965) Rundzelleninfiltrate des Endometrium und ihre nosologische Bewertung. Zentralbl Gynäkol 87:737
Ramadan M, Goudie RB (1986) Epithelial antigens in malignant mixed Müllerian tumors of endometrium. J Pathol 148:13
Ramsey EM (1949) The vascular pattern of the endometrium of the pregnant rhesus monkey (*Macaca mulatta*). Carneg Instn Wash Publ 583. Contrib Embryol 33:113
Ramsey EM (1955) Vascular patterns in the endometrium and the placenta. Angiology 6:321
Randall CL (1943) Sarcoma of the uterus. Am J Obstet Gynecol 45:445
Randall CL (1945) Recognition and management of the woman predisposed to uterine carcinoma. JAMA 127:20
Randall CL, Birtch PK, Harkins JL (1957) Ovarian function after the menopause. Am J Obstet Gynecol 74:719
Randall JH, Goddard WB (1956) A study of 531 cases of endometrial carcinoma. Surg Gynecol Obstet 103:221
Randall JH, Mirick DF, Wieben EE (1951) Endometrial carcinoma. Am J Obstet Gynecol 61:596
Randall LM (1935) Endometrial biopsy. Proc Mayo Clin 10:143
Rao BR, Wiest WG (1970) Progesterone binding in rabbit uterus. Excerpta Med Int Congr Ser 210:153

Rao BR, Wiest WG, Allen WM (1973) Progesterone "receptor" in rabbit uterus. Endocrinology 92:1229
Rao BR, Wiest WG, Allen WM (1974) Progesterone "receptor" in human endometrium. Endocrinology 95:1275
Rappaport F, Rabinovitz M, Toaff R, Krochik N (1960) Genital listeriosis as a cause of reapeated abortion. Lancet I:1273
Ratner M, Schneiderman C (1948) Metastase to endometrium and skin from carcinoma of kidney; report of case and review of literature. J Urol 60:389
Ratzenhofer M, Schmid KO (1954) Über die Involutionsvorgänge am Drüsenepithel bei in Blüte befindlicher glandulär-cystischer Hyperplasie. Beitr Pathol Anat 114:417
Ratzenhofer M, Schmid KO (1954) Über die Beziehungen zwischen Proliferationszustand des Drüsenepithels und Drüsenform bei glandulär-cystischer Hyperplasie der Corpusmucosa. Beitr Pathol Anat 114:441
Rauramo L, Grönroos M, Kivikoski A (1964) The significance of oestrogen activity in postmenopausal genital carcinoma. Ann Chir Gynaecol Fenn 53:110
Rauscher H, Leeb H (1965) Untersuchungen über den Effekt von Äthinyl-Nor-Testosteronazetat auf das innere Genitale der Frau. Fortschr Geburtshilfe Gynäkol 21:165
Ravinsky E (1984) Ovarian hyperthecosis associated with pseudosarcomatous changes in the endometrial stroma. Am J Surg Pathol 8:939
Reeves KO, Kaufman RH (1977) Exogenous estrogens and endometrial carcinoma. J Reprod Med 18:297
Reicher NB, Phillips RS (1961) Carcinoma of the endometrium. Am J Obstet Gynecol 82:457
Reifenstein EC (1971) Hydroxyprogesterone caproate therapy in advanced endometrial cancer. Cancer (Philad) 27:485
Reiffenstuhl G, Kroemer H (1965) Endometriumtransplantationen mit nachfolgenden Schwangerschaften. Geburtshilfe Frauenheilkd 25:1070
Remotti G (1956) Osservazioni sul comportamento dell'acido ribonucleinico (RNA) dei mucopolisaccaridi Hotchkiss-positivi nelle iperplasia endometriali. Ann Ostet Ginecol 78:653
Reyniak JV, Gordon M, Stone ML, Sedlis A (1975) Endometrial regeneration after voluntary abortion. Obstet Gynecol 45:203
Rice-Wray E, Aranda-Rosell A, Maqueo M, Goldzieher JW (1963) Comparison of the long-term endometrial effects of synthetic progestins used in fertility control. Am J Obstet Gynecol 87:429
Rice-Wray E, Corren S, Gorodovsky J et al. (1967) Resumption of ovulation after discontinuing oral contraception. Proc 5th World Congr Fertil Steril Stockholm 1966. Excerpta Medica, Amsterdam, p 1061
Richter R (1909) Ein Mittel zur Verhütung der Konzeption. Dtsch Med Wochenschr 35:1525
Rickers K, Krone HA (1969) Zur nukleolären Stoffabgabe der Endometriumepithelzelle im elektronenmikroskopischen Bild. Z Geburtshilfe Gynäkol 170:137
Riehm H, Stoll P (1952) Korpuskarzinom nach 17jähriger Follikelhormon-Medikation. Geburtshilfe Frauenheilkd 12:985
Rifkin I, Nachtigall LE, Beckman EM (1972) Amenorrhea following use of oral contraceptives. Am J Obstet Gynecol 113:420
Ringertz N (1970) Hydatidiform mole, invasive mole and choriocarcinoma in Sweden 1958–1965. Acta Obstet Gynecol Scand 49:195
Risse EKJ, Beerthuizen RJ, Vooijs GP (1981) Cytologic and histologic findings in women using an IUD. Obstet Gynecol 58:569
Ritchie DA (1965) The vaginal maturation index and endometrial carcinoma. Am J Obstet Gynecol 91:578
Ritzmann H, Hillemanns HG (1977) Die Hyperplasieformen des Endometriums und ihre Beziehungen zum Endometriumkarzinom. Arch Gynäkol 223:345
Roach WR, Guderian AM, Brewer JI (1960) Endometrial gland cell atypism in the presence of trophoblast. Am J Obstet Gynecol 79:680
Robboy SJ, Bradley R (1979) Changing trends and prognostic features in endometrial cancer associated with exogenous estrogen therapy. Obstet Gynecol 54:269

Roberts DK, Horbelt DV, Powell LC (1975) The ultratructural reponse of human endometrium to medroxyprogesterone acetate. Am J Obstet Gynecol 123:811

Robertson DM, Mester J, Beilby J et al. (1971) The measurement of high-affinity oestradiol receptors in human uterine endometrium and myometrium. Acta Endocrinol (Kbh) 68:534

Robey M, Herve R, de Brux J, Sergent P (1968) Action de l'acétate de noréthistérone sur la muqueuse utérine. Gynécol Obstét 67:425

Robinson CR (1964) Endometrial ossification following a recent abortion. Can Med Assoc J 90:1317

Rochefort H, Garcia M (1976) Androgens on the estrogen receptor. I. Binding and in vivo nuclear translocation. Steroids 28:549

Rochefort H, Lignon F, Capony F (1972) Effect of antiestrogens on uterine estradiol receptors. Gynecol Invest 3:43

Rock J, Bartlett MK (1937) Biopsy studies of human endometrium. Criteria of dating and information about amenorrhea, menorrhagia and time of ovulation. JAMA 108:202

Rock J, Hertig AT (1944) Information regarding the time of human ovulation derived from a study of 3 unfertilized and 11 fertilized ova. Am J Obstet Gynecol 47:343

Rockenschaub A (1960) Der menstruelle Zyklus. Z Geburtshilfe Gynäkol 155:105

Roddick JW, Greene RR (1957) Relation of ovarian stromal hyperplasia to endometrial carcinoma. Am J Obstet Gynecol 73:843

Rodriguez J, Hart WR (1982) Endometrial cancers occurring 10 or more years after pelvic irradiation for carcinoma. Int J Gynecol Pathol 1:135

Rodriguez J, Sen KK, Seski JC et al. (1979) Progesterone binding by human endometrial tissue during the proliferative and secretory phases of menstrual cycle and by hyperplastic and carcinomatous endometrium. Am J Obstet Gynecol 133:660

Rodriguez M, Okagaki T, Richart RM (1972) Mycotic endometritis due to candida. Obstet Gynecol 39:292

Rodriguez M, Rubin A, Koss LG, Harris J (1974) Evaluation of endometrial jet wash technic (Gravlee) in 303 patients in a community Hospital. Obstet Gynecol 43:392

Roemer H (1941) Karzino-Sarkom des Endometriums mit Knorpelbildung. Zentralbl Gynäkol 65:1497

Roland M (1967) Clinical value of synthetic progestagens in luteal deficiency. Proc 5th World Congr Fertil Steril Stockholm 1966. Excerpta Medica, Amsterdam, p 461

Roland M, Clyman MJ, Decker A, Ober WB (1964) Classification of endometrial response to synthetic progestagen-estrogen compounds. Fertil Steril 15:143

Roland M, Clyman MJ, Decker A, Ober WB (1966) Sequential endometrial alterations during one cycle of treatment with synthetic progestagen-estrogen compounds. Fertil Steril 17:338

Roman C, Labaeye M (1964) L'insuffisance lutéale de l'endomètre dans la stérilité. Ann Endocrinol (Paris) 25:229

Romeis B (1968) Mikroskopische Technik. Oldenbourg, München

Romney SL, Hertig AT, Reid DE (1950) The endometria associated with ectopic pregnancy. A study of 115 cases. Surg Gynecol Obstet 91:605

Rorat E, Wallach RC (1984) Papillary metaplasia of the endometrium: clinical and histopathologic considerations. Obstet Gynecol 64:90S

Rorat E, Ferenczy A, Richart RM (1974) The ultrastructure of clear cell adenocarcinoma of endometrium. Cancer (Philad) 33:880

Rosado A, Hernández O, Aznar R, Hicks JJ (1976) Comparative glycolytic metabolism in the normal and in the Copper treated human endometrium. Contraception 13:17

Rosado A, Mercado E, Gallegos AJ et al. (1977) Subcellular distribution of lysosomal enzymes in the human endometrium. I. Normal menstrual cycle. Contraception 16/3:287

Rosenberg RJ, García C-R (1975) Endometrial biopsy in the cycle of conception. Fertil Steril 26:1088

Rosenberg RJ, García C-R (1976) A comparison of endometrial histology with simultaneous plasma progesterone determinations in infertile women. Fertil Steril 27:1256

Rosenberg RJ, Sarkar AK, Pekala SJ (1964) Endometrial stromaloma. Obstet Gynecol 23:708
Rosenfeld DL, Chodow S, Bronson RA (1980) Diagnosis of luteal phase inadequacy. Obstet Gynecol 56:193
Rosenwaks Z, Wentz AC, Jones GS et al. (1979) Endometrial pathology and estrogens. Obstet Gynecol 53:403
Ross JC, Eifel PJ, Cox RS et al. (1983) Primary mucinous adenocarcinoma of the endometrium. Am J Surg Pathol 7:715
Roth E, Taylor HB (1966) Heterotopic cartilage in the uterus. Obstet Gynecol 27:838
Roth LM (1974) Clear cell adenocarcinoma of the female genital tract. Cancer (Philad) 33:990
Roth LM, Pride GL, Sharma HM (1976) Müllerian adenosarcoma of the uterine cervix with heterologous elements. Cancer (Philad) 37:1725
Rott H-D, Richter E, Rummel W-D, Schwanitz G (1972) Chromosomenbefunde bei Ehepaaren mit gehäuften Aborten. Arch Gynäkol 213:110
Rotter W, Eigner J (1949) Über Degenerationsformen der „hellen Zellen" des Endometriums. Frankfurt Z Pathol 61:92
Rozin S, Sacks MI, Shenker JG (1967) Endometrial histology and clinical symptoms following prolonged retention of uterine contraceptive devices. Am J Obstet Gynecol 97:197
Ruck CJ (1952) Über Endometritis. Rückblick auf ein Jahrhundert Schleimhautdiagnostik. Zentralbl Allg Pathol 88:317
Rudel HW, Maqueo M, Martinez-Manautou J (1964) Correlation between the state of growth of the human endometrium and its response to a synthetic progestagen (Chlormadinone). J Reprod Fertil 8:305
Rudel HW, Manautou JM, Topete MM (1966) Comparison of the antiestrogenic activity of several progestogens in women. J New Drugs 6:126
Ruffolo EH, Metts NB, Sanders HL (1969) Malignant mixed Müllerian tumors of the uterus: a clinicopathologic study of 9 patients. Obstet Gynecol 33:544
Ruge IC (1918) Epithelveränderungen und beginnender Krebs am weiblichen Genitalapparat. Arch Gynäkol 109:102
Rumbolz L, Greene G (1957) Observations on metachromatic granules in human endometrium. Am J Obstet Gynecol 73:992
Runge H, Ebner H (1954) Die Bedeutung der Histochemie für die Gynäkologie. In: Antoine (ed) Klinische Fortschritte: Gynäkologie. Urban & Schwarzenberg, Wien
Runge H, Ebner H, Lindenschmidt W (1956) Vorzüge der kombinierten Alcianblau-PAS-Reaktion für die gynäkologische Histopathologie. Dtsch Med Wochenschr 81:1525
Ruppert H (1949) Zur Genese der Schleimhautsarkome des Uterus. Zentralbl Gynäkol 71:629
Russell P, Bannatyne P, Shearman RP et al. (1982) Premature hypergonadotropic ovarian failure: clinicopathological study of 19 cases. Int J Gynecol Pathol 1:185
Rust T (1979) Die Basaltemperatur der Frau. Geburtshilfe Frauenheilkd 39:947
Rutherford RN, Hertig AT (1945) Noninvolution of the placental site. Am J Obstet Gynecol 49:378
Rutledge F, Kotz HL, Chang SC (1965) Mesonephric adenocarcinoma of the endometrium. Report of a case and a review of the literature. Obstet Gynecol 25:362
Rüttner JR, Leu HJ (1954) Die Bedeutung der „Grenzfallveränderungen" der Corpusmucosa. Schweiz Med Wochenschr 84:531
Ryan GM, Craig J, Reid DE (1964) Histology of the uterus and ovaries after long-term cyclic norethynodrel therapy. Am J Obstet Gynecol 90:715
Rybo G (1966) Plasminogen activators in the endometrium. II. Clinical activators during the menstrual cycle and its relation to menstrual blood loss. Acta Obstet Gynecol Scand 45:97
Ryden ABV (1952) Cancer of the corpus uteri and the ovary in the same patient. Acta Radiol (Stockh) 37:49
Ryder DE (1982) Verrucous carcinoma of the endometrium: a unique neoplasm with long survival. Obstet Gynecol 59:78S

Sachs H (1968) Quantitative histochemische Untersuchung des Endometrium in der Schwangerschaft und der Placenta (cytophotometrische Messungen). Arch Gynäkol 205:93

Saksela E, Lampinen V, Procope B-J (1974) Malignant mesenchymal tumors of the uterine corpus. Am J Obstet Gynecol 120:452

Saksena KC, Arora MM, Gupta JC, Rangam CM (1965) Histochemical studies in histologically normal endometrium. Indian J Med Sci 19:121

Sakuma S (1970) Glykogengehalt und -verteilung in der Uterusschleimhaut der Frau während des normalen Zyklus im elektronenmikroskopischen Bild. Beitr Pathol Anat 140:454

Salaverry G, Mendez MC, Zipper J, Medel M (1973) Copper determination and localization in different morphologic components of human endometrium during the menstrual cycle in copper contraceptive device wearers. Am J Obstet Gynecol 115:163

Salazar OM, De Papp EW, Bonfiglio TA et al. (1977) Adenosquamous carcinoma of the endometrium. Cancer (Philad) 40:119

Salazar OM, Bonfiglio TA, Patten SF et al. (1978) Uterine sarcomas. Natural history, treatment and prognosis. Cancer (Philad) 42:1152

Salazar OM, Feldstein ML, De Papp EW et al. (1978) The management of clinical stage I endometrial carcinoma. Cancer (Philad) 41:1016

Sall S, Sonnenblick B, Stone ML (1970) Factors affecting survival of patients with endometrial adenocarcinoma. Am J Obstet Gynecol 107:116

Salm R (1962) Mucin production of normal and abnormal endometrium. Arch Pathol 73:30

Salm R (1962) Macrophages in endometrial lesions. J Pathol Bacteriol 83:405

Salm R (1969) Superficial intrauterine spread of intraepithelial cervical carcinoma. J Pathol 97:719

Salm R (1972) The incidence and significance of early carcinomas in endometrial polyps. J Pathol 108:47

Sandstrom RE, Welche WR, Green TH (1979) Adenocarcinoma of the endometrium in pregnancy. Obstet Gynecol 53:73S

Sanhueza H, Sivin I (1975) The Dalcon Shield in four Latin American countries. Contraception 11:711

Sarbach W (1955) Über helle Zellen im Endometrium unter besonderer Berücksichtigung der glandulär-zystischen Hyperplasie. Gynaecologia (Basel) 139:356

Sasagawa M, Watanabe S, Ohmormo Y et al. (1986) Reactivity of 2 monoclonal antibodies (Troma 1 and CAM 5,2) on tumor tissue sections: analysis of their usefulness as a histological trophoblast marker in normal pregnancy and trophoblastic disease. Int J Gynecol Pathol 5:345

Sato N, Mori T, Orenstein JM, Silverberg SG (1984) Ultrastructure of papillary serous carcinoma of the endometrium. Int J Gynecol Pathol 2:337

Saw EC, Smale LE, Einstein H, Huntington RW (1975) Female genital coccidioidomycosis. Obstet Gynecol 45:199

Sawaragi I, Wynn RM (1969) Ultrastructural localization of metabolic enzymes during the human endometrial cycle. Obstet Gynecol 34:50

Schaefer G, Marcus RS, Kramer EE (1972) Postmenopausal endometrial tuberculosis. Am J Obstet Gynecol 112:681

Scheffey LC (1942) Malignancy subsequent to irradiation of the uterus for benign conditions. Am J Obstet Gynecol 44:925

Scheffey LC, Thudium WJ, Farrell DM (1943) Further experience in the management and treatment of carcinoma of the fundus of the uterus with five year end results in seventy-five patients. Am J Obstet Gynecol 46:786

Schiller W (1927) Über Xanthomzellen im Uterus. Arch Gynäkol 130:346

Schindler AE (1977) Endometriumkarzinom und extraglanduläre Östrogenbiosynthese. Geburtshilfe Frauenheilkd 37:242

Schinkele O (1947) Ein Angiomyom des Endometriums. Wien Klin Wochenschr 617

Schlagenhaufer F (1912) Pathologisch-anatomische Kasuistik. Arch Gynäkol 95:1

Schmid KO (1968) Über ungewöhnliche Epithelveränderungen und Rückbildungsvorgänge der Corpusmucosa infolge abnormer Hormonzufuhr. Arch Gynäkol 205:466

Schmidt-Elmendorff H, Kaiser E (1967) Zur Ovulationsauslösung mit Gonadotropinen bei anovulatorischen Cyclen. Arch Gynäkol 204:286

Schmidt-Matthiesen H (1962) Histochemische Untersuchungen der Endometrium-Grundsubstanz. Acta Histochem (Jena) 13:129

Schmidt-Matthiesen H (1962) Die Vascularisierung des menschlichen Endometriums. Arch Gynäkol 196:575

Schmidt-Matthiesen H (1963) Histochemische Studien am Sekret der Endometriumdrüsen. Acta Histochem (Jena) 16:28

Schmidt-Matthiesen H (1963) Das normale menschliche Endometrium. Thieme, Stuttgart

Schmidt-Matthiesen H (1965) Die dysfunktionelle uterine Blutung. Histochemie und Mechanismus. Gynaecologia (Basel) 160:197

Schmidt-Matthiesen H (1967) Die fibrinolytische Aktivität von Endometrium und Myometrium, Dezidua und Plazenta, Kollum- und Korpuskarzinomen. Physiologie, Pathologie und klinisch-therapeutische Konsequenzen. Fortschr Geburtshilfe Gynäkol 31:1

Schmidt-Matthiesen H (1968) Endometrium und Nidation beim Menschen. Z Geburtshilfe Gynäkol 168:113

Schmitt K, Schäfer A (1977) Intraepitheliale Ausbreitung des Plattenepithelcarcinoms der Cervix uteri auf das Corpusendometrium. Z Krebsforsch Klin Onkol 89:45

Schneider GT, Bechtel M (1956) Ovarian cortical stromal hyperplasia. Obstet Gynecol 8:713

Schneider ML (1985) Möglichkeiten und Grenzen eines zytologischen Früherkennungsprogramms beim Endometrium-Carcinom. Geburtshilfe Frauenheilkd 45:831

Schneider V, Behm FG, Mumaw VR (1982) Ascending herpetic endometritis. Obstet Gynecol 59:259

Schopper W, Pliess G (1949) Über Chorionepitheliosis. Ein Beitrag zur Genese. Diagnostik und Bewertung ektopischer chorionepithelialer Wucherungen. Virchows Arch Pathol Anat 317:347

Schrader WT, O'Malley BW (1978) Molecular structure and analysis of progesterone receptors. In: O'Malley BW, Birnbaumer L (eds) Receptors and hormone action, vol 2. Academic Press, New York, p 189

Schröder R (1913) Der normale menstruelle Zyklus der Uterusschleimhaut. Hirschwald, Berlin

Schröder R (1914) Über das Verhalten der Uterusschleimhaut um die Zeit der Menstruation. Monatsschr Geburtshilfe Gynäkol 39:3

Schröder R (1915) Anatomische Studien zur normalen und pathologischen Physiologie des Menstruationszyklus. Arch Gynäkol 104:55, 82

Schröder R (1920) Über die Pathogenese der Uterustuberkulose. Monatsschr Geburtshilfe Gynäkol 15:15

Schröder R (1928) Der menstruelle Genitalzyklus des Weibes und seine Störungen. In: Stoeckel (ed) Handbuch der Gynäkologie, vol I/2. Bergmann, München

Schröder R (1954) Endometrial hyperplasia in relation to genital function. Am J Obstet Gynecol 68:294

Schröder R (1920) Hillejahn A (1920) Über einen heterologen Kombinationstumor des Uterus. Zentralbl Gynäkol 44:1050

Schüller E (1961) Epithelien und Stromazellen des menschlichen Endometriums. Arch Gynäkol 196:49

Schüller E (1968) Cilated epithelia of the human uterine mucosa. Obstet Gynecol 31:215

Schüller E (1973) Ultrastructure of ciliated cells in the human endometrium. Obstet Gynecol 41:188

Schumacher H (1956) Das Talkumgranulom des Endometriums. Geburtshilfe Frauenheilkd 16:1082

Schümmelfeder N (1950) Die Fluorochromierung des lebenden, überlebenden und toten Protoplasmas mit dem basischen Farbstoff Acridinorange und ihre Beziehung zur Stoffwechselaktivität der Zelle. Virchows Arch Pathol Anat 318:119

Schümmelfeder N, Ebschner KJ, Krogh E (1957) Die Grundlage der differenten Fluoro-

chromierung von Ribo- und Desoxyribonukleinsäure mit Acridinorange. Naturwissenschaften 44:467
Schwabe C, Steinetz B, Weiss G et al. (1978) Relaxin. Recent Prog Horm Res 34:123
Scommegna A, Lee AW, Borushek S (1970) Evaluation of an injectable progestin-estrogen as a contraceptive. Am J Obstet Gynecol 107:1147
Scommegna A, Pandya GN, Christ M et al. (1970) Intrauterine administration of progesterone by a slow releasing device. Fertil Steril 21:201
Scommegna A, Avila T, Luna M et al. (1974) Fertility control by intrauterine release of progesterone. Obstet Gynecol 43:769
Scully RE (1953) Hyperestrinism in old women. Am J Obstet Gynecol 65:1248
Scully RE, Young RH (1981) Trophoblastic pseudotumor. A reappraisal. Am J Surg Pathol 5:75
Scully RE, Aguirre P, De Lellis RA (1984) Argyrophilia, serotonin, and peptide hormones in the female genital tract and its tumors. Int J Gynecol Pathol 3:51
Sedlis A, Kim NG (1971) Significance of the endometrial subepithelial collagen band. Obstet Gynecol 38:264
Segal SJ (1967) Regulatory action of estrogenic hormones. Dev Biol 1:264
Sehrt E (1905) Uterussarkom mit sekundärer multipler Carcinombildung. Beitr Geburtshilfe Gynäkol 10:43
Seitz A (1923) Beiträge zur Pathogenese der Meno- und Metrorrhagien. Arch Gynäkol 116:252
Sekiba D (1924) Zur Morphologie und Histologie des Menstruationszyklus. Arch Gynäkol 121:36
Seltzer VL, Klein M, Beckman EM (1977) The occurrence of squamous metaplasia as a precursor of squamous cell carcinoma of the endometrium. Obstet Gynecol 49:34s
Sen DK, Fox H (1967) The lymphoid tissue of the endometrium. Gynaecologia (Basel) 163:371
Sengel A, Stoebner P (1970) (1972) Ultrastructure de l'endomètre humain normal. Z Zellforsch 109:245, 260; 133:47
Shahani SM, Dandekar PV, Chikhlikar AR (1967) Intra-uterine devices: clinical effectiveness and changes in the genital tract. Proc 5th World Congr Fertil Steril Stockholm 1966. Excerpta Medica, Amsterdam, p 1138
Shapiro SS, Dyer RD, Colas AE (1980) Progesterone-induced glycogen accumulation in human endometrium during organ culture. Am J Obstet Gynecol 136:419
Shapiro S, Kelly JP, Rosenberg I et al. (1985) Risk of localized and widespread endometrial cancer in relation to recent and discontinued use of conjugated estrogens. N Engl J Med 313:969
Sharf M, Eibschitz I, Eylan E (1973) Latent toxoplasmosis and pregnancy. Obstet Gynecol 42:349
Sharman A (1955) La fonction tubaire et ses troubles. In: Colloques sur la fonction tubaire. Masson, Paris
Sharman A (1967) Ovulation in the post partum period. Int J Fertil 12:14
Shaw ST, Macaulay LK, Hohman WR (1979) Vessel density in endometrium of women with and without intrauterine contraceptive devices: A morphometric evaluation. Am J Obstet Gynecol 135:202
Shaw ST, Macaulay LK, Aznar R et al. (1981) Effects of a progesterone-releasing intrauterine contraceptive device on endometrial blood vessels: a morphometric study. Am J Obstet Gynecol 141:821
Shaw W, Dastur B (1949) The association of certain ovarian cells with endometrial cancer. Br Med J 4619:113
Shearman RP (1971) Prolonged secondary amenorrhoea after oral contraceptive therapy. Lancet II:64
Shearman RP (1973) Post-coital contraception. A review. Contraception 7:459
Shearman RP (1975) Secondary amenorrhoea after oral contraceptives-treatment and follow-up. Contraception 11:123
Sheehan JF, Schmitz HE (1950) Histologic changes produced by radiation in adenocarcinomas of the uterus. Comparison with changes produced in squamous cell carcinomas of the cervix. Am J Clin Pathol 20:241

Sheffield H, Soule SD, Herzog GM (1969) Cyclic endometrial changes in response to monthly injections of an estrogen-progestogen contraceptive drug. Am J Obstet Gynecol 103:828
Sherman AI (1966) Progesterone caproate in the treatment of endometrial cancer. Obstet Gynecol 28:309
Sherman AI (1969) Chromosome constitution of endometrium. Obstet Gynecol 34:753
Sherman AI, Brown S (1979) The precursors of endometrial carcinoma. Am J Obstet Gynecol 135:947
Sherman AI, Woolf RB (1959) An endocrine basis for endometrial carcinoma. Am J Obstet Gynecol 77:233
Shute E (1963) Late results of the irradiation menopause. J Obstet Gynaecol Br Cwlth 70:833
Sibley CH, Tomkins GM (1974) Mechanisms of steroid resistance. Cell 2:221
Sica F, Bresciani F (1979) Estrogen-binding proteins of calf uterus. Purification to homogeneity of receptor from cytosol by affinity chromatography. Biochemistry 18:2369
Siegal GP, Taylor LL, Nelson KG et al. (1983) Characterization of a pure heterologous sarcoma of the uterus: rhabdomyosarcoma of the corpus. Int J Gynecol Pathol 2:303
Siegel P, Heinen G (1965) Die Reaktion des Endometriums auf die cyklische Behandlung mit Ovulationshemmern. Geburtshilfe Frauenheilkd 25:312
Siegel P, Heinen G (1965) Endometriumbefunde bei Ovulationshemmern. Arch Gynäkol 202:248
Siegert F (1938) Follikelhormon und Plattenepithelmetaplasie der Corpusschleimhaut. Arch Gynäkol 165:135
Siegler AM (1962) Synechiae of the uterine cavity after curettage. Am J Obstet Gynecol 83:1595
Siiteri PK (1978) Steroid hormones and endometrial cancer. Cancer Res 38:4360
Sillo-Seidl G (1967) Die Endometriumbiopsie im Dienste der Sterilitätsdiagnose. Zentralbl Gynäkol 89:488
Sillo-Seidl G (1971) The analysis of the endometrium of 1000 sterile women. Hormones 2:70
Sillo-Seidl G, Dallenbach-Hellweg G (1974) Uterusschleimhaut-Polypen und Sterilität. Fortschr Med 92:825
Silverberg SG (1971) Malignant mixed mesodermal tumor of the uterus: an ultrastructural study. Am J Obstet Gynecol 110:702
Silverberg SG, De Giorgi LS (1973) Clear cell carcinoma of the endometrium. Cancer (Philad) 31:1127
Silverberg SG, Makowski EL (1975) Endometrial carcinoma in young women taking oral contraceptive agents. Obstet Gynecol 46:503
Silverberg SG, Makowski EL, Roche WD (1977) Endometrial carcinoma in women under 40 years of age. Comparison of cases in oral contraceptive users and non-users. Cancer (Philad) 39:592
Silverberg SG, Wilson MA, Board JA (1971) Hemangiopericytoma of the uterus: an ultrastructural study. Am J Obstet Gynecol 110:397
Silverberg SG, Haukkamaa M, Arko H et al. (1986) Endometrial morphology during long-term use of levonorgestrel-realising intrauterine devices. Am J Obstet Gynecol 5:235
Simon WE, Hölzel F (1979) Hormone sensitivity of gynecological tumor cells in tissue culture. J Cancer Res Clin Oncol 94:307
Singh RP, Carr DH (1967) Anatomic findings in human abortions of known chromosomal constitution. Obstet Gynecol 29:806
Sirtori C (1969) Some ultrastructural aspects of human uterine physiopathology; cyclosenility, senility, antisenile and antitumoral therapies and contraceptive drugs. Proc Int Sympos Obstet Gynecol. Erba, Milano
Sjöstedt S, Strandh J (1971) Effect of polyestriol phosphate on the vaginal cytology and uterine endometrium of postmenopausal women. Acta Obstet Gynecol Scand 50:30
Sjövall A (1938) Untersuchungen über die Schleimhaut der Cervix uteri. Acta Obstet Gynecol Scand [Suppl 4] 18

Skaarland E (1985) Morphometric analysis of nuclei in epithelial structures from normal and neoplastic endometrium: a study using the Isaaks cell sampler and endoscan instruments. J Clin Pathol 38:496

Skaarland E (1986) New concept in diagnostic endometrial cytology: diagnostic criteria based on composition and architecture of large tissue fragments in smears. J Clin Pathol 39:36

Sledge GW, Ramzy I, Dressler LG et al. (1985) Presence of an estrogen-regulated protein in endometrial cancer. Obstet Gynecol 66:423

Slunsky R (1976) Histologische Untersuchungen über die Blutstillung beim Abbruch der Schwangerschaft im II.–III. Lunarmonat. Vergleich mit der postpartalen Hämostase. Arch Gynäkol 220:325

Smith DC, Prentice R, Thompson DJ, Herrmann WL (1975) Association of exogenous estrogen and endometrial carcinoma. N Engl J Med 293:1164

Smith FR, Bowden L (1948) Cancer of the corpus uteri following radiation therapy for benign uterine lesions. Am J Roentgenol 59:796

Smith GV (1941) Carcinoma of the endometrium. N Engl J Med 225:608

Smith GV, Johnson LC, Hertig AT (1942) Relation of ovarian stromal hyperplasia and thecoma of the ovary to endometrial hyperplasia and carcinoma. N Engl J Med 226:364

Smith OW, Smith GV, Gavian NG (1959) Urinary estrogens in women. Am J Obstet Gynecol 78:1028

Snoden R, Williams M (1975) The United Kingdom Dalkon Shield trial: two years of observation. Contraception 11:1

So-Bosita JL, Lebherz TB, Blair OM (1970) Endometrial jet washer. Obstet Gynecol 36:287

Söderlin E (1975) Factors affecting prognosis of endometrial carcinoma. Acta Obstet Gynecol Scand [Suppl] 38

Sommers SC, Hertig AT, Bengloff H (1949) Genesis of endometrial carcinoma. Cancer (Philad) 2:957

Sommers SC, Meissner WA (1957) Endocrine abnormalities accompanying human endometrial cancer. Cancer (Philad) 10:516

Song J, Mark MS, Lawler MP (1970) Endometrial changes in women receiving oral contraceptives. Am J Obstet Gynecol 107:717

Sorvari TE (1969) A histochemical study of epithelial mucosubstances in endometrial and cervical adenocarcinomas with reference to normal endometrium and cervical mucosa. Acta Pathol Microbiol Scand [Suppl] 207:1

Soules MR, Wiebe RH, Aksel S, Hammond CB (1977) The diagnosis and therapy of luteal phase deficiency. Fertil Steril 28:1033

Soutter WP, Hamilton K, Leake RE (1979) High affinity binding of oestradiol-17β in the nuclei of human endometrium cells. J Steroid Biochem 10:529–534

Spechter HJ (1953) Über die Deziduabildung ohne Schwangerschaft. Münch Med Wochenschr 982

Speert H (1948) Corpus cancer. Clinical, pathological, and etiological aspects. Cancer (Philad) 1:584

Speert H (1949) The endometrium in old age. Surg Gynecol Obstet 89:551

Speert H (1958) The uterine decidua in extrauterine pregnancy: its natural history and some biologic interpretations. Am J Obstet Gynecol 76:491

Speert H, Peightal TC (1949) Malignant tumors of the uterine fundus subsequent to irradiation for benign pelvic conditions. Am J Obstet Gynecol 57:261

Spickmann F (1947) Atypische Regelblutungen bei abnormen Lebensbedingungen der Frau. Zentralbl Gynäkol 69:1077

Spirtos NJ, Yurewicz EC, Maghissi KS et al. (1985) Pseudocorpus luteum insufficiency: a study of cytosol progesterone receptors in human endometrium. Obstet Gynecol 65:535

Stadtmüller A (1950) Die verlängerte menstruelle Abstoßung und verzögerte Regeneration der Korpusschleimhaut und ihre klinische Bedeutung. Arch Gynäkol 177:392

Staemmler M (1953) Untersuchung über die Bedeutung der Gitterfasern im Stroma der Uterusschleimhaut. Arch Gynäkol 182:445

Staffeldt K, Lübke F (1967) Endometrial findings in the investigation of sterility. Proc 5th World Congress Fertil Steril Stockholm 1966. Excerpta Medica, Amsterdam, p 489
Stähler F (1950) Cytometrie der Uterusmucosa. Med Klin 366
Stanley MA (1969) Chromosome constitution of human endometrium. Am J Obstet Gynecol 104:99
Stanley MA, Kirkland JA (1968) Cytogenetic studies of endometrial carcinoma. Am J Obstet Gynecol 102:1070
Starup J (1967) Endometrial histology and vaginal cytology during oral contraception. Acta Obstet Gynecol Scand 46:419
Starup J (1972) Amenorrhoea following oral contraception. Acta Obstet Gynecol Scand 51:341
State D, Hirsch EF (1941) The distribution of the nerves to the adult endometrium. Arch Pathol 32:939
Steele SJ, Scott JM, Stephens TW (1968) Endometrial stromal sarcoma. Report of a case with a pulmonary metastasis extending through the heart. Br J Surg 55:943
Stemmermann GN (1961) Extrapelvic carcinoma metastatic to the uterus. Am J Obstet Gynecol 82:1261
Sternberg WH, Clark WH, Smith RC (1954) Malignant mixed müllerian tumor (mixed mesodermal tumor of the uterus). A study of twenty-one cases. Cancer (Philad) 7:704
Stevenson CS (1965) The endometrium in infertile women: prognostic significance of the initial study biopsy. Fertil Steril 16:208
Stevenson TC, Taylor DS (1972) The effect of methyl cyanocrylate tissue adhesive on the human Fallopian tube and endometrium. J Obstet Gynaecol Br Cwlth 79:1028
Stieve H (1928) Die Enge der menschlichen Gebärmutter, ihre Veränderungen während der Schwangerschaft, der Geburt und des Wochenbettes und ihre Bedeutung. Z Mikrosk Anat Forsch 14:549
Stieve H (1952) Angeblich sterile Zeiten im Leben geschlechstüchtiger Frauen. Z Geburtshilfe Gynäkol 136:117
Stoerk quoted in Schiller (1927) S-B Akad Wiss Wien, math-nat Kl 1906
Stohr G (1942) Granulosa cell tumor of the ovary and coincident carcinoma of the uterus. Am J Obstet Gynecol 43:586
Stokes EM (1948) The association of estrogenic administration and adenocarcinoma of the endometrium. West J Surg 56:494
Stoll P (1949) Die Zusammenarbeit des behandelnden Arztes mit dem Histologen bei der Diagnose gynäkologischer Blutungen. Med Klin 44:564
Stoll P (1957) Frühdiagnose gynäkologischer Carcinome. Therapiewoche 7:231
Stoll P (1969) Gynecological vital cytology. Springer, Berlin Heidelberg New York
Stoll P, Bach HG (1954) Zur Bedeutung der Blutung in der Menopause. Dtsch Med Wochenschr 79:1559
Stoll P, Dallenbach-Hellweg G (1981) Systematik der gynäkologischen Morpholigie II. Fortschr Med 99:981
Stoll P, Pecorari D (1962) Die hormonale Aktivität im Vaginalsekret bei Patientinnen im Senium (über 65 Jahre) mit und ohne gynäkologische Tumoren. First Int Congr of Exfol Cytol. Lippincott, Philadelphia, p 22
Stoll P, Riehm L (1954) Über die statistische Erfassung histologischer Befunde in der Gynäkologie. Zentralbl Gynäkol 76:452
Stoll P, Ebner H, Lindenschmidt W (1954) Die Bedeutung histochemischer Methoden für die gynäkologische Histo- und Zytodiagnostik. Geburtshilfe Frauenheilkd 14:1065
Stolz J, Schönfeld V, Kafka V (1964) Über einen weiteren Fall von Gehirngewebebefund im Endometrium. Zentralbl Gynäkol 86:274
Strakosch W, Wurm H (1951) Talkum-Endometritis nach intrauteriner Anwendung von Marbadalglobuli und -Styli. Geburtshilfe Frauenheilkd 11:1109
Strauss F (1964) Die Ovoimplantation beim Menschen. Gynäkol Rundsch 1:3
Strauss G (1962) Zur Histochemie der Kohlenhydrate in den Endometriumdrüsen des Menschen. Arch Gynäkol 197:524
Strauss G (1963) Die Anwendung von Aldehydfuchsin und Methylviolett in der histologischen Abrasionsdiagnostik. Zentralbl Gynäkol 85:644

Strauss G, Hiersche HD (1963) Zur Frage der sogenannten Plattenepithelknötchen im Endometrium. Geburtshilfe Frauenheilkd 23:142

Stray-Pedersen B, Lorentzen-Styr AM (1977) Uterine toxoplasma infections and repeated abortions. Am J Obstet Gynecol 128:716

Stumpf WE (1970) Localization of hormones by autoradiography and other histochemical techniques. A critical review. J Histochem Cytochem 18:21

Stumpf WE, Baerwaldt C, Sar M (1971) Autoradiographic cellular and subcellular localization of sexual steroids. In: Basic actions of sex steroids on target organs. Karger, Basel

Stüper R (1955) Glandulär-zystische Hyperplasie und Tuberkulose der Gebärmutterschleimhaut. Geburtshilfe Frauenheilkd 15:122

Sturgis SH, Meigs JV (1936) Endometrial cycle and mechanism of normal menstruation. Am J Surg 33:369

Stutzer JM (1947) Über einen Fall von Uterussarkom in der Gravidität. Zentralbl Gynäkol 69:350

Suchowsky GK, Baldratti G (1964) Relationship between progestational activity and chemical structure of synthetic steroids. J Endocrinol 30:159

Sutherland AM (1958) Tuberculosis of endometrium. Obstet Gynecol 11:527

Sutherland AM (1982) Postmenopausal tuberculosis of the female genital tract. Obstet Gynecol 59:54S

Suzuki A, Konishi I, Okamura H, Nakashima N (1984) Adenocarcinoma of the endometrium associated with intrauterine pregnancy. Gynecol Oncol 18:261

Swan RW, Woodruff JD (1969) Retained products of conception. Obstet Gynecol 34:506

Swerdloff RS, Odell WD (1968) Gonadotropins: present concepts in the human. Calif Med 109:467

Sylven B (1945) The occurrence of ester sulfuric acids of heigh molecular weight and of mast cells in the stroma of the normal uterine corpus mucosa. Acta Obstet Gynecol Scand 25:189

Symmers WS (1959) On the differential diagnosis of thrombotic microangiopathy in endometrial curettings. J Clin Pathol 12:557

Symmonds RE, Dockerty MB (1955) Sarcoma and sarcoma-like proliferations of the endometrial stroma. II. Carcinosarcoma. Surg Gynecol Obstet 100:322

Symmonds RE, Dockerty MB, Pratt JH (1957) Sarcoma and sarcoma-like proliferations of the endometrial stroma. III. Stromal hyperplasia and stromatosis (stromal endometriosis). Am J Obstet Gynecol 73:1054

Szegvary M, Szereday Z, Ormos J (1963) In die Gebärmutter metastasierender Brustkrebs. Arch Geschwulstforsch 21:208

Szulman AE, Buchsbaum HJ (eds) (1987) Gestational trophoblastic disease. Springer, Berlin Heidelberg New York

Szulman AE, Surti U (1978) The syndromes of hydatidiform mole. I. Cytogenetic and morphologic correlations. II. Morphologic evolution of the complete and partial mole. Am J Obstet Gynecol 131:665; 132:20

Szulman AE, Surti U (1982) The clinicopathologic profile of the partial hydatidiform mole. Obstet Gynecol 59:597

Szulman AE, Surti U (1984) Complete and partial hydatidiform moles: cytogenetic and morphological aspects. In: Patillo Ra, Hussa RO (eds) Human trophoblast neoplasms. Plenum, New York, p 135

Taki I, Iijima H (1963) A new method of producing endometrial cancer in mice. Am J Obstet Gynecol 87:926

Taki I, Iijima H, Doi T et al. (1966) Histochemistry of hydrolytic and oxidative enzymes in the human and experimentally induced adenocarcinoma of the endometrium. Am J Obstet Gynecol 94:86

Tamada T, Okagaki T, Maruyama M, Matsumoto S (1967) Endometrial histology associated with an intrauterine contraceptive device. Am J Obstet Gynecol 98:811

Tang C, Toker C, Ances IG (1979) Stromomyoma of the uterus. Cancer (Philad) 43:308

Tase T, Toki T, Oikawa N et al. (1985) Flow cytometric DNA analysis of human endometrial carcinoma. Tohoku J Exp Med 146:429

Tatum HJ (1973) Metallic copper as an intrauterine contraceptive agent. Am J Obstet Gynecol 117:602
Tatum HJ (1977) Clinical aspects of intrauterine contraception: circumspection 1976. Fertil Steril 28:3
Tatum HJ, Schmidt FH, Jain AK (1976) Management and outcome of pregnancies associated with the Copper T intrauterine contraceptive device. Am J Obstet Gynecol 126:869
Taubert HD (1969) Die medikamentöse Auslösung der Ovulation mit Clomiphen. Gynäkologe 1:139
Tausk M (1969) The mechanism of action of oral contraceptives. Acta Obstet Gynecol Scand [Suppl 1] 48:41
Tavassoli F, Kraus FT (1978) Endometrial lesions in the uteri resected for atypical endometrial hyperplasia. Am J Clin Pathol 70:770
Tavassoli FA, Norris HJ (1981) Mesenchymal tumors of the uterus. VII. A clinicopathologic study of 60 endometrial stromal nodules. Histopathology 5:1
Taylor AB (1960) Sarcoidosis of the uterus. J Obstet Gynaecol Br Emp 67:32
Taylor CW (1958) Mesodermal mixed tumours of the female genital tract. J Obstet Gynaecol Br Cwlth 65:177
Taylor CW (1972) Müllerian mixed tumour. Acta Pathol Microbiol Scand [A] [Suppl] 233:48
Taylor ES, McMillan JH, Greer BE et al. (1975) The intrauterine device and tubo-ovarian abscess. Am J Obstet Gynecol 123:338
Taylor HC (1938) The pathology of the ovarian hormone. Am J Obstet Gynecol 36:332
Taylor HC (1944) Endocrine factors in the origin of tumors of the uterus. Surgery 16:91
Taylor HC, Becker WF (1947) Carcinoma of the corpus uteri. End results of treatment in 531 cases from 1926–1940. Surg Gynecol Obstet 84:129
Taymor ML (1961) Laboratory and clinical effects of nortestosterone. II. The endometrial response. Am J Obstet Gynecol 81:95
Tchernitchin A, Hasbun J, Pena G, Vega S (1970) Autoradiographic study of the in vitro uptake of estradiol by eosinophils in human endometrium. Proc Soc Exp Biol Med 137:108
Tekelioğlu-Uysal M, Edwards RG, Kişnişçi HA (1975) Ultrastructural relationship between decidua, trophoblast and lymphocytes at the beginning of human pregnancy. J Reprod Fertil 42:431
Ten Berge BS (1936) Primäre Amenorrhoe. Zentralbl Gynäkol 60:2149
Teng CS, Hamilton TH (1968) The role of chromatin in estrogen action in the uterus. I. The control of template capacity and chemical composition and the binding of H^3-estradiol-17β. Proc Nat Acad Sci USA 60:1410
Tenhaeff D (1971) Gezielter Einsatz von Ovulationshemmern. Ärztl Prax 23:3351
Terasaki O (1928) Beiträge zur Frage der Metrorrhagie. Beitr Pathol Anat 79:819
Terruhn V (1977) Polypen der Cervix uteri in der kindlichen hormonalen Ruheperiode. Geburtshilfe Frauenheilkd 37:35
Terzakis JA (1965) The nucleolar channel system of human endometrium. J Cell Biol 27:293
Themann H, Schünke W (1963) Die Feinstruktur der Drüsenepithelien des menschlichen Endometriums. Elektronenoptische Morphologie. In: Schmidt-Matthiesen H (ed) Das normale menschliche Endometrium. Thieme, Stuttgart, p 111
Thiede HA, Lund CJ (1962) Prognostic factors in endometrial adenocarcinoma. Obstet Gynecol 20:149
Thiery M (1955) Irregular shedding of the endometrium. Gynaecologia (Basel) 139:1
Thiery M, Willighagen RGJ (1967) Enzyme histochemistry of adenocarcinoma of the endometrium including hormone induced changes. Am J Obstet Gynecol 99:173
Thiessen P (1952) Die hormonrezeptorische Tumorentstehung als Ausdruck einer dienzephalhypophysären Regulationsstörung und Grundlage einer gerichteten Hormontherapie. Z Geburtshilfe Gynäkol 137:138
Thiessen P (1952) Hormonale Behandlungen genitaler Tumoren. Therapiewoche 3:47
Thiessen P (1956) Über Genese, Therapie und Prophylaxe hormonal gesteuerter Tumoren. Zentralbl Gynäkol 78:1625

Thom H (1952) Über die Genitaltuberkulose der Frau. Geburtshilfe Frauenheilkd 12:651
Thom MH, Davies KJ, Senkus RJ et al. (1981) Scanning electron microscopy of the endometrial cell surface in postmenopausal women receiving oestrogen therapy. Br J Obstet Gynaecol 88:904
Thomas WO, Harris HH, Enden JA (1969) Postirradiation malignant neoplasms of the uterine fundus. Am J Obstet Gynecol 104:209
Thomas W, Sadeghieh B, Fresco R et al. (1977) Malacoplakia of the endometrium, a probable cause of postmenopausal bleeding. Am J Clin Pathol 69:637
Thompson M, Husemyer R (1981) Carcinofibroma – a variant of the mixed Müllerian tumor. Br J Obstet Gynaecol 88:1151
Thomsen K (1955) Zur Fehlentwicklung junger Placentarzotten. Arch Gynäkol 185:807
Thrasher TV, Richart RM (1972) Ultrastructure of the Arias-Stella reaction. Am J Obstet Gynecol 112:113
Thrasher TV, Richart RM (1972) An ultrastructural comparison of endometrial adenocarcinoma and normal endometrium. Cancer (Philad) 29:1713
Tietze K (1934) Die Follikelpersistenz mit glandulärer Hyperplasie des Endometriums in klinischer und anatomischer Beziehung. Arch Gynäkol 155:525
Tillson SA, Marian M, Hudson R et al. (1975) The effect of intrauterine progesterone on the hypothalamic-hypophyseal-ovarian axis in humans. Contraception 11:179
Tiltman AJ (1980) Mucinous carcinoma of the endometrium. Obstet Gynecol 55:244
Tobon H, Watkins GJ (1985) Secretory adenocarcinoma of the endometrium. Int J Gynecol Pathol 4:328
Topkins P (1949) The histologic appearance of the endocervix during the menstrual cycle. Am J Obstet Gynecol 58:654
Topkins P (1962) Traumatic intrauterine synechiae. Am J Obstet Gynecol 83:1599
Toth F, Gimes R (1964) Senile changes in the female endocrine glands and internal sex organs. Acta Morphol Acad Sci Hung 12:301
Toth F, Gimes R, Horn B, Kerenyi T (1972) Suche neuer Wege mit „low dose" Kontrazeptivemitteln. Z Ärztl Fortbild 66:957
Tracy SL, Askin FB, Reddick RL et al. (1985) Progesterone secreting Sertoli cell tumor of the ovary. Gynecol Oncol 22:85
Trams G, Maass H, Tross J (1971) Some evidence for binding of ^{3}H progesterone in the rat uterus. Horm Metab Res 3:135
Treloar AE, Boynton RE, Behn BG (1967) Variation of the human menstrual cycle through reproductive life. Int J Fertil 12:77
Tseng L, Gusberg SB, Gurpide E (1977) Estradiol receptor and 17β-Dehydrogenase in normal and abnormal human endometrium. Ann NY Acad Sci 286:190
Tseng L, Mazella J, Funt MI et al. (1984) Preliminary studies of aromalose in human neoplastic endometrium. Obstet Gynecol 63:150
Tseng P-Y, Gurpide E (1974) Estradiol and 20α-dihydroprogesterone dehydrogenase activities in human endometrium during the menstrual cycle. Endocrinology 94:419
Tseng P-Y, Jones HW (1969) Chromosome constitution of carcinoma of the endometrium. Obstet Gynecol 33:741
Tsuji K, Nakano R (1978) Chromosome studies of embryos from induced abortions in pregnant women age 35 and over. Obstet Gynecol 52:542
Turnbull AC (1956) Radiation menopause or hysterectomy. Part. II – Mortality, Reliability and subsequent pelvic cancer. J Obstet Gynaecol Br Emp 63:179
Turunen A (1966) Zur traumatischen Amenorrhoe. Gynaecologia (Basel) 164:13
Tuttle SE, O'Toole RV, O'Shaughnessy RW, Zuspan FP (1985) Immunohistochemical evaluation of human placental implantation: an inital study. Am J Obstet Gynecol 153:239
Tweeddale DN, Early LS, Goodsitt ES (1964) Endometrial adenoacanthoma. A clinical and pathologic analysis of 82 cases, with observations on histogenesis. Obstet Gynecol 23:611
Twombly GH, Scheimer S, Levitz M (1961) Endometrial cancer, obesity, and estrogenic excretion in women. Am J Obstet Gynecol 82:424
Twombly GH, Bassett M, Meisel D, Levitz M (1967) Estrogen storage in fat. Am J Obstet Gynecol 99:785

Ueda G, Yamasaki M, Inoue M et al. (1986) Immunohistochemical demonstration of HNK-1-defined antigen in gynecologic tumors with argyrophilia. Int J Gynecol Pathol 5:143

Ueda S, Tsubura A, Izumi H et al. (1983) Immunohistochemical studies on carcinoembryonic antigen in adenocarcinomas of the uterus. Acta Pathol Jpn 33:59

Ulbright TM, Roth IM (1985) Metastatic and independent cancers of the endometrium and ovary: a clinico-pathologic study of 34 cases. Hum Pathol 16:28

Ulesko-Stroganowa K (1925) Die Endotheliome des Uterus. Arch Gynäkol 124:802

Ulm R (1965) Die Diagnostik des Uterus-Korpus-Karzinoms aus klinischer und histologischer Sicht. Krebsarzt 20:317

Ulm R (1970) Dysfunktionelle Blutung aus pathologisch-histologischer Sicht. Zentralbl Gynäkol 92:1068

Urbanke A (1962) Proliferating glia in the endometrium. Gynaecologia (Basel) 153:349

Vacek Z (1965) Die Topochemie der Enzyme in der Sekretionsphase des Endometriums und in der Dezidua im 1. bis 3. Schwangerschaftsmonat. Acta Histochem (Jena) 20:8

Vaczy L, Scipiades E (1949) New Considerations in histologic examinations of the endometrium in connection with sterility. Gynaecologia (Basel) 128:260

Valdez VA, Planas AT, Lopez VF et al. (1979) Adenosarcoma of uterus and ovary. A clinicopathologic study of two cases. Cancer (Philad) 43:1439

Valicenti JF, Priester SK (1977) Psammoma bodies of benign endometrial origin in cervicovaginal cytology. Acta Cytol 21:550

Van Campenhout J, Choquette P, Vauclair R (1980) Endometrial pattern in patients with primary hypoestrogenic amenorrhea receiving estrogen replacement therapy. Obstet Gynecol 56:349

Vanderick G, Beernaert J, de Muylder E, Ferin J (1975) Hormonal contraception. Sequential formulations and the endometrium. Contraception 12:655

Vanecko RM, Yao ST, Schmitz RL (1967) Metastasis to the fibula from endometrial carcinoma. Obstet Gynecol 29:803

Vanek J, Lane V (1963) Gliagewebe im Endometrium. Gynaecologia (Basel) 156:193

Van Santen MR, Haspels AA (1980) Interfering with implantation by postcoital estrogen administration. Prog Reprod Biol 7:310

Vara P (1962) Über die Funktion der Mastzellen im Endometrium und ihre Beteiligung an der Ungerinnbarkeit des Menstrualblutes. Geburtshilfe Frauenheilkd 22:989

Varela-Duran J, Nochomovitz LE, Prem KA, Dehner LP (1980) Postirradiation mixed müllerian tumors of the uterus. A comparative clinicopathologic study. Cancer (Philad) 45:1625

Varga A, Henriksen E (1961) Clinical and histopathologic evaluation of the effect of 17-alpha-hydroxyprogesterone-17-n-caproate on endometrial carcinoma. Obstet Gynecol 18:658

Varga A, Henriksen E (1963) Urinary excretion assays of pituitary luteinizing hormone (LH) related to endometrial carcinoma. Obstet Gynecol 22:129

Varga A, Henriksen E (1965) Histologic observations on the effect of 17α-hydroxyprogesterone-17n-caproate on endometrial carcinoma. Obstet Gynecol 26:656

Vasek V (1947) Zur Pathogenese der Blutung aus dem pathologisch proliferierten Endometrium. Zentralbl Gynäkol 69:1095

Vassilakos P, Wyss R, Wenger D, Riotton G (1975) Endometrial cytohistology by aspiration technic and by Gravlee jet washer. A comparative study. Obstet Gynecol 45:320

Vassilakos P, Riotton G, Kajii T (1977) Hydatidiform mole: two entities. A morphologic and cytogenetic study with some clinical considerations. Am J Obstet Gynecol 127:167

Vellios F, Stander RW, Huber CP (1963) Carcinosarcoma (malignant mixed mesodermal tumor) of the uterus. Am J Clin Pathol 39:496

Vellios F, Ng ABP, Reagan JW (1973) Papillary adenofibroma of the uterus – A benign mesodermal mixed tumor of Müllerian origin. Am J Clin Pathol 60:543

Venkataseshan KS, Woo TH (1985) Diffuse viral papillomatosis (condyloma) of the uterine cavity. Int J Gynecol Pathol 4:370

Verhagen A, Themann H (1965) Elektronenmikroskopische Endometriumbefunde nach Behandlung mit ovulationshemmenden Stoffen. Arch Gynäkol 202:253

Verhagen A, Themann H (1970) Elektronmikroskopische Untersuchungen am menschlichen Endometrium unter Einwirkung von Ovulationshemmern mit gleichzeitiger Oestrogen- und Gestagenwirkung. Arch Gynäkol 209:162

Vihko R, Jänne O, Kauppila A (1980) Steroid receptors in normal, hyperplastic and malignant human endometria. Ann Clin Res 12:208

Villa-Santa U (1964) Tumors of mesonephric origin in the female genital tract. Am J Obstet Gynecol 89:680

Villee CA (1961) Die Beeinflussung von Enzymen in Uterus und Placenta durch Oestrogene. Klin Wochenschr 39:173

Vogel M (1969) Placentabefunde beim Abort. Ein Beitrag zur Patho-Morphologie placentarer Entwicklungsstörungen. Virchows Arch Pathol Anat [A] 346:212

Vokaer R (1951) Observations sur l'histologie, l'histométrie et l'histophotométrie de l'endomètre humain. Gynécol Obstét 50:372

Vokaer R (1956) La régénération de l'endomètre humain au cours du post-partum. Arch Biol (Liège) 67:529

Vokaer R (1964) La progestérone et les progestifs des synthése. Ann Endocrinol (Paris) 25:151

Vollmann RF (1967) The length of the premenstrual phase by age of women. Proc 5th World Congr Fertil Steril Stockholm 1966. Excerpta Medica, Amsterdam, p 1171

Vorys N, Ullery JC, Stevens V (1965) The effects of sex steroids on gonadotropins. Am J Obstet Gynecol 93:641

Waard F de, Oettle AG (1967) A propos des facteurs exogènes et endogènes dans les états oestrogéniques postménopausiques. Arch Anat Pathol 15:26

Wagner D, Richart RM (1968) Polyploidy in the human endometrium with the Arias-Stella reaction. Arch Pathol 85:475

Wagner D, Richart RM, Terner JY (1967) Deoxyribonucleic acid content of precursors of endometrial carcinoma. Cancer (Philad) 20:1067

Wagner D, Richart RM, Terner JY (1968) DNA content of human endometrial gland cells during the menstrual cycle. Am J Obstet Gynecol 100:90

Wagner H, Pfautsch M, Beller FK (1976) Bakteriologische, raster- und transmissionselektronenmikroskopische Untersuchungen an Dalcon Shields. Arch Gynäkol 221:17

Waidl E, Fikentscher H, Brückner W (1968) Die interzellulären Strukturen des Endometriums bei der oralen Kontrazeption. Geburtshilfe Frauenheilkd 28:159

Wajntraub G (1970) Fertility after removal of the intrauterine ring. Fertil Steril 21:555

Wakonig-Vaartaja R, Hughes DT (1967) Chromosome studies in 36 gynaecological tumours: of the cervix, corpus uteri, ovary, vagina and vulva. Eur J Cancer 3:263

Wall JA, Franklin RR, Kaufman RH (1964) Reversal of benign and malignant endometrial changes with clomiphene. Am J Obstet Gynecol 88:1072

Wall JA, Franklin RR, Kaufman RH, Kaplan AL (1965) The effects of clomiphene citrate on the endometrium. Am J Obstet Gynecol 93:842

Wall JA, Collins VP, Kaplan AI, Hudgins PT (1967) Adenocarcinoma of the endometrium. Am J Obstet Gynecol 97:787

Wall RL, Hertig AT (1948) Habitual abortion. A pathologic analysis of 100 cases. Am J Obstet Gynecol 56:1127

Wallau F (1948) Untersuchungen über die funktionelle Amenorrhoe unter Kriegsverhältnissen. Arch Gynäkol 176:320

Walser H, Margulis R, Ladd J (1964) Effects of prolonged administration of progestins on the endometrium and the function of the pituitary, thyroid and adrenal glands. Int J Fertil 9:189

Walters D, Robinson D, Park RC, Pattow WE (1975) Diagnostic outpatient aspiration curettage. Obstet Gynecol 46:160

Walthard B (1933) Sepsis und Miliartuberkulose nach künstlicher Unterbrechung der Schwangerschaft. Arch Gynäkol 153:26

Walther O (1934) Über die Lymphosarkomatose der weiblichen Genitalorgane. Arch Gynäkol 157:44

Wan LS, Hsu Y-C, Ganguly M, Bigelow B (1977) Effects of the Progestasert on the menstrual pattern, ovarian steroids and endometrium. Contraception 16:417

Warhol MJ, Rice RH, Pinkus GS, Robboy SJ (1984) Evaluation of squamous epithelium in adenoacanthoma and adenosquamous carcinoma of the endometrium: immunoperoxidase analysis of involucrin and keratin localization. Int J Gynecol Pathol 3:82
Waterman EA, Benson RC (1967) Medrogestone therapy in advanced endometrial adenocarcinoma. Obstet Gynecol 30:626
Way S (1954) The aetiology of carcinoma of the body of the uterus. J Obstet Gynaecol Br Emp 61:46
Webb MJ, Gaffey TA (1976) Outpatient diagnostic aspiration curettage. Obstet Gynecol 47:239
Weber E (1961) Beitrag zur Klinik des Corpuscarcinoms. Gynaecologia (Basel) 151:232
Weber M (1954) Die hormonale Therapie der durch „verzögerte Abstoßung" bedingten Blutungsstörung. Geburtshilfe Frauenheilkd 14:710
Weingold AB, Boltuch SM (1961) Extragenital metastases to the uterus. Am J Obstet Gynecol 82:1267
Weisbrot IM, Janovski NA (1963) Endometrial stromal sarcoma. Am J Clin Pathol 39:273
Weiss G, Beller FK (1969) Tissue activator of the fibrinolytic enzyme in the female reproductive system. Obstet Gynecol 34:809
Welch WR, Scully RE (1977) Precancerous lesions of the endometrium. Hum Pathol 8:503
Wentz AC (1980) Endometrial biopsy in the evaluation of infertility. Fertil Steril 33:121
Wentz WB (1964) Effects of a progestational agent on endometrial hyperplasia and endometrial cancer. Obstet Gynecol 24:370
Wentz WB (1966) Treatment of persistent endometrial hyperplasia with progestins. Am J Obstet Gynecol 96:999
Werbin H, Leroy GV (1954) Cholesterol, a precursor of tetrahydrocortisone in man. J Am Chem Soc 76:5260
Wermbter F (1924) Über die Bindegewebsfibrillen der Uterusschleimhaut mit besonderer Berücksichtigung der Hyperplasia glandularis. Virchows Arch Pathol Anat 253:735
Werner H, Hoffbauer H, Struck E, Voss H (1968) Die latente Toxoplasmainfektion des Uterus und ihre Bedeutung für die Schwangerschaft. Zentralbl Bakteriol I Abt Orig 205:517
Wessel W (1959) Die menschlichen Deciduazellen und ihre „Kollageneinschlüsse" im Elektronenmikroskop. Virchows Arch Pathol Anat 332:224
Wessel W (1960) Das elektronenmikroskopische Bild menschlicher endometrialer Drüsenzellen während des menstruellen Zyklus. Z Zellforsch 51:633
Wessel W (1961) Die glandulär-cystische Hyperplasie des menschlichen Endometrium im elektronmikroskopischen Bild. Virchows Arch Pathol Anat 334:181
Wessel W (1965) Endometriale Adenocarcinoma verschiedener Differenzierungsgrade und ihr Stroma im elektronenmikroskopischen Bild. Z Krebsforsch 66:421
Wetzstein R, Wagner H (1960) Elektronenmikroskopische Untersuchungen am menschlichen Endometrium. Anat Anz 108:362
Wewer UM, Faber M, Liotta LA, Albrechtsen R (1985) Immunochemical and ultrastructural assessment of the nature of the pericellular basement membrane of human decidual cells. Lab Invest 53:624
Wheelock JB, Krebs HB, Schneider V, Goplerud DR (1985) Uterine sarcoma: analysis of prognostic variables in 71 cases. Am J Obstet Gynecol 151:1016
Wheelock MC, Strand CM (1953) Endometrial sarcoma. Relationship to certain instances of stromal endometriosis. Obstet Gynecol 2:384
White AJ, Buchsbaum HJ, Macasaet MA (1973) Primary squamous cell carcinoma of the endometrium. Obstet Gynecol 41:912
White TH, Glover JS, Peete CH, Parker RT (1965) A 34-year clinical study of uterine sarcoma, including experience with chemotherapie. Obstet Gynecol 25:657
Whitehead MI, McQueen J, Beard RJ et al. (1977) The effects of cyclical oestrogen therapy and sequential oestrogen/progestogen therapy on the endometrium of postmenopausal women. Acta Obstet Gynecol Scand 65:91
Whitelaw MJ, Grams LR, Stamm WJ (1964) Clomiphene citrate: Its uses and observations on its probable action. Am J Obstet Gynecol 90:355

Whitelaw MJ, Kalman CF, Grams LR (1970) The significance of the high ovulation rate versus the low pregnancy rate with clomid. Am J Obstet Gynecol 107:865

Wied GL (1953) Zytologische Untersuchungen beim Adenokarzinom des corpus uteri. Geburtshilfe Frauenheilkd 13:492

Wiegand R (1930) Systematische histologische Untersuchungen über die Arterien des Uterus. Z Mikrosk Anat Forsch 20:433

Wiele RC van de, Turksoy RN (1965) Treatment of amenorrhoea and of anovulation with human menopausal and chorionic gonadotropins. J Clin Endocrinol 25:369

Wienke EC, Cavazos F, Hall DG, Lucas FV (1968) Ultrastructure of the human endometrial stroma cell during the menstrual cycle. Am J Obstet Gynecol 102:65

Wienke EC, Cavazos F, Hall DG, Lucas FV (1969) Ultrastructural effects of norethynodrel and mestranol on human endometrial stroma cell. Am J Obstet Gynecol 103:102

Wildner GP, Klein K (1967) Die Sarkome der primären und sekundären weiblichen Geschlechtsorgane. Arch Geschwulstforsch 30:78

Wilkin PG (1960) La vascularisation de l'endomètre humain au cours de la phase progrestative du cycle menstrual et au cours de la nidation ovulaire. In: Ferin, Gaudefroy (eds) Les fonctions de nidation utérine et leurs troubles. Masson, Paris, p 331

Wilkinson EJ, Andrasko KP, Stafl A (1980) Endometrial involvement by cervical intraepithelial neoplasia. Obstet Gynecol 55:378

Wilkinson EJ, Friedrich EG, Mattingly RF et al. (1973) Turner's syndrome with endometrial adenocarcinoma and stilbestrol therapy. Obstet Gynecol 42:193

Willén R, Stendahl U, Willén H, Tropé C (1983) Malakoplakia of the cervix and corpus uteri: a light microscopic, electron microscopic and X-ray microprobe analysis of a case. Int J Gynecol Pathol 2:201

Williams AO (1967) Pathology of schistosomiasis of the uterine cervix due to S. haemtobium. Am J Obstet Gynecol 98:784

Williams GL (1965) Adenoacanthoma of the corpus uteri. J Obstet Gynaecol Br Cwlth 72:674

Williamson EO, Christopherson WM (1972) Malignant mixed Müllerian tumors of the uterus. Cancer (Philad) 29:585

Willson JR, Ledger WJ, Andros GJ (1965) The effect of an intrauterine contraceptive device on the histologic pattern of the endometrium. Am J Obstet Gynecol 93:802

Wilson EW (1976) Some properties of human endometrial alkaline phosphatase. Fertil Steril 27:299

Wilson EW (1977) The effect of copper on lactic dehydrogenase isoenzymes in human endometrium. Contraception 16:367

Wilson L, Kurzrok R (1938) Cystic endometrial changes in ovulatory cycles: The mixed endometrium. Am J Obstet Gynecol 36:302

Winkler B, Reumann W, Mitao M et al. (1984) Chlamydial endometritis. A histological and immunohistochemical analysis. Am J Surg Pathol 8:771

Winter G (1950) Glandulär-cystische Hyperplasie und Korpuskarzinom. Zentralbl Gynäkol 72:880

Winter G (1955) Über Varianten des Endometriums. Z Geburtshilfe Gynäkol 143:86

Winter G (1956) Über die Beziehungen zwischen Lebensalter und Curettagebefund. Dtsch Gesundheitswes 26

Winter G, Pots P (1956) Morphologische Untersuchungen über die medikamentöse Transformation des Endometriums. Z Geburtshilfe Gynäkol 147:44

Wislocki GB, Dempsey EW (1945) Histochemical reactions of the endometrium in pregnancy. Am J Anat 77:365

Wislocki GB, Streeter GL (1938) On the placentation of the macaque (Macaca mulatta), from the time of implantation until the formation of the definitive placenta. Carnegie Inst Wash Publ 496. Contrib Embryol 27:1

Wislocki GB, Bunting H, Dempsey EW (1950) The chemical histology of the human uterine cervix with supplementary notes on the endometrium. In: Engle ET (ed) Menstruation and its disorders. Thomas, Springfield, p 23

Witt H-J (1963) Strukturelemente und funktionelle Gesamtheit des Endometriums. Karyometrie. In: Schmidt-Matthiesen H (ed) Das normale menschliche Endometrium. Thieme, Stuttgart, p 26, 96

Wittlinger H, Hilgenfeldt J, Dallenbach-Hellweg G (1975) Korrelation morphologischer und biochemischer Befunde bei Frauen in der Peri- und Postmenopause. Fortschr Med 93:24

Woll E, Hertig AT, Smith GVS, Johnson LC (1948) The ovary in endometrial carcinoma, with notes on the morphological history of the aging ovary. Am J Obstet Gynecol 56:617

Wollner A (1937) The physiology of the human cervical mucosa. Surg Gynecol Obstet 64:758

Woodruff JD, Julian CG (1969) Multiple malignancy in the upper genital canal. Obstet Gynecol 103:810

Wright CJE (1973) Solitary malignant lymphoma of the uterus. Am J Obstet Gynecol 117:114

Wynder EL, Escher GC, Mantel N (1966) An epidemiological investigation of cancer of the endometrium. Cancer (Philad) 19:489

Wynn RM (1967) Intrauterine devices: effects on ultrastructure of human endometrium. Science 156:1508

Wynn RM (1967) Current problems in uterine cellular biology, chap 13. In: Cellular biology of the uterus. North-Holland, Amsterdam

Wynn RM (1968) Fine structural effects of intrauterine contraceptives on the human endometrium. Fertil Steril 19:867

Wynn RM (1974) Ultrastructural development of the human decidua. Am J Obstet Gynecol 118:652

Wynn RM, Harris JA (1967) Ultrastructural cyclic changes in the human endometrium. I. Normal preovulatory phase. Fertil Steril 18:632

Wynn RM, Harris JA (1967) Ultrastructure of trophoblast and endometrium in invasive hydatidiform mole. (Chorioadenoma destruens.) Am J Obstet Gynecol 99:1125

Wynn RM, Woolley RS (1967) Ultrastructural cyclic changes in the human endometrium. II. Normal postovulatory phase. Fertil Steril 18:721

Wyss RH, Heinrichs WL, Herrmann WL (1968) Some species differences of uterine estradiol receptors. J Clin Endocrinol 28:1227

Yamamoto KR, Alberts BM (1976) Steroid receptors: elements for modulation of eukaryotic transcription. Annu Rev Biochem 45:721

Yamamoto M, Fujimori R, Ito T et al. (1975) Chromosome studies in 500 induced abortions. Humangenetik 29:9

Yamashina M, Kobara TY (1986) Primary squamous cell carcinoma with its spindle cell variant in the endometrium. Cancer (Philad) 57:340

Yaneva H, Lumbroso P, Netter A (1965) Étude histochimique des endomètres soumis à certaines progestoides de synthèse. Minerva Ginecol [Suppl 78] 17

Yoonessi M, Hart WR (1977) Endometrial stromal sarcomas. Cancer (Philad) 40:898

Young PCM, Ehrlich CE, Cleary RE (1976) Progesterone binding in human endometrial carcinomas. Am J Obstet Gynecol 125:353

Young RH, Kleinman GM, Scully RE (1981) Glioma of the uterus. Am J Surg Pathol 5:695

Young RH, Harris NL, Scully RE (1985) Lymphoma-like lesions of the lower female genital tract: a report of 16 cases. Int J Gynecol Pathol 4:289

Young RH, Gregor T, Scully RE (1986) Atypical polypoid adenomyoma of the uterus. A report of 27 cases. Am J Clin Pathol 86:139

Zador G, Nilsson BA, Sjöberg NO et al. (1976) Clinical experience with the uterine progesterone system (Progestasert). Contraception 13:559

Zaldivar A, Gallegos AJ (1971) Metabolism and tissue localization of [14–15^{3}H]d-Norgestrel in the human. Contraception 4:169

Zaloudek CJ, Norris HJ (1981) Adenofibroma and adenosarcoma of the uterus: a clinicopathologic study of 35 cases. Cancer (Philad) 48:354

Zaloudek CJ, Norris HJ (1982) Mesenchymal tumors of the uterus. Prog Surg Pathol 3:1

Zander J (1949) Pathologisch-anatomische Untersuchungen zur Tuberkulose des Endometriums. Virchows Arch Pathol Anat 317:201

Zander J (1954) Progesterone in human blood and tissues. Nature (Lond) 174:406
Zander J, Wiest WG, Ober KG (1962) Klinische, histologische und biochemische Beobachtungen bei polycystischen Ovarien mit gleichzeitiger adenomatöser, atypischer Hyperplasie des Endometriums. Arch Gynäkol 196:481
Zarrow MX, Holmstrom EG, Salhanick HA (1955) The concentration of relaxin in the blood serum of normal pregnant women. Endocrinology 15:22
Zettergren L (1956) So-called glioma of the uterus. Acta Obstet Gynecol Scand 35:375
Zettergren L (1973) Glial tissue in the uterus. Am J Pathol 71:419
Ziel HK, Finkle WD (1976) Association of estrone with the development of endometrial carcinoma. Am J Obstet Gynecol 124:735
Ziel HK, Finkle WD (1975) Increased risk of endometrial carcinoma among users of conjugated estrogens. N Engl J Med 293:1167
Zielske F, Becker K, Knauf P (1977) Schwangerschaften bei Intrauterinpessaren in situ. Geburtshilfe Frauenheilkd 37:473
Zipper JA, Medel M, Prager R (1968) Experimental suppression of fertility by intrauterine copper and zinc in rabbits. In: Abstracts of the sixth World Congress on Fertil and Steril, Tel Aviv, Israel, p 154
Zondek B (1940) The effect of prolonged administration of estrogen. JAMA 114:1850
Zondek B (1947) Placental hormones after death of foetus with viable placenta. Lancet I:178
Zucker PK, Kasdon EJ, Feldstein ML (1985) The validity of PAP smear parameters as predictors of endometrial pathology in menopausal women. Cancer (Philad) 56:2256
Zuckerman S (1949) The menstrual cycle. Lancet I:1031

Subject Index

Abortion, Arias-Stella phenomenon 144, 304, 306
—, chromosome abnormalities in 301, 313
—, decidual changes in 303, 304
—, due to delayed ovulation 302
—, du to endometrial abnormalities 302
—, due to oral contraceptives 302, 303
—, due to trophoblast abnormalities 301, 312
—, fetal structures, diagnosis of from curettings 19, 326
—, habitual 301
—, induced 298, 300
—, infectious causes of 303, 308
—, maternal factors 302, 309
—, retained remnants of 324
—, spontaneous 300
—, therapeutic 298
Abortive secretion 104, 106, 137, 153, 169, 180, 189
Acid mucopolysaccharides in adenocarcinoma 249
— —, fibrinolytic inhibitors 44
— — in glandular epithelium 14, 27, 66, 139
— — in glandular lumen 68
— — in ground substance 36, 44
— phosphatase 32, 43, 56, 112, 127, 139, 182, 249, 250
Acridine orange, fluorochromation with 15, 79, 88
Actinomycosis 210
Adaptation hyperplasia 324, 330, 335, 336
Adenoacanthoma 229, 235, 236, 282, 294
—, development of 117, 263
—, prognosis of 236
Adenoacanthosis 245
Adenocarcinoma arising from adenomatous hyperplasia 127, 129, 229, 255, 256, 270
— — —, characteristics of 230
— — —, decrease in ribonucleic acid 270
— — —, histochemical studies 127, 245
— — —, irreversible change 257, 270

Adenocarcinoma, cervical 294, 295, 296
—, endometrial (see also carcinoma) 232, 282, 294
—, —, ciliated cell 229, 235
—, —, glandular 229, 232, 233, 244
—, —, secretory 229, 234, 235
—, —, solid 229, 233, 234
—, —, with squamous metaplasia 229, 235
—, mucinous 229, 238, 239, 282, 294
—, mucoepidermoid 229, 238, 240, 282, 294
Adenofibroma 224, 288
—, malignant 288
Adenomatous hyperplasia 90, 117, 120
— —, architectural changes of glands 124, 125
— —, change to carcinoma 127, 129, 229, 231, 255
— —, cytological atypia in 124, 125, 126, 127
— —, distinction from carcinoma 127, 128, 230
— —, — from metaplasia 128, 214
— —, DNA of 120, 126, 245
— — of endocervical mucosa 186, 187
— — due to exogenous estrogen 123, 160, 263
— — due to unopposed estrogen 268
— —, foam cells of 122, 123
— —, grade 1: 121, 124, 128
— —, grade 2: 123, 124, 128
— —, grade 3: 124, 125, 127, 129
— —, juvenile 123, 124, 245, 246, 247, 270
— —, misdiagnosed as cancer 245
— —, oral contraceptives and 177, 180
— —, persistent anovulation with 124
— —, precursor of carcinoma 254, 270
— and stromal hyperplasia, combined 135
— polyp 130, 131, 223
Adenomyoma, polypoid 225
Adenosarcoma 282, 288, 289
Adenosquamous carcinoma 229, 237, 282, 294
Adhesions, endometrial 199
Alcian blue stain for acid mucopolysaccharides 14, 36

Aldehyde-fuchsin reaction for polysaccharides 14
Alkaline phosphatase 27, 42, 50, 51, 56
— —, in anovulatory cycle 104
— —, in deficient secretory phase 139
— — in endometrial carcinoma 249, 250
— — after hormones 181
— — in hyperplasia 112, 127, 249
Amenorrhea, from adhesions 199
—, causes for 155, 174
—, endometrial changes associated with 101, 155
— after oral contraceptives 174, 182
— in ovarian tumors 158
—, tests in 162
—, types of 101
Aminopeptidase 43
Androblastoma 158
Androstendione 268
Angiomyoma 224
Angiosarcoma 281
Anovulation 88
Anovulatory cycle, after oral contraceptives 175
— —, diagnosis of 103
— —, endometrial changes in 104, 105, 153, 155
— —, intermediate type 106
— —, persistent follicle 102, 105
— —, types of 103
— — withdrawal bleeding of 107
Antiestrogen 188
Antifertility agents, see oral contraceptives
— —, intrauterine device 190
Antigonadotropin 189
Antiprolaktin 137
Apoplexia uteri 97
APUD cells 250
Argyrophilic cells, in carcinomas 250
Arias-Stella phenomenon, causes 144, 304
— — in extrauterine pregnancy 329, 331
— —, gonadotropin in 305
— —, histochemistry of 306
— —, in hydatidiform mole 318
— —, incidence in abortions 306
— — with intrauterine device 190
— — with irregular shedding 144, 330
Arrested proliferation 162
Arrested secretion 148, 153, 162, 163, 331
— —, focal, after intrauterine device 192, 194
Artefacts in currettings 20
Artefacts, histological 8
Arterioles, spiral 39, 51, 173, 178

Arteriosclerosis 97
Asherman's syndrome 199
Asynchronous cycle 152, 153, 155
Atrophy, cystic 90, 91
—, endometritis atrophicans 204
— from estrogen therapy 160, 185
—, infertility with 137, 153, 155,
—, from non-functioning ovaries 99, 101
— after oral contraceptives 174–176, 180, 185
— with ovarian tumors 158
—, postmenopausal 90, 91
—, pressure, from intrauterine device 190
—, —, from submucosal leiomyoma 100
— after progesterone therapy 162, 180, 185, 272
— with refractory state 183, 275
—, simple 90, 91
Atypical hyperplasia 124

Basalis, characteristics of 18
β-glucuronidase 44, 182
Biopsy, techniques of 5–6
Blastocyst, implantation of 36, 37, 53, 153
Blastomyces dermatitidis 208
Bleeding, with anatomic disturbances 93, 96, 101
—, breakthrough 113, 160, 170, 173, 174
— in climacterium 156
—, estrogen withdrawal type 103, 107, 113, 160
— with functional disturbances 93
— in glandular-cystic hyperplasia 113
— after hormonal therapy 160
— with intrauterine devices 195
— after oral contraceptives 170, 173, 174
—, ovulatory 66
—, caused by polyps 134
—, postmenopausal 92, 204, 211, 268
—, post partum 333, 336
—, —, and adaptation hyperplasia 336
—, caused by systemic diseases 93, 97
—, withdrawal 103, 107, 113, 160, 162
Blighted ovum 301, 312
Blood vessels, changes in due to relaxin 39
— — after oral contraceptives 173
Bony parts, in curettings 19, 201, 326
Breakthrough bleeding 113, 160
— — after gestagen 170, 173
— — after oral contraceptives 160, 170, 173, 174
Brenner tumors and endometrial carcinoma 261

Candida infection 210
Capillaries, hormonal changes in 39
Carbonic anhydrase 45, 182
Carcinofibroma 282, 288, 290
Carcinoma, adenosquamous 237
—, aneuploidy 126
—, argyrophilic cells in 250
— in castrated patients 264
— of cervix 292, 294
— —, differentiated from endometrial carcinoma 238, 249, 295
—, chromosome studies 245
—, classification 227, 229
—, clear-cell type 238, 242, 244, 282, 294
—, — —, of endocervix 295, 297
— in climacterium 156
—, constitutional factors 226, 267
—, cytoplasmic constituents of 249, 250
—, distinction from adenomatous hyperplasia 127, 128, 230, 231
—, early 231, 232, 249
—, endocrine disturbances 226, 262, 266, 267
— with endometrial differentiation 232, 244
— and estrogen therapy 262, 267
—, etiological concepts 259, 268
—, extension to endocervix 228
— and foam cells 251, 252, 253
—, frequency 226, 229
—, gross appearance of 11, 227
—, histochemical studies of 245, 273
—, histogenesis 229
—, histological grading 229, 230
—, — typing 229, 294
—, hormone receptors of 245, 248, 273
— from hyperplasia of basalis 129
—, increased estrogen levels with 260, 268
— and liver cirrhosis 262
—, metastases 228
— with Müllerian differentiation 238
—, nuclear DNA of 245, 273
— and oral contraceptives 180, 263
—, ovarian changes in 260, 267
—, after ovariectomy 264
—, pituitary disturbances in 267
— in polyps 259
—, preceding hyperplasia 127, 255
—, precursors 229, 254, 266, 270
—, problems in diagnosis 245
—, progesterone therapy for 272
—, prognosis 251
—, prophylaxis against 275
—, risk factors for 226, 256, 263, 267
—, in senile patients 230
—, serous-papillary 241, 282, 294

—, sites of predilection 5, 227
—, squamous cell 244, 282
—, stages of 228
—, statistical studies of 226, 254
—, stroma of 251
—, suction biopsy of 6
—, survival rates 229, 251
—, therapy of 272–275
—, in young women 226, 245
— after X-ray therapy 264, 267, 275
Carcinosarcoma 282, 284, 286
Cartilaginous metaplasia 222
Cataloguing specimens 23, 24
— —, system used, advantages of 23, 24
CEA, in carcinomas 250
Cell proliferation after estrogen 50
Cellular proteins, staining for 13
Cervical carcinoma 294
Cervical mucosa (see endocervical mucosa)
Chlamydial endometritis 210
Cholesterol, staining for, with Schulz's method 14
Chondrosarcoma 281, 282
Choriocarcinoma 321, 322
—, diagnosis of 322
—, prognosis of 323
—, trophoblasts of 321
Chorionepitheliosis 323
Chorionic invasion, of decidua 309, 310
Chorionic villi, disturbed development of 301, 303, 312
— —, hydropic change of 303, 312, 313
— —, non vascularized 312
— —, regressive changes of 309, 312
— —, retained 326
— —, stages in development 299
— —, staining for 309
Chromosomal anomalies in abortions 301, 313
— — after clomiphene 189
— — after oral contraceptives 302
Chromosomes, analysis 17
— in carcinomas 245
— in normal endometrium 25
Chronic passive hyperemia 96
Ciliated cells of glandular epithelium 27, 180, 218, 220, 229
Circulatory disorders 93, 94
— disturbances causing uterine bleeding 96
Clear cell carcinoma of endocervix 295, 297
— — — endometrium 229, 242, 244, 282
Clear cells of endometrial carcinoma 238
— — in hyperplasia 110, 229

Clear cells, types 27, 28, 222
Climacterium 86, 90, 156
—, treatment of symptoms 161, 275
Clinical report, importance in diagnosing abnormal cycles 152
— —, — — irregular shedding 146
— —, — of for pathologist 3
Clomiphene, therapy with 137, 186, 274
Coagulation disturbances 93, 97
Collagen inclusions 79, 306, 307
— —, demonstration of 12, 306
— — in extrauterine pregnancy 329
— —, origin 306
Collision-tumor 282, 283
Combination-tumor 282, 283
Compacta, beginning dissociation of 81
— of functionalis 75
—, predecidual reaction of 70, 73, 76
Composition-tumor 282, 283
Computer programs 17
Connective tissue, formed by stromal cells 29
— —, Goldner stain for 12
— —, reticulum fibers 12
— —, special stains for 12
Contaminants of curettings 20
Contraceptive agents, intrauterine devices 190
— —, see oral contraceptives 166
Copper "T" devices 191, 195, 196
Corpus luteum insufficiency 136, 153
Corpus luteum, persistent, causes of 143
— —, premature regression of 136
Cryostat, use of 8
Cryosurgery 200
Cryptococcus glabratus 208
Curettage, in abnormal bleeding 2, 157
— for anovulatory cycle 104
— for carcinoma 5
—, complete 5
—, complications of 199
—, endocervical 5, 158, 228
—, guide lines for 3
— for hydatidiform mole 6
— in hypomenorrhea 3
— for incomplete abortion 5
—, indications for 1–2
— for infertility 152, 154
— for irregular shedding 3
—, post partum 333
—, procedures for 4
—, regeneration after 198
—, selection of proper time for 2
— by suction 6
—, technique of 5–6
—, in tuberculosis 207
—, value of repeated 152

— for various conditions 3
Curettings, in abortion 19, 298
—, artefacts of 20–22
—, bony parts in 19, 201, 326
—, carcinoma of cervix in 294
—, choriocarcinoma in 321
—, components of 17, 294, 334
—, contamination of 20
—, diagnosis of basalis 18
—, — of leiomyoma from 18, 93, 135
—, — of pregnancy 298, 309, 325, 328
—, diseases diagnosed from 93
—, extensive necrosis of, causes 19, 201
— of extrauterine pregnancy 328
—, histological diagnoses of 21, 22
—, myometrial component 18, 334
—, pathological changes in 94
—, products of conception 19
—, re-orientation of, for sectioning 10
Cystadenofibroma 224
Cystomas of ovary 157
Cytomegalovirus endometritis 210
Cytometry 16
Cytokeratin filaments, markers for 16
Cytoskeleton, markers for 15, 16
Cytotrophoblast 299

Dating the endometrium 17, 55, 64, 84
— —, in infertility 152
— —, problems after oral contraceptives 174, 182
— —, selection of criteria for 56, 64
Decidua, of abortions 304, 306
—, after death of fetus 328
—, development of 30, 53, 299
— of extrauterine pregnancy 328
—, ground substance 300
—, hyaline remnants distinguished from hyaline thrombi 19, 324
— with intrauterine device 190–194, 331
—, involving after abortion 79, 304, 306
—, mens II 79
—, PAS stain for 11
— due to persistent corpora lutea 148
— without pregnancy 330
— after progesterone therapy 148, 162, 163, 170, 180
—, remnants of 11, 324
—, retained products of conception 19
—, reticulum fibers of 36, 329
Decidual cast 148
— — after oral contraceptives 170
— cells 30–32, 53, 299
— —, collagen inclusions of 306, 307, 329
— change with ovarian tumors 157, 158
—, necroses of 300, 308

Subject Index

Deficient proliferation 105, 106, 137, 153, 155
Deficient secretory phase 136, 137, 153, 155, 189
Dehydrogenases 45
— in carcinoma 250
—, after hormones 182
Delayed ovulation 154, 302
Desmoplastic stromal reaction 230
Desoxyribonucleic acid, of carcinomas 245
— — in functional diagnosis 13, 25
— — in hyperplasias 110, 120
— — during menstrual cycle 25
— — of stromal cells 29, 30
Diagnosis of functional changes 50, 55, 86, 149, 182
Dysmenorrhea membranacea 148, 170

Early carcinoma 232, 249
Edema, stromal, mechanical causes of 96
—, —, patchy, after oral contraceptives 94, 96, 170
—, —, pathological 94, 95
—, —, physiological 58, 60, 70, 72
Embedding techniques 10
Endocervical mucosa 18
— —, functional disturbances of 158
— —, after contraceptive agents 184, 186, 187
—, polyps 133, 134
Endocervicitis 213
—, post abortum 326
Endocrine disturbances, and carcinoma 226, 262, 266, 267
— — and endometrial hyperplasias 262, 266, 267
Endodermal sinus tumor 291
Endolymphatic stromal myosis 280
Endometrial atrophy (see atrophy)
— biopsy, suction-biopsy 6
— —, technique of 5
— cytology 7
— granulocytes, action on blood vessels 173
— —, action of, during implantation 36, 39, 53
— —, characteristics of 30–33
— —, differentiation from leukocytes 13, 14, 33, 77, 202, 300
— —, enzyme contents of 43
— —, fibrinolytic enzymes in 43
— —, formation of 30, 52, 70
— — at implantation site 33, 36, 53
— — at menstruation 79
— — among precidual cells 75, 76, 78
— —, staining for 13, 14, 79

— involution, first signs of 75
— stromal sarcoma 276, 282
— tissue, preparation of 7
Endometriosis, gestagen therapy for 162
Endometritis, acute 201
— atrophicans 204
—, caused by polyps 134
—, causes of 201
—, causing infertility 156
—, chronic 203
—, criteria of 203, 205
—, cyclic changes in 203
—, diagnosis of 203
—, distinction from lymphoma 205
— due to actinomycosis 210
— due to blastomyces 208
— due to candida 210
— due to chlamydia 210
— due to cryptococcus 208
— due to cytomegalovirus 210
— due to herpes simplex virus 210
— due to mycoplasma 210, 308
— due to schistosomiasis 211
— due to toxoplasmosis 210
— due to viruses 210
—, foreign body granuloma 212
—, gonorrheal 211
—, granulomatous 208
—, healing of 203
—, histology of 201, 203
—, incidence 201, 203
— from intrauterine device 213
—, menstrual cycle and 200
—, plasma cells in 203
—, pneumococcal 211
—, pneumopolycystic 211
— post abortum 201, 308, 324, 325
—, postmenopausal 203
—, post partum 333, 334
—, regeneration of endometrium in 203
—, sarcoidosis 208, 209
—, senile 204
—, specific, due to rare microorganisms 208
— tuberculous, complications of 207
—, —, demonstration of bacteria 205
—, —, diagnosis of 205
—, —, incidence 205
—, —, infertility in 156, 207
—, —, symptoms of 156, 208
Endometrium adhesions of 199
—, arteriosclerosis of 97
—, changes seen in amenorrhea 101
—, — associated with persistent follicle 102
—, — in, causing infertility 137, 149
— in the climacterium 86, 90, 156

Endometrium, cystic atrophy 90, 91
—, dating of 17, 55, 64, 84
—, endocrine function of 30
—, estrogen production in 30
—, in extrauterine pregnancy 328
—, fetal 54
—, fibrinolytic activity of 44
—, foreign tissues in 326
—, functional disturbances 99
—, glial tissues in 326
—, histiocytes of 34
—, hormonal effects on 45, 50 158, 165
—, iatrogenic changes of 158
— during implantation 36, 38, 53
—, layers of 17, 62
—, lymphocytes of 34
— after the menopause 86
— during menstrual cycle 55
—, after menstruation 79, 85
—, methods of obtaining, preparing and interpreting 1
—, morphometry of 16
—, necrosis of 19
— in newborns 54
—, normal histology 25, 55
—, — variations in 84
—, polymorphonuclear leukocytes in 35
—, post partum 331
—, precancerous changes 124–129, 254, 267
—, pressure atrophy of 100
—, progesterone effect 51
—, proliferation 50, 57
—, pseudomelanosis of 98
— before puberty 54
—, regeneration of 84, 85, 198
—, regions of 17
—, resting 101
—, steroid receptors 16, 45–47, 48, 140
—, study of whole uteri 7
—, tissue culture 7, 16
—, transitional 88
—, transplantation 200
Endothelial proliferation caused by relaxin 39, 40, 300, 308, 309, 332
Enzyme-histochemistry 42
Enzymes and hormones 42, 51, 181
—, localization of 42
—, proteolytic 43, 44, 53
Eosinophilic metaplasia 219, 220, 222
Eosinophils 34
Epithelial metaplasia 214
Epithelial surface antigens 16
Epithelium, glandular 25
—, superficial 29
ER-ICA assay 16, 49, 248
Esterase 43

— in carcinoma 249, 250
— in endometrial granulocytes 32, 43
— in hyperplasias 112, 249
Estrogen, "-carcinoma" 263
— as cocarcinogens 268
—, causing "clear cells" 28
—, — edema 94
—, cell proliferation 47, 50
—, effects on cilia formation 28, 222
—, — of different compounds 108, 159
—, — on endocervix 158
—, — on endometrium 50, 54, 160, 165
—, — on fibrinolytic activity 44
—, — of hypoestrogenism 101
—, — on stromal cells 29, 251
—, — of unopposed 120, 260, 268
— and endometrial carcinoma 262, 268
—, genetic disposition 268
—, glandular-cystic hyperplasia 108, 117
—, histamine release 50
—, hyperemia 50, 94
—, ovarian tumors producing 157, 260, 261
—, potency 50, 159
—, priming 137, 162
—, produced by adrenals 264
—, — by endometrium 30
— receptors 45, 48, 140
— — affinity 45
— —, in anovulatory cycle 103
— —, in carcinoma 245, 273
— —, clomiphene effect on 160, 188
— —, detection of 16, 49
— —, exhaustion of 160, 174, 185
— —, in hyperplasia 127
— —, in irregular proliferation 106
—, RNA increase 26, 50, 62
—, stimulation of DNA synthesis 50, 120
—, stored in fat 267
—, stromal cells of ovary 260
—, synthetic 159
— therapy and endometrial carcinoma 265, 267
— — and squamous metaplasia 117
— —, thromboses after 98
— withdrawal bleeding 113, 160, 173
— withdrawal test 162
Estrophilin 49

Fatty metaplasia 222
Fetal parts (see abortion) 19, 326
Feulgen stain 13
Fibrinolytic acitvity of endometrium 39, 44, 112
— — at implantation 53
— enzymes, release of 44, 53

— inhibitors 44
Fibroleiomyosarcoma 283
Fixatives 7
—, coagulants, non-coagulants 8
—, mixtures of 9
Foam cells, in adenomatous hyperplasia 122, 123, 124, 249, 266, 271
— —, autofluorescence of 123
— — in carcinoma 249, 251, 253, 265
— — after estrogen therapy 30, 160, 266
— — in polyps 134
— —, staining for 14, 123
— — from stromal cells 30
Foreign bodies, in curettings 20
Foreign body granuloma 212
Formalin fixation, advantages of 8, 9
Freezing artefacts 20, 22
Frozen sections 8
— —, advantages 8
— —, selection of tissue for 10
Functional abnormalities, iatrogenic 158
— bleeding, treatment of 166
— diagnosis, importance of DNA in 13
— disturbances 93
— —, definition 156
— — during climateric 156
— —, in endocervix 158
— — in endometritis 203
— —, in infertility 137, 149, 153
— —, importance of enzyme-histochemistry 42
— —, statistical analysis of 23, 24
— — in tuberculous endometritis 207
Functionalis, diagnostic value of 17
—, division of, into compacta and spongiosa 70
—, — of into layers, failure of 88
—, reticulum fibers of 36

Galactosidase 44
Gestagens, effects of 161
—, —, on blastocyst 181
—, —, on endocervix 186, 187
—, —, on endometrium 161, 180, 183, 184
—, —, on nucleoli 170, 180
— potency 161, 173
—, predecidual change 162, 163, 170
—, causing pseudosarcomatous proliferation 135, 178, 283
—, sarcomas after 178, 283
—, use in carcinoma 162, 272
—, use in endometriosis 162
Glands, changes in, after oral contraceptives 168, 174, 176, 178, 180

—, cystic dilatation of 86, 87
—, — — with anovulatory cycles 105
—, discordant development of 138, 139
—, normal variations in 84–88
—, secretion of 27, 64
— without secretory activity 86
—, tortuosity of 58, 60, 61, 65
Glandular cells, changes in, during secretory phase 64
— —, ciliated cells, "clear cells" 27, 28, 220, 222
— —, cytoplasm of 26
— —, nuclei of 25
— —, pseudostratified 56, 58, 61
— —, secretion of 27
— —, secretory vacuoles of 64–68
— -cystic hyperplasia (see also hyperplasia, glandular cystic) 108
Glial tissue 326, 328
Glioma 224
Glucosaminidase 44
Glucose-6-Phosphatase 43, 44
Glycogen phosphorylase 44
Glycogen synthetase 44
Glycogen vacuoles 8, 11, 58, 64
— —, disappearance of 66
— —, early secretion of 26, 27, 64
— —, fluorochromation of 15, 58
— — after oral contraceptives 168
— —, PAS reaction for 11, 58
— —, post-ovulatory 64, 66
Goldner stain, advantages of 12
Gonadal dysgenesis 137, 153
Gonadotropin-resistent ovary syndrome 103, 137, 153
Gonadotropins, in abortion 305
— with Arias-Stella phenomenon 144, 306
— in choriocarcinoma 323
— after contraceptive agents 183
—, with decidual change 331
—, with hydatidiform mole 318
—, reduced secretion of 183
—, therapy with 137, 186
Granulocytes, differentiated from leukocytes 13, 14, 30, 33, 77, 201, 300 (see endometrial granulocytes)
Granuloma, foreign body, talcum 212
—, mucus 134
—, sarcoidosis 208
—, tuberculous 205
Granulosa-cell tumor 108, 157, 260
Ground substance, of decidua 300
— —, during implantation 53
— —, of menstrual cycle 36
Gynandroblastoma 158

Hemangioendothelioma 281
Hemangioma 223
Hemangiopericytoma 224
Hematometra 98, 199
Herpes virus infection 210
Hilar-cell hyperplasia, ovarian 108, 261
Histiocytes of endometrium 34
Histiocytic storage disease 198
Histochemical reactions, advantages of 12, 42
Histological diagnosis, correlation with clinical history and tests 4, 94, 185
— —, importance of clinical report 3, 21, 22
— —, limiting factors 21, 22
— —, reporting of 21, 22
— —, statistical analysis of 23
— techniques, embedding 10
— —, fixation 7
— —, orientation of tissue 10
— —, staining 11
Hofbauer cells 313
Hormonal disturbances 99
— imbalance, detection of, by histological studies 57, 167
— preparations 166, 167, 174, 178, 180
— stimuli, local unresponsiveness to 86, 100, 185
Hormone therapy for castrates 165
Hormones, changes induced in endometrium by 45, 165, 185, 275
— and enzymes 42
Hyaline thrombi of glandular-cystic hyperplasia 19, 112, 113, 324
Hydatidiform mole, complete 317
— —, —, and choriocarcinoma 321
— —, —, curettage of 6
— —, —, gonadotropin by 318
— —, —, histological characteristics of 318, 319
— —, —, malignant transformation of 318, 321
— —, —, prognosis of 318
— —, invasive 320, 321
— —, partial 314, 315
— —, —, differential diagnosis 312, 317
— —, —, prognosis of 317
— —, —, trophoblast of 315–317
Hydropic change of villi, cause of 303, 312, 313
Hydroxysteroid dehydrogenases 45
Hyperemia, caused by estrogen 50, 94
—, passive 96
Hyperestrogenism and endometrial carcinoma 260, 265, 266, 268
—, foam cells in 14, 251, 265, 271

—, glandular-cystic hyperplasia 108, 117
—, importance of 117, 265, 268
—, in polycystic ovary syndrome 136
Hypermenorrhea 155
Hyperplasia, "adaptation" 324, 335, 336
—, —, causing postpartum bleeding 336
—, —, in extrauterine pregnancy 330
—, adenomatous 120, 270
—, —, fate of 128, 129, 256, 270
—, atypical 124
— of basalis 128, 129
—, associated with carcinoma 255, 270
—, causing infertility 155
—, complex 124
—, electron-microscopic studies 112
—, of endocervix 186, 187
—, endocrine disturbances 266, 267
—, focal 128, 129, 258
—, glandular-cystic 108
—, —, in animals 108
—, —, bleeding in 113
—, —, causes of 103, 108, 255, 269
—, —, changes in, after therapy 114
—, —, "clear cells" of 28, 110
—, —, in climacterium 156
—, —, "discharged" 114
—, —, after estrogen therapy 108, 119
—, —, foam cells in 124
—, —, gross appearance of 11, 109
—, —, histochemical characteristics of 110, 112, 249
—, —, histology of 109
—, —, homologous 108
—, —, hyaline thrombi and necroses in 19, 98, 112, 113, 324
—, —, incidence 108
—, —, oral contraceptives and 177, 180
—, —, with ovarian tumors 157
—, —, with persistent follicle 108
—, —, polypoid changes of 129
—, —, as precursor of adenomatous hyperplasia 117
—, —, as precursor of carcinoma 254, 255, 269
—, —, recurrence of 114
—, —, secretory changes in 114, 116
—, —, special forms 117, 129
—, —, squamous metaplasia in 114, 118
—, —, and tuberculous endometritis 207
—, heterologous 108
—, histochemical studies 249
—, with intrauterine device 191
—, microglandular, of endocervix 186, 187
—, polypoid 129
—, precursor of carcinoma 127, 129, 255, 270

−, regressive 90, 117
−, resting 117
− stromal 108, 134, 178, 179, 223
−, types of 108
Hyperprolactinemia 137
Hypertrophy, secretory 149, 150, 151, 157
Hypomenorrhea and endometrial atrophy 101

Iatrogenic changes of endometrium 158
Ichthyosis uteri 204, 210, 215, 240
− −, carcinomas from 240
Immunocytochemistry, techniques 15, 16
− for receptor proteins 49
Implantation, biochemical and histological changes of endometrium during 53, 153, 299
−, changes in ground substance during 39, 300
−, disturbance of 302
−, polypoid 302
−, relaxin effect during 39, 40, 52
Infections, causing sterility 156
 (see also endometritis)
Infertility from adhesions 199
−, anovulatory cycles 103, 153, 154
−, atrophy with 153
−, causes of 152, 153
−, curettage in 152
−, endometrial disturbances in 152, 153
−, histochemical changes in endometrium 154
−, polyps with 155
− from tuberculous endometritis 156, 208
Innervation of endometrium 41
Intermediate filaments, markers for 15, 16
Intrauterine adhesions 199
Intrauterine device, action of 190
− −, complications of 193, 194, 195, 325
− −, endometritis 191, 213
− −, histological reaction to 190, 194, 195, 213
− −, inert types 190
− −, medicated types 194
− −, pregnancy rates with 193, 194, 197
− −, types of 191
− instillation 197, 213
Invasive mole 320, 321
In vitro fertilization, effect of follicular puncture 200
− − −, after hormonal stimulation 189

Irregular cycles 86
Irregular proliferation 105, 106, 137, 153, 155, 270
− shedding 143
− −, advanced 147
− −, with Arias-Stella phenomenon 144, 306, 329
− −, causes of 143, 146, 329
− −, diagnosis of 144, 146
− −, dysmenorrhea membranacea 148
− −, granulocytes in 144
− −, histological characteristics 144
− −, with hypomenorrhea 102
− −, lack of relaxin 144
− −, mechanisms in 143
− −, occurrence of 143, 329
− −, with oral contraceptives 146, 182
− −, post partum 336
− −, reticulum fibers in 12, 144, 145, 329
Ischemia in menstruation, causes for 79
Isthmic endometrium 17

Jet washings 6
Juvenile adenomatous hyperplasia 123, 124, 245
Juvenile cervical polyp 134

Karyometry 16

Laminin, in decidual cells 53
Lectins, studies with 53
Leiomyoma, submucosal 100
−, −, in curettings, distinguished from myometrium 18, 135
Leiomyosarcoma 281
Leukemic infiltration 281
Lipids in glandular epithelium 27, 249
−, staining for 14
− in stromal cells 14, 30, 123, 251, 266
Listeriosis 308
Luteal phase: see secretory phase
Luteinized unruptured follicle syndrome 103, 137, 154
Luteoma 157
Lymphatics 41
−, cysts 96
Lymphocytes of endometrium 34
 (see also endometritis, chronic)
Lymphoid follicles 34, 35
Lymphoma 224
−, distinction from endometritis 205
Lymphosarcoma 281
Lysosomes, effect of progesterone on 33, 43, 52

Malakoplakia 211
Malignant mixed tumors 281, 282, 283
— — mesenchymal 281, 282
— — mesodermal 282, 283
— — Müllerian 282, 283, 285, 286
Marker proteins 15, 16
Mast cells 34
Menopause, definition 88
Menorrhagia, due to extragenital disease 93, 97
— in glandular-cystic hyperplasia 113
— from malakoplakia 211
— post partum 333
— from talcum granulomata 212
Menstrual cycle, abnormal duration 152
— —, asynchronous 152, 153, 155
— —, changes of glandular cells during 25
— —, — in ground substance 36
— —, — of stromal cells during 29
— —, fifteenth day 64
— —, sixteenth day 64, 65
— —, seventeenth day 66, 67
— —, eighteenth day 66, 68
— —, nineteenth day 66, 69
— —, twentieth day 68, 70
— —, twenty-first day 70, 71
— —, twenty-second day 70, 72
— —, twenty-third day 70, 73
— —, twenty-fourth day 70, 74
— —, twenty-fifth day 75, 76
— —, twenty-sixth day 75, 77
— —, twenty-seventh day 75, 80
— —, twenty-eighth day 75, 81
— —, irregular 86
— —, phases of 57
— —, its variations 55, 64, 84, 152
Menstruation, cause of 77
—, early leukocytic infiltration 33
—, first day of 77, 82
— with irregular shedding 143
—, ischemia in 79
—, lack of, with normal ovarian function 101
— processes of 79
—, release of relaxin 33, 79
—, second day of 77, 83
Mesodermal tumors, mixed, benign 224
— —, —, malignant 283
Metachromasia, of glandular secretion 27
— of ground substance 36
Metachromatic cells 33
Metaplasia 214
—, distinction from malignant epithelium 215, 216, 223
—, of endocervix 134, 186
—, eosinophilic 219, 220, 222

—, epithelial 214
—, mucinous (endocervical) 216, 229
—, myogenic 222
—, serous papillary 217, 219, 229
—, squamous 215, 229
—, —, in adenoacanthoma 117, 235, 236
—, —, in atrophic endometrium 204, 215
—, —, after hormone therapy 178
—, —, in hyperplastic endometrium 114, 118, 245
—, stromal 222
Metastatic tumors 291
Metrorrhagia 93
Microvilli of glandular cells 27
Minipill 167
Mitoses, induced by estrogen 50
Monoclonal antibodies against receptor proteins 49
— — techniques with 15, 16
Monosomies 301, 314
Morphometry 16
Morules 114, 117, 118, 215, 229, 236, 245
Mucinous adenocarcinoma 229, 238, 239, 282
— —, distinction from endocervical carcinoma 249
— metaplasia 216, 229
Mucoepidermoid adenocarcinoma 216, 229, 238, 240, 282
Mucopolysaccharides 14, 27, 36, 51, 249
Mucus granuloma 134
Müllerian adenosarcoma 282, 288, 289
Müllerian epithelium, tumors arising from 228, 238, 282
— tumors 282, 283
Mycoplasma 210, 308
Myelogenous leukemia 281
— sarcoma 281
Myogenic metaplasia 222
Myxometra 219

Necrosis, in curettings 19, 98, 112, 113, 201
—, hemorrhagic 107, 112, 113, 173
Neometaplasia 250
Neoplasms, benign 223
—, carcinoma (see under carcinoma) 226
—, leiomyoma 100, 135
—, malignant mixed mesodermal 283
—, metastatic 291
—, ovarian 157
—, sarcomas 275
Nerves of endometrium 41
Neurofibroma 224
Nidation, changes in endometrium during (see implantation)

Nuclei, estrogen receptor content of 47, 49
- of glandular cells 25
Nucleic acids, demonstration of 13
Nucleoli of glandular cells 26
Nucleolar channel-system 26, 51, 140, 170, 180

Oocytes, abnormal, effect of 136
Oral contraceptives 166
- -, chromosomal damage from 302
- -, combination agents 167
- -, effect on endocervix 186, 187
- -, - on endometrial blood vessels 173
- -, - on endometrium 167, 183
- -, - on ovaries 184
- -, - after prolonged use 174, 178, 182
- -, - on reticulum fibers 12, 171, 183
- -, electron-microscopic studies 170, 180
- -, enzyme-histochemical studies 181
- -, functions of 166, 183
- -, injectable long-acting gestagens 167, 174
- -, irregular shedding from 143, 146, 182
- -, late consequences 178, 325
- - and malformed blastocyst 302
- -, mode of action 183
- -, pathologic edema from 94, 96, 170
- -, postcoital pills 181
- -, potency 159, 161, 173
- -, progestagen alone 180
- -, pseudomelanosis of endometrium 98
- -, R2323 agent 181
- - resumption of fertility 182
- - sequential agents 178
- -, side-effects 167, 182, 325
- -, in tissue culture 182
- -, types 166
Osseous metaplasia 222
Osteosarcoma 282
Ovarian atrophy after contraceptive agents 183, 184
- changes, seen with endometrial carcinoma 260
- dysfunction 94, 99, 101
- -, staining for 14
- function, changes in, detected histologically 57
- -, climacteric decline of 88, 90
- - in climacterium 156, 157

- -, effect of insufficiency on endometrium 99, 101
- hormones 45
- - in climacterium 156
- -, control of menstrual cycle 55
- -, implantation 53
- tumors, androgen secreting 158
- -, decidual effect 157
- -, seen with endometrial carcinoma 157, 260, 261
- -, endometrial hyperplasia 157
- -, hormone-producing 157
- -, progesterone secreting 157
Ovary, hilar-cell hyperplasia of 261
-, stromal hyperplasia of 260
Ovulation, detection of 64
-, delayed 137, 153, 154, 155, 302
-, premature 153
Ovulatory bleeding 66
Ovum, "blighted" 301, 312

Papillary proliferations of glands 218, 220
Papillomatosis 210, 216
PAS reaction, advantages of 11
Persistent follicle 102, 137, 153
Phloxine-tartrazine stain for endometrial granulocytes 14
- - for squamous epithelium 14
Phosphatases, staining for 42
Phosphoamidase 44
Pituitary and hyperestrogenism 267
Placental polyp 325, 327
- site trophoblastic tumor 323
- tissue 298, 325
- - in curettings 19, 309, 325
- -, necrotic 309, 311
- -, retained 5, 19, 325, 334
Plasma cells 34, 203
Plasmacytoma 281
Polycystic ovary syndrome 103, 108, 136, 137, 153
Polyps, carcinoma arising in 130, 257
-, changes in 134
- in climacterium 157
-, clinical symptoms of 134
-, definition 129, 131, 223
-, detection of, with van Gieson stain 12, 130
-, of endocervix, decidual change in 134
-, with infertility 155
-, juvenile 134
-, occurrence of 130
-, placental 325, 327
- of portio vaginalis 134
-, sites of predilection 130

Polyps of transitional epithelium 134
— with tuberculosis 208
—, types 129–134, 223
Polypoid adenomyoma 225
Polysaccharides, stains for 14
Postcoital pills 181
Post-menstrual regeneration 84, 85
Postmenopausal endometrium 88–92
Postpartum endometrium 331
Precancerous changes 269, 270
— —, development from hyperplasias 270
— — in polyps 130
Preclimacteric endometrium 86, 90
Predecidual cells 30, 33, 38, 51
— reaction 70, 73, 74
— — around spiral arterioles 74, 79
— —, beginning 70, 73
— —, with gestagens 162, 163, 170, 178
— — with intrauterine devices 191–194
Pregnancy, changes in cervical epithelium during 325
—, early, intrauterine 298
—, —, —, disturbances in 300
—, extrauterine, diagnosis of 329
—, steroid receptors 48
Pressure atrophy 100
PR-ICA assay 16, 249
Progesterone, action of 48, 51, 57, 161
—, deficiency of 136
—, effect on fibrinolytic activity 44
—, — on lysosomal membranes 43, 44
—, — on mitochondria 51
—, — on nucleic acids 48, 51, 273
—, — on nucleoli 26, 51
—, — on spiral arterioles 39, 70
—, endometrial reaction to 165, 184
—, influence on relaxin release (see relaxin) 33, 36, 39, 173
—, ovarian tumors producing 157
—, receptors 48, 53
— —, in anovulatory cycle 103
— —, detection of 16, 152
— —, in hyperplasia 127
— —, in infertility 137
—, secretion of, before ovulation 58
— test 162, 187
— therapy for endometrial carcinoma 272
— — for hyperplasias 264
— — for infertility 137, 143
— — during proliferative phase 161
— withdrawal test 160, 162
Proliferation markers, techniques 15
Proliferative phase, changes during 57
— —, cytoplasmic changes of glandular cells 26

— —, deficient 105, 106
— —, early stage 57, 59
— —, enzyme studies 42
— —, glandular cells 25–28
— —, iatrogenic 158, 166
— —, irregular 105, 106
— —, late stage 58, 61
— —, mid stage 58, 60
— —, stages of 57
— —, steroid receptors 48
Prostaglandins 190
Proteolytic enzymes 43
Psammoma bodies in carcinoma 241, 251
Pseudo-corpus luteum insufficiency 137, 143
Pseudomelanosis of endometrium 98
"Pseudopregnancy" 102
Pseudosarcomatous proliferation 135, 178, 283
Pyometra 205, 207

R2323-steroid 181
Receptors, defect 137
—, hormone 16, 45, 48, 140, 245, 273
Regenerative phase, post-menstrual 84, 85
Regions of endometrium, diagnostic value of 17
Registry of diagnoses 23, 182
Regressive hyperplasia 91, 117
Relaxin, absence of, in dysmenorrhea membranacea 148
—, — of, in irregular shedding 144
—, actions of 33, 36, 38, 51, 53
—, chemistry of 52
—, effect on blood vessels 39, 40, 52
—, — on endometrium 33
—, — during implantation 33, 36, 39
— in endometrial granulocytes 33, 52
—, experimental studies with 39, 40, 51
—, fibrinolytic activity of 43, 53
—, formation of 52
—, at menstruation 79
— secretion, dependent on progesterone 33, 39, 52, 79
— in trophoblasts 334, 336
  (see also implantation)
Reserve cell hyperplasia, of endocervical glands 134, 158, 186, 187
Resting endometrium 101
Reticulum fibers, characteristics of 36
— —, dissolution of 36, 38, 52
— —, formation of 36
— —, functional variations of 36
— —, in implantation 53
— —, in irregular shedding 144, 145

− −, in menstrual cycle 37, 52
− −, staining for 12
− network, importance of, in functional diagnoses 36
− − after oral contraceptives 172
Retrosteroid 189
Rhabdomyoblasts 286
Rhabdomyosarcoma 281, 282
RIA assay 16
Ribonucleic acid, criterion of estrogen effect 13, 15
− − during menstrual cycle 26, 56, 57, 79
− − in hyperplasia and carcinoma 110, 120, 249
− −, increase after estrogen 50

Salpingitis, causing infertility 208
−, tuberculous 205
Sarcoidosis 208
Sarcoma 275
− botryoides 134, 282, 288
−, endometrial stromal 276, 282
−, − −, clear cell type 279
−, − −, high-grade 276
−, − −, homologous type 276, 277
−, − −, low-grade 280
−, − −, polymorphic type 279
−, etiology 134, 276, 283, 284
−, after gestagens 283
−, heterologous 282
−, homologous 282
− in situ 276
−, metastases 280
− and pregnancy 276
−, prognosis 280, 285
− and stromal hyperplasia 276, 283
−, types 275, 282
Schistosomiasis 211
Secretion, arrested 148, 153, 162, 163, 331
Secretions of glandular cells 27
Secretory endometrium, height of 84
− hypertrophy 149, 150, 151, 157
− −, cause 149, 157
− phase, abnormalities of 136
− −, changes in endometrium during 49, 56, 64
− −, − in glandular cells 26, 27
− −, − in stromal cells 30, 56, 64, 70
− −, deficient 136, 137, 153, 154, 155
− −, −, causes of 136, 153, 168, 169, 179
− −, −, clinical aspects of 138
− −, −, gestagen therapy of 143, 162
− −, −, histology 137–140
− −, −, incidence of 138

− −, −, types 138–140
− −, enzyme studies 42
− −, iatrogenic 168, 169, 179, 190
− −, lipids of 27
− −, pre-implantation 52, 53
− −, socalled leukocytic infiltration of 13, 33, 201
− −, steroid receptors 48
Senile atrophy 90, 91
Sequential agents, see oral contraceptives 178
Serous papillary carcinoma 229, 241, 243, 282
− − metaplasia 217, 219, 229
"Silent ovulation" 100
Sinusoidal capillaries of decidua 39, 300, 308
Spiral arterioles, changes during implantation 39, 53
− −, − during secretory phase 70
− −, characteristics of 39
− − in menstruation 79
Squamous-cell carcinoma 229, 244, 282
Squamous cell metaplasia (see also metaplasia), of endometrium 114, 118, 215, 229, 236, 240, 245
− − −, of endocervix 134, 186
Staining, advantages of special methods 11
−, aldehyde-fuchsin reaction for polysaccharides 13
− for cellular proteins 13
−, enzyme-histochemical techniques 15
−, ER-ICA assay for receptor proteins 16, 49
−, Feulgen stain 13
−, fluorochromation 15
−, gallocyanin-chromalum method 13
−, van Gieson method 12
−, Goldner stain 12
−, Gomori method 12
−, immunocytochemical techniques 15–16
− for lipids with Sudan black 14
−, Masson-trichrome 12
−, methyl green-pyronin stain 13
−, PAS reaction 11
−, phloxine-tartrazine of Lendrum 13, 14, 79
− for phosphatides 14
− for polysaccharides 14
−, tetrazonium reaction 13
−, thionine-"enclosure" 28
Statistical analysis of histological diagnoses 23
Stein-Leventhal syndrome 124, 188
− − and carcinoma 262, 287
Sterility = see Infertility

Steroid hormones 45
– –, molecular biology of 45
– –, receptors for 16, 45, 48
Stromal cells, changes in, during menstrual cycle 29, 70
– –, – in, during proliferative phase 64
– –, – in, during secretory phase 64, 70
– –, characteristics of, in normal endometrium 29, 30, 33
– –, differentiation of 29, 30, 33, 70
– –, enzyme systems of 30, 181
– changes after oral contraceptives 162, 163, 170, 172, 178, 179
– edema after oral contraceptives 96, 170, 178
– –, pathological 94
– –, physiological 58, 60, 70, 72
– hyperplasia 108, 134, 223, 276, 283
– –, focal (nodular) 178, 179
– – and sarcoma 135, 178, 276, 283
– metaplasia 222
– nodule 223
– sarcoma (see also sarcoma) 276, 282
– tumor with epithelial differentiation 224
Stromaloma 223
Stromatosis 280
Suction-biopsy, limitations of 6
Sudan black stain 14
Superficial epithelium, characteristics of 29
Syncytiotrophoblasts 299, 309, 318, 321
Systemic diseases, causing uterine bleeding 93, 97

Tachyphylaxis 46
Talcum granuloma 212
Tamoxifen 47, 273
Target cells 16

Target organs 46
Teratoma 225, 226, 326
Theca cells, characteristics of 260
Thecoma 108, 157, 260
Three sequence preparations 167
Thrombotic thrombocytopenia 98
Thromboses 98, 173
Tissue culture of endometrium 7, 16, 182, 273
Toxoplasmosis 210, 308
Triploidies 301, 314
Trisomies 301, 314
Trophoblasts 298, 299, 308, 309
–, abnormalities of 312
–, action on vessels 336
–, of blighted ova 313
–, with decidua 308, 310
–, of hydatidiform mole 315, 316, 319
–, intermediate 323
–, retained 324, 325, 334, 336
Tuberculosis 156, 205
Tumors, metastatic 291

Uterine bleeding, atypical 93
  (see also bleeding)
– – – due to extragenital diseases 93, 97

Vacuum aspiration 6
Van Gieson stain, advantages of 12
Veins, hormonal changes in 39
Vessels of endometrium 39, 173
Villi, see chorionic villi
Vimentin filaments 16
– –, in carcinomas 250

Withdrawal bleeding, cause of 103, 107, 113
– –, estrogen 113, 160, 162, 173
– –, in glandular-cystic hyperplasia, causes of 113
– –, progesterone 160, 162, 173

G. Dallenbach-Hellweg, Mannheim;
H. Poulsen, Kopenhagen

Atlas der Histopathologie des Endometrium

1985. 260 meist farbige Abbildungen. 225 Seiten.
ISBN 3-540-13666-5

Inhaltsübersicht: Technische Bemerkungen. Das normale Endometrium. – Metaplastische Veränderungen. – Kreislaufstörungen. – Funktionsstörungen. – Iatrogene Veränderungen. – Endometritis. – Tumoren.

Die histopathologische Diagnostik des Endometriums ist durch den schnellen zyklischen Wandel von Form und Funktion besonders erschwert. Morphologische Krankheitsbilder gestalten sich vor diesem Hintergrund dynamisch und wechselhaft, sie sind stets eine Synthese aus Funktionszustand und aufgepfropfter Läsion. Die Vielfalt der resultierenden morphologischen Bilder läßt sich in einem Textbuch nur in den Grundzügen beschreiben, in einem Atlas dagegen präziser darstellen.

Mit dem vorliegenden Bildatlas erhält der Pathologe die Möglichkeit, unter dem Mikroskop erkennbare Veränderungen einzuordnen und differentialdiagnostisch abzugrenzen. Neben der knappen Darstellung des Krankheitsbildes werden die in Frage kommenden Ursachen und deren Unterscheidung sowie die klinische Bedeutung und Therapiemöglichkeiten erörtert. Dabei geht der Atlas von den histologischen Krankheitsbildern aus und setzt diese in Beziehung zu den möglichen Ursachen, d. h. er geht den Weg des diagnostizierenden Pathologen und erspart ihm die Suche nach vergleichbaren Krankheitsbildern in verschiedenen Kapiteln. Dadurch erübrigen sich Doppelabbildungen gleicher morphologischer Bilder bei verschiedener Genese.

Der Atlas betont den ständigen Dialog zwischen Pathologen und behandelnden Gynäkologen, der ganz besonders auf diesem Gebiet Voraussetzung für eine exakte Diagnosestellung und eine erfolgreiche Therapie ist.

Springer-Verlag
Berlin Heidelberg New York
London Paris Tokyo

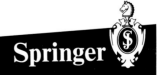

G. Dallenbach-Hellweg, Universität Mannheim (Hrsg.)

Ovarialtumoren

1982. 152 Abbildungen, 38 Tabellen.
IX, 306 Seiten. (163 Seiten in Englisch).
ISBN 3-540-11327-4

Inhaltsübersicht: Einführung. – Epidemiologie. – Klinische Symptomatik. – Morphologie. – Experimentelle Erzeugung. – Neue Aspekte der Chemotherapie.

Die Ovarialtumoren gehören heute zu den häufigsten Tumoren des weiblichen Genitale. Ihre morphologische Differentialdiagnostik und die sich darauf aufbauende gezielte Therpaie ist aufgrund der Vielfalt dieser Tumoren ungleich viel komplizierter als bei Tumoren anderer Organe.
Dieses Buch gibt einen umfassenden Überblick über die gesamte Problematik der Ovarialtumoren, angefangen von der Epidemiologie, über die klinische Diagnostik bis hin zur ausführlichen morphologischen Differentialdiagnostik. Diese baut auf der modernen, derzeit weltweit anerkannten histogenetischen Klassifikation der WHO auf, welche anhand der Erfahrungen an drei deutschen großen Frauenkliniken kleine Ergänzungen und Variationen erfährt. Der abschließende Teil befaßt sich ausführlich mit den modernen Möglichkeiten einer gezielten Therapie der Ovarialtumoren auf der Grundlage der histologischen Diagnostik. Dabei steht die Chemotherapie im Vordergrund. Diskutiert werden außerdem die modernen Möglichkeiten eines Rezeptornachweises im Tumorgewebe im Hinblick auf die Frage einer Hormonbehandlung.

Springer-Verlag
Berlin Heidelberg New York
London Paris Tokyo

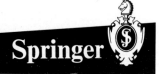